cat owner's encyclopedia of veterinary medicine

ISBN 0-87666-856-2

cat owner's encyclopedia of veterinary medicine

BY

JOAN O. JOSHUA

F.R.C.V.S.

t.f.h.

Distributed in the U.S. by T.F.H. Publications, Inc., 211 West Sylvania Avenue, P.O. Box 427, Neptune, N.J. 07753; in England by T.F.H. (Gt. Britain) Ltd., 13 Nutley Lane, Reigate, Surrey; in Canada to the book store and library trade by Beaverbooks, 953 Dillingham Road, Pickering, Ontario L1W 1Z7; in Canada to the pet trade by Rolf C. Hagen Ltd., 3225 Sartelon Street, Montreal 382, Quebec; in Southeast Asia by Y.W. Ong, 9 Lorong 36 Geylang, Singapore 14; in Australia and the South Pacific by Pet Imports Pty. Ltd., P.O. Box 149, Brookvale 2100, N.S.W., Australia; in South Africa by Valiant Publishers (Pty.) Ltd., P.O. Box 78236, Sandton City, 2146, South Africa; Published by T.F.H. Publications, Inc., Ltd., The British Crown Colony of Hong Kong.

CONTENTS

FOREWORD

This book is a partially up-dated version of the work previously entitled "The Clinical Aspects of Some Diseases of Cats", 1965. It is not claimed that it is a complete second edition. Much of the text remains valid but revision of sections in which considerable advances have been made such as anaesthesia, virus diseases and urolithiasis has been undertaken. Two chapters have been deleted as they were no longer considered of value to an international readership, but a chapter on the functional anatomy of the cat has been added which should prove invaluable to a wide readership in view of the dearth of published material in this field hitherto.

The prime object of the book is still to provide a readable, practical yet informative text for the veterinary undergraduate, but it is realised that it will have appeal to the cat owning public as well.

It is appreciated that the book may attract some criticism as not being a fully revised edition but it is hoped the compromise presented will nonetheless be of value.

The main author (Joan O. Joshua) is grateful to her co-authors for their work in various sections and is appreciative of their willingness to participate in a project which some may not find wholly acceptable.

Chapter 1

THE CAT; PET AND PATIENT

Relationship with Man

Cats have lived in a close association with the human race from ancient times and have been variously esteemed, revered or reviled as vermin.

This relationship is almost unique in the sphere of animal owning by man since the cat is the only animal kept by man which produces nothing in the way of animal products or work. If one excepts rodent control which, after all, is merely the pursuit of natural instincts even though extremely valuable the relationship is different from that with cage birds or other exotic pets usually kept caged, such as rabbits, hamsters, bush babies and so on. Companionship of a kind is offered by cats but has nothing in common with the subservient affectionate behaviour of dogs. Indeed most cats give the impression of a tolerant acceptance of human company together with the comforts which can be obtained by contact with man resulting in a type of mutual respect. Exceptions to this general rule occur in some particular breeds, notably the Siamese and to some extent the Burmese and Abyssinian, in which a more dog-like attachment to the owners is often evident with resultant greater dependence on human contacts. It is this unusual pattern of behaviour that appeals to many cat owners but it is this same pattern which can present so many problems to the veterinary surgeon in dealing with feline patients.

Unless kept by cat breeders, most cats live a life of freedom from physical control; they are seldom confined to houses and flats and it is accepted in law that control of the kind possible with other animals is not possible with cats. Hence cat owners can seldom, if ever, be held responsible for any nuisance caused by their pets.

Although freedom-loving and highly athletic, cats are, somewhat paradoxically, lazy by nature and the amount of exercise taken, once the playful stages of kittenhood are passed, is minimal except in the pursuit of sexual activities or hunting.

These facts need to be appreciated by anyone who proposes to deal at all closely with the domestic cat.

As Patients

Cats present peculiar problems to the veterinary surgeon, owner and nursing attendant.

First and foremost it must be remembered that, although a domestic animal, the cat is probably nearer to the wild than most other domesticated species; the veneer of civilised behaviour is thin and can easily be breached by interferences which would evoke little response from many animals. This can result in outbursts of savage temper which makes the cat the most dangerous animal with which the veterinary surgeon has to deal. Weapons of offence are teeth and claws both of which can inflict potentially serious injury and neither of which can be adequately controlled by the routine methods applied, for example, to dogs.

Additionally there is the fact that the normal bacterial flora of the cat's mouth includes two types of organisms, *Pasteurellas* and *Streptococci*, which are highly pathogenic when introduced into wounds, which makes any damage inflicted by cats on handlers potentially serious. For this reason in addition to protecting himself from injury it is the veterinary surgeon's duty to instruct the owner in the correct way of holding the cat during treatment and to advise prompt medical attention should he be bitten in spite of all precautions.

On the other hand the feline patient has many advantages. It seldom runs a 'surgery' or excitement temperature. Its surgical anatomy is ideal for many operative techniques and it is usually possible to carry out abdominal palpation easily and fully. Despite the development of numerous breeds, the basic conformation of cats is uniform. Hence departures from the normal can be recognised more easily, dose rates of therapeutic agents cover a small range and radiographic techniques can be standardised far more easily than in canine patients.

As patients to be nursed, cats present some problems. They retain certain instincts which domestication has done little to eradicate. One of these is the desire to seek solitude and concealment when ill; this means that sick cats cannot be allowed much freedom. Failure of careful supervision often results in the disappearance of the patient which causes much distress to the owner and the necessity to presume death.

Cats are also difficult subjects to dose and tend to resent and resist the forced administration of drugs or nutrients. Considerable patience, perseverance and dexterity is required by owners or nursing attendants to ensure the regular medication occasionally called for. Ancillary nursing procedures such as temperature taking, cleansing of discharge from eyes and nose, grooming, application of heat etc. are at best tolerated, at worst forcibly resisted and seldom welcomed as seems to be the case with many canine patients. Considerable skill and discretion are called for in deciding whether the procedure desired is likely to do more harm than good to a resisting patient.

As an inmate, whether boarder or patient

Immediately a cat is accepted as an inmate of a veterinary surgeon's premises, whether for a short stay of a few hours for some minor procedure or for a period of several weeks, the safety of the animal becomes the responsibility of the veterinary surgeon.

Safety must be regarded as an all-embracing term covering security from escape, maintenance of health, avoidance of infection and safe transport.

Security

Cats can be most expert escapologists and it is essential that this fact be recognised and all precautions taken to minimise the risk. This means first and foremost that there must always be at least two barriers between the cat and freedom so that one is always closed, e.g. if the cage door is open the door of the room must be closed and vice versa. It is an extraordinary fact that this simple and obvious precaution can never be impressed upon students and staff until disaster or near disaster has occurred.

The greatest care must always be taken in transporting a cat from one place to another. This should preferably be in a secure container such as a cat basket but if for any reason this is not desirable or possible the cat must be carried in such a manner that the risk of its being able to get away is minimal. In view of the fact that cats will suddenly panic and make violent efforts to escape if faced with a frightening situation it is better that the animal should be held with its head away from the direction in which it is being carried; this is especially true on veterinary surgeon's premises when dogs may be met at any time. A good method is for the cat's scruff to be grasped in one hand, the forequarters of the animal tucked under the opposite arm, head facing backwards, when the hand on this side can be used to control the hind limbs. Similarly when it is necessary to remove a cat from a cage in a room where a dog is loose the cat's head should be kept turned away from the dog during removal.

These suggestions will be obvious to many yet it is surprising how often these simple precautions which can obviate so much trouble are neglected even by experienced people.

When it is necessary to have a cat loose in a surgery for purposes of examination, e.g. of movement, it is essential that all windows be closed or protected with wire guards and that chimneys should be blocked off at the fireplace; the number of times cats have escaped into chimneys is too great for peace of mind and their recovery is often extremely difficult. Precautions should also be taken to guard against the cat's escape if the door is opened unexpectedly.

Transport

When it is necessary to move a cat any distance it is preferable to put it in a safe container. Cat baskets are designed for this purpose and are of a variety of types and material. The container should not be too large; it is not a kindness to allow cats much room to move about during transport. The container should be of sufficient size to permit the cat to lie in the sternal position, with limbs flexed in comfort, and to allow the animal to turn round. Whatever the material of the container a thick layer of newspaper should be provided as cats frequently urinate or defaecate when frightened on a journey. Cats are fastidious creatures in personal habits and much dislike being forced to lie in their own excrement, hence if it is found that a cat arriving at the surgery has fouled its container it is a humane as well as cleanly act to change the paper.

Owners often need advice on how to bring their cats to the surgery. They should be advised that it is essential they should be under proper restraint, preferably in a suitable container but if this is not available the cat should be wrapped securely in a piece of blanket. Cats not under proper restraint in a veterinary surgeon's waiting room are a danger to themselves, their owners and other people, as they may escape and get lost or maul their owners or other people in a desperate bid to escape. The veterinary surgeon is the person who knows the propensity of cats to do this and is thus under a duty to ensure so far as lies in his power that accidents do not happen through lack of insistence on proper control of feline patients on his premises.

If the owner has not a suitable basket, an excellent substitute is a leather or canvas travelling bag with a zip fastener. The zip may be fastened completely or left one inch open only; a larger opening allows the cat to get its muzzle into the aperture, force the zip back and so escape. These bags properly used are secure and easy to carry: they are lighter and less bulky than a basket. Other alternatives are laundry baskets or boxes of wood or cardboard suitably secured with rope or twine.

Owners frequently find difficulty in putting their cat into the container and will require to be advised of the correct method, controlling the forehand of the cat by holding the neck or scruff, supporting the hindquarters by the other hand under the rump and dropping the cat gently, hind end first, into the basket, keeping control of the head with the second hand while the lid is closed or the zip fastened.

Loan of baskets

Veterinary surgeons are frequently asked to lend baskets for transport purposes. This is a request the author has consistently refused except in exceptional circumstances. Quite apart from the obvious risk of loss and damage to baskets, which will necessitate a large stock being kept it can result in much unpleasantness between practitioner and client; there is the worse danger of transmission of infection in cases of ecto-parasitism, virus diseases and sepsis, a risk which is so great that it is necessary that every basket should be rigidly disinfected either by scrubbing with hot soda water and exposure to sun and air for several days or by blow-lamp every time it has been used to transport a cat which has not already been examined by the veterinary surgeon. Exceptions may be made in the case of clients well known to the veterinary surgeon whose cat is suffering from a condition known to be non-transmissible. Only by strict adherence to such rules will transmission of virus diseases such as panleukopenia and respiratory conditions and the avoidance of infection of spay and castration wounds by pyogenic bacteria be avoided.

Sedation for Travelling

Veterinary surgeons are often consulted regarding cats being taken on journeys and are asked to dispense or prescribe suitable sedatives. Advice should include information as to a suitably sized container, as previously described, and most careful consideration given to the question of sedation. Cats are seldom subject to travel sickness, in marked contrast to dogs, so anti-emetic drugs are rarely needed. The reaction of cats to small doses of the tranquillising (ataractic) drugs is so variable and idiosyncracy so common that these are best avoided; similarly, response to sedative doses of barbiturates is somewhat irregular. A perfectly safe and reasonably effective drug is potassium bromide and the best recommendation is to give a dose of 150–600 mg. ($2\frac{1}{2}$–10 gr.) pot. bromide 1 hour before the start of the journey. Small doses of the same drug may be continued for 1–2 weeks when it is desirable to assist a cat to accept a new and strange environment, e.g. 150 mg. ($2\frac{1}{2}$ gr.) twice daily.

In-patient or Boarder

Contrary to the usual belief, cats are far more liable to fret after admission to kennels than dogs. The latter are more extrovert in outlook and so quickly become interested in kennel routine and tend to forget themselves, but cats are introspective by nature and can rarely be persuaded to take an interest in routines which do not involve them and which they often find frightening; because of this reason cats may refuse to eat for several days after admission and may require much cajoling to get them started. To be called by name means less to cats than dogs but the offering of some article of diet of which the cat is particularly fond or the use of a particular method of fondling normally used by the owner will often get results. For these reasons any help the owner can give on diet and management should be noted and not regarded as a mere pandering to whims.

Cats very rapidly assume territorial rights and quickly learn to regard their cage or even basket as a place of security. For this reason changes of cage are to be deplored; once installed the cat should remain in occupation of the same compartment throughout its stay unless exceptional circumstances arise; similarly the owner's offer to supply an article of bedding familiar to the cat should not be lightly rejected although it may be discarded and replaced with routine bedding as soon as the cat has settled down.

Despite normally fastidious habits and the desire to seek solitude and concealment for excretory functions, cats adapt themselves remarkably quickly to whatever facilities are available in their cages provided these are kept scrupulously clean.

To minimise the risk of air-borne infection by the various respiratory viruses it is desirable that individual cage units should be as widely separated as is reasonable with free circulation of air throughout the cattery block. A minimum of 3 feet between cages has recently been suggested by Thomson (1963) as the ideal. For boarding of healthy cats the pleasure afforded by allowing some freedom in wired runs has to be balanced against the risk of spread of infection and must be decided by the veterinary surgeon.

In-patients often need to be admitted without much regard to ecto-parasitism or immune status but in the case of boarders it is open to the veterinary surgeon to impose whatever conditions he may think fit in an attempt to avoid introduction of infection.

Whilst immunisation will be dealt with in more detail in relevant sections some mention of vaccination is desirable under the present heading.

Feline Enteritis—Panleukopenia

For this, vaccination is available. It should be a requirement that all cat boarders are vaccinated. The vaccine is a formalised tissue suspension; booster doses are necessary to maintain immunity at an effective level and the veterinary surgeon may reasonably require evidence of recent boosting before admission.

Feline Respiratory Viruses

In the light of recent work and the recognition of many strains of virus causing disease of the respiratory tract, together with the evidence that immunity may last weeks only, it is clear that effective long term vaccination is not feasible. It is, however, possible to obtain autogenous vaccine prepared from cases of infection which have occurred on the premises and to require that all cats admitted as boarders should receive this vaccine during the week preceding or on admission; by this means a serviceable level of immunity is afforded to cover an average stay in kennels.

Parasites

Lay staff should be trained to examine every cat on admission for evidence of heavy ecto-parasitism as well as obvious disease. Cats heavily infested with fleas or lice may be refused admission or admitted only on the clear understanding that appropriate treatment will be immediately instituted. Lesions of ringworm are often not apparent but reasonable care should be taken to look for obvious signs.

If long-haired cats are presented for admission with the coat in a neglected state this should be pointed out to the owner and a suitable note made on the admission record.

The foregoing are but some of the considerations the veterinary surgeon will have in mind to ensure that the worries and risks inseparable from having cat inmates on his premises are reduced to a minimum.

Longevity

The normal expectation of life varies considerably and is probably an inherited factor. Some cats are aged and suffering senile changes in vital organs at 9 or 10 years whilst others are still symptom free at 20 or more. In a series of cats destroyed for neoplasia the following is the age distribution for those patients where a reasonably accurate age was available.

Years	Number
4	2
5	–
6	6
7	5
8	8
9	9
10	12
11	8
12	11
13	9
14	9
15	7
16	4
17	2
18	–
19	2
20	1
20+	1

Clients often ask to what age they may expect their cats to live, an impossible question to answer unless a fairly full knowledge of close relations is available from which a rough estimate may be hazarded. It is often justifiable to undertake major therapeutic techniques in cats of 14 years of age and more if the general health of the patient is good apart from the condition under immediate consideration.

Many old cats lose weight without any obvious evidence of defective health and this *per se* should not be taken as evidence of failure. The feline skeleton is less subject to degenerative changes such as osteoarthritis than that of the dog. Chronic nephritis is also less common. Two reasons for euthanasia frequent in dogs are thus eliminated.

REFERENCE

Thomson, A. (1963) *Vet. Rec.* **75**, 1206.

SUGGESTED FURTHER READING

Worden, A. N. (1959) *Vet. Rec.* **71**, 966. (Abnormal behaviour in the dog and cat.)

Comfort, A. (1957) *J. Mammal.* **37**, 118. (Maximum ages reached by domestic cats.)

Thomas, J. (1964) *Prakt. Tierarzt* **45**, 206. (In German). (Behaviour of domestic cats in various situations.)

Knappe, H. (1964) *Wiss. Z.* Humboldt Univ. **13**, 205. (In German). (Prey-catching behaviour in domestic cats.)

Morris, M. L. (1963) *Cornell Vet.* **53**, 157. (Breeding, housing and management of cats.)

Todd, N. B. (1963) *Cornell Vet.* **53**, 99. (Behaviour and genetics of the domestic cat.)

Pierson, G. & Senior, C. (1963) *J. Anim. Tech. Ass.* **13**, 79. (Establishment and maintenance of an outdoor cat colony.)

Chapter 2

THE FUNCTIONAL ANATOMY OF THE CAT
G.C. Skerritt, B.V. Sc., M.R.C.V.S.

In a single chapter it would be impossible to make an exhaustive survey of the anatomy of the cat. There are a number of textbooks available which deal solely with either feline or carnivore anatomy and the reader is recommended to consult the references following this chapter if more detailed information is required.

. An attempt is made here to give a broad outline of feline gross anatomy whilst emphasising those aspects that are of particular functional or clinical significance.

It is appreciated that few readers will be fully conversant with modern anatomical terminology. However, it is the author's belief that the use of colloquial or outdated terms is unnecessary and leads to the perpetuation of errors and confusion. Accordingly the terminology used here is the anglicised version of that adopted by Nomina Anatomica Veterinaria (1973).

A systematic approach to feline anatomy is employed because it allows convenient division of the subject. Although each system is described separately, it is important to realise that the mammalian body is a highly integrated organism. All systems show a functional association with one another, and this is the basis of symptomatology.

The Skeleton

Bones of all shapes and sizes provide a framework which supports and protects the soft tissues of the body. In addition the bones function as a system of levers under the control of the muscles, resulting in movement of the cat or its appendages.

Bone is a particularly hard and strong tissue. It consists of a calcified matrix in which are embedded living bone cells, the osteoblasts. The remarkable regenerative properties of bone are due to its vascularity and the activity of its component cells.

The internal architecture of bone is such that it very efficiently resists forces both of tension and compression. That this arrangement of the tissue is restored during healing is an essential requirement in the return to normality following a fracture. According to engineering principles the maximum forces acting on a bone develop in the outermost areas. Solidity of form would convey no mechanical advantage and would result in unnecessary weight. The hollow structure of bones

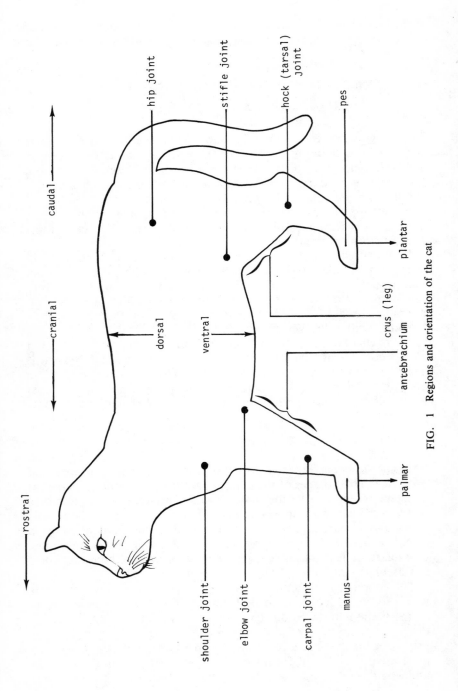

FIG. 1 Regions and orientation of the cat

20

is thus a significant design feature. The medullary cavities of the bones are not wasted spaces but are filled with the blood-producing bone marrow.

The axial skeleton comprises the skull, vertebrae, ribs and sternum. (fig. 2).

The appendicular skeleton is represented by the bones of the pectoral and pelvic limbs (see fig. 2).

The Skull

The bones of the head include the skull, the lower jaw, the hyoid apparatus and the bones of the ears.

The skull itself comprises the neurocranium, enclosing the brain and the splanchnocranium, or facial portion. The relative sizes and shapes of these two parts of the skull is a major factor in determining head shape in the cat; the long-haired breeds possess a dome-shaped neurocranium and a rostro-caudally flattened splanchnocranium contrasting markedly with the elongated nasal area of the Siamese.

The bones of the skull tend to be flattened, plate-like structures closely apposed to their neighbours by immovable joints called sutures. There are numerous perforations of the skull bones, known as foramina; many of these are the exits for nerves arising from the brain.

The large foramen at the rostral end of the skull is the piriform aperture and gives access to the nasal cavity in which are contained the delicate scroll-like ethmoturbinate bones. At the caudal end of the skull the foramen magnum allows continuity of the brain with the spinal cord.

The two large concavities, on either side of the splanchnocranium, are the orbits and contain the eyeballs. The two bulbous structures situated on the caudo-ventral aspect of the skull are the tympanic bullae; each encloses the tympanic cavity of the middle ear.

The two mandibular bones are united in the midline, rostrally, at the mandibular synchondrosis. The fibrocartilage of this articulation normally never becomes ossified and so remains most vulnerable to trauma.

The Vertebral Column

The vertebral column functions as an axial support for the body and also almost completely encloses the spinal cord.

There are 51 to 54 vertebrae in the vertebral column of the cat. They are classified according to their characteristic shape at the various levels of the vertebral column. There are 7 cervical vertebrae, 13 thoracic vertebrae, 7 lumbar vertebrae, 3 sacral vertebrae and 21-24 coccygeal vertebrae.

The first cervical, or atlas, vertebra articulates with the occipital

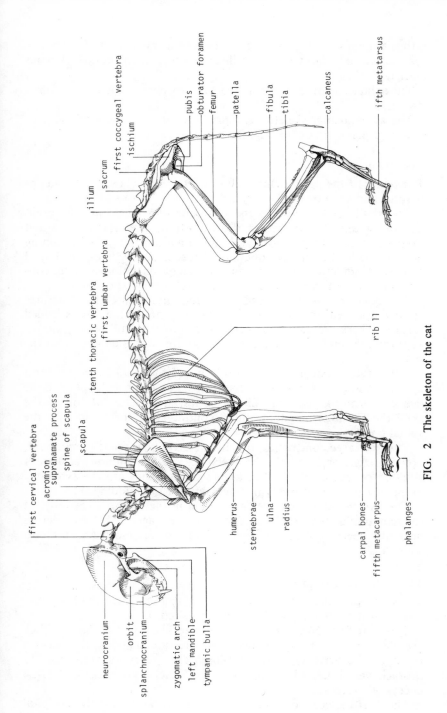

FIG. 2 The skeleton of the cat

first cervical vertebra
acromion
supranamate process
spine of scapula
scapula
tenth thoracic vertebra
first lumbar vertebra

ilium
sacrum
first coccygeal vertebra
ischium
pubis
obturator foramen
femur
patella
fibula
tibia
calcaneus
ifth metatarsus

neurocranium
orbit
splanchnocranium
zygomatic arch
left mandible
tympanic bulla

humerus
sternebrae
ulna
radius
carpal bones
fifth metacarpus
phalanges

rib 11

22

condyles of the skull. The flattened lateral projections of the atlas vertebra are the wings.

The thoracic vertebrae are characterised by their long dorsal spinous processes and articular processes for the ribs, whereas the lumbar vertebrae possess prominent transverse processes.

The 3 sacral vertebrae are fused together as the sacrum, although the dorsal spinous processes remain separate.

Between the bodies of adjacent vertebrae lie the intervertebral discs. These comprise an outer fibrous anulus and the inner jelly-like nucleus pulposus. This construction provides an efficient shock-absorption apparatus for the vertebral column.

It is suggested (King, et al., 1958) that older cats are prone to protrusions of the intervertebral discs into the vertebral canal since the discs undergo senile changes which render them less able to absorb shocks.

The Ribs and Sternum

There are 13 pairs of ribs in the cat. Dorsally the ribs articulate with the thoracic vertebrae and ventrally the first nine pairs have a direct attachment to the sternum. The 13th pair are termed floating ribs as they are free distally; the 10th to 12th ribs are attached distally to the costal cartilage of the ninth rib.

The sternum comprises eight sternebrae, the most rostral of these is the manubrium and the most caudal sternebra is the xiphoid process.

The ribs and sternum protect the thoracic viscera and provide a framework capable of expansion and contraction during breathing.

The Forelimb Skeleton

The most proximal bone of the forelimb is the scapula. It is a flattened semi-circular shaped bone with a spine on its lateral aspect. The spine ends distally as the acromion which, in the cat bears a caudal projection, the suprahamate process. The scapula does not articulate with the axial skeleton but is attached to the ribs and vertebrae by muscles.

Distally the scapula articulates at the shoulder joint (fig. 3) with the humerus, the long bone of the brachium. Just cranial to the proximal humerus is the clavicle, a small rod-shaped bone within the brachiocephalicus muscle. In the cat there is a supracondyloid foramen just proximal to the medial condyle of the distal humerus.

At the elbow joint (fig. 4) the humerus articulates with the bones of the antebrachium, the radius and ulna. The olecranon process is the proximal extremity of the ulna and projects caudally beyond the elbow joint. The forepaw, including the bones of the carpus is called the manus. In the cat there are seven carpal bones, the radial and ulnar carpal bones articulating with the distal radius and ulna. The palpable bone on the caudal aspect of the carpus is the accessory carpal bone.

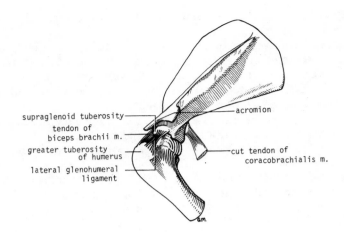

supraglenoid tuberosity
tendon of
biceps brachii m.
greater tuberosity
of humerus
lateral glenohumeral
ligament

acromion

cut tendon of
coracobrachialis m.

FIG. 3 The shoulder joint

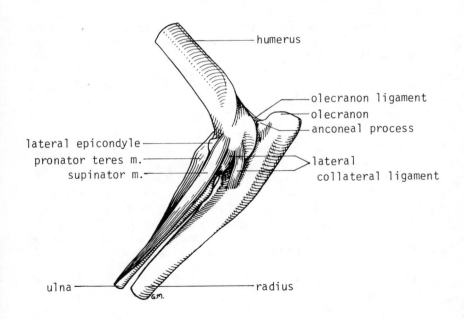

humerus

olecranon ligament
olecranon
anconeal process

lateral epicondyle
pronator teres m.
supinator m.

lateral
collateral ligament

ulna

radius

FIG. 4 Lateral view of left elbow joint

There are five metacarpal bones, that of the first digit being much shorter than the other four. The four main digits comprise proximal, middle and distal phalanges, whereas the first digit lacks a middle phalanx. The ungual process is the projection of the distal phalanx into the claw.

The Hindlimb Skeleton

The ilium, pubis and ischium are fused together to comprise the os coxae. The left and right ossa coxarum are united in the ventral midline at the pelvic symphysis, a cartilaginous joint in the young cat but often ossified in the older animal. The two ilia articulate with the sacrum, contrasting with the forelimb skeleton which has no articulation with the axial skeleton. On either side of the pelvic symphysis there is an oval-shaped foramen about 1.5 cm in length; these are the obturator foramina. Each os coxae bears, on its lateral aspect, a cup-shaped depression, the acetabulum, which accommodates the head of the femur (see fig. 5).

The femur is a long slender bone bearing the palpable greater trochanter immediately lateral to the hip joint and, distally, two condyles which articulate with the proximal tibia at the stifle joint (see figs. 6 and 7).

The patella, or knee-cap, is about 0.5 cm in diameter and lies in the tendon of the quadriceps muscle where this passes over the cranial aspect of the femoral condyles.

The fibula is a long thin bone on the lateral aspect of the tibia, with which it articulates both proximally and distally. The tibia is a substantial bone, triangular in cross-section at its proximal end, the

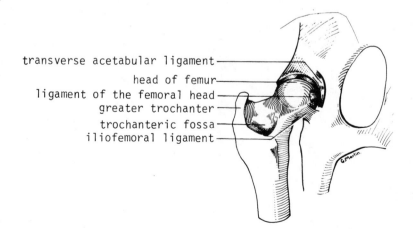

transverse acetabular ligament
head of femur
ligament of the femoral head
greater trochanter
trochanteric fossa
iliofemoral ligament

FIG. 5 Caudo-ventral view of the left hip joint

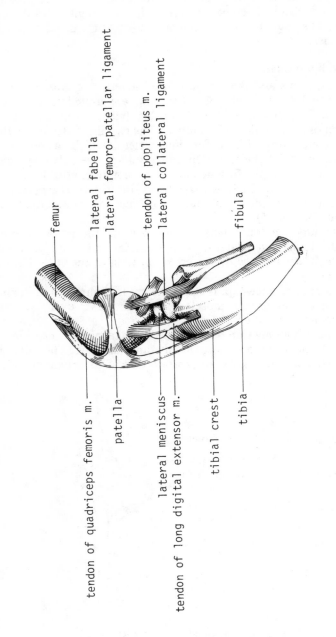

femur

lateral fabella

lateral femoro-patellar ligament

tendon of popliteus m.

lateral collateral ligament

fibula

tendon of quadriceps femoris m.

patella

lateral meniscus

tendon of long digital extensor m.

tibial crest

tibia

FIG. 6   Lateral view of the left stifle joint

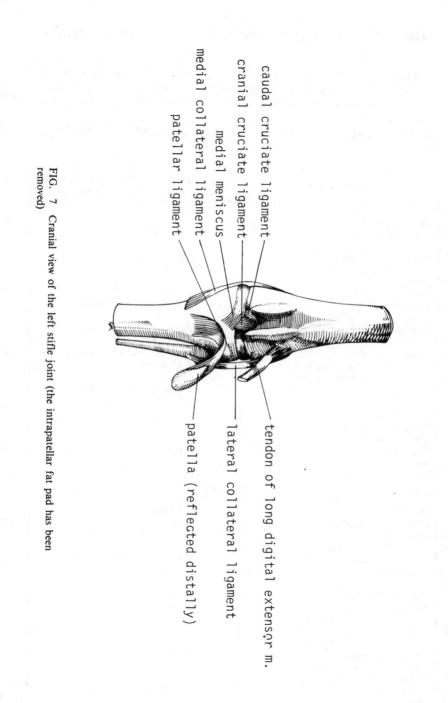

caudal cruciate ligament

cranial cruciate ligament

medial meniscus

medial collateral ligament

patellar ligament

tendon of long digital extensor m.

lateral collateral ligament

patella (reflected distally)

FIG. 7 Cranial view of the left stifle joint (the intrapatellar fat pad has been removed)

Table I
Ossification Times of Growth Plates in the Limbs of the Cat

Radiographs of the limbs of young cats reveal the presence of radiolucent areas between the epiphyses and diaphyses of the bones. These areas consist of cartilage and are known as growth plates; they ossify at varying ages.

Most of the data in the table below was recorded by Smith (1969).

FORELIMB	EARLIEST AGE AT WHICH FUSION WITH DIAPHYSIS IS APPARENT.
Scapula	
Supraglenoid tubercle	16 weeks
Coracoid process	16 weeks
Humerus	
Proximal epiphysis	58 weeks
Distal epiphysis	16 weeks
Radius	
Proximal epiphysis	28 weeks
Distal epiphysis	58 weeks (up to 88 weeks)
Ulna	
Olecranon	38 weeks (always complete by 52 weeks)
Distal epiphysis	58 weeks (up to 100 weeks)
Accessory carpal bone	16-18 weeks
Metcarpals II-V	
Distal epiphysis	29 weeks (complete by 40 weeks)
Phalanges of digits II-V	
Proximal epiphysis of proximal phalanx	18 weeks
Proximal epiphysis of distal phalanx	18 weeks
HINDLIMB	
Femur	
Head of femur	30-40 weeks
Greater trochanter	28-36 weeks
Lesser trochanter	34-44 weeks
Tibia	
Tibial tuberosity	50 weeks
Proximal epiphysis	50 weeks
Fibula	
Proximal epiphysis	54-72 weeks
Distal epiphysis	40-56 weeks
Calcaneus	
Tuber calcis	30-52 weeks
Metatarsals II-V	
Distal epiphyses	32 weeks
Phalanges	
Similar to forelimb	

Table II
The Muscles and Nerves of the Limbs

The following two tables summarise the main actions of the more important muscles of the fore and hindlimbs. It must be emphasized that many muscles have more than one action (e.g. the gastrocnemius muscle is a flexor of the stifle joint as well as an extensor of the tarsal joint). Often the movement produced in a limb is the net result of the contraction of several muscles.

FORELIMB			
NERVE	SOMATIC AFFERENT COMPONENT	SOMATIC EFFERENT COMPONENT	
		MUSCLE	MAIN ACTION
Accessory	None	Trapezius Omotransversarius Rhomboideus Brachiocephalicus	Protraction and elevation of the limb
Suprascapular	None	Supraspinatus Infraspinatus	Extension and stabilisation of the shoulder joint
Subscapular	None	Subscapularis	Extension and stabilisation of the shoulder joint
Axillary	Sensory to lateral brachium and proximal antebrachium	Deltoideus Teres major Teres minor	Flexion of the shoulder joint
Radial	Sensory to cranial and lateral antebrachium and dorsal aspect of paw	Triceps brachii Anconeus Tensor fasciae antebrachium	Extensions of the elbow joint
		Brachioradialis Supinator	Supination of the antebrachium
		Extensor carpi radialis	Extension of the carpal joint
		Ulnaris lateralis	Flexion of the carpal joint
		Common digital extensor Lateral digital extensor Abductor pollicis longus	Extension of the joints of the digits

Table II continued

Musculo-cutaneous	Sensory to medial antebrachium	Coracobrachialis	Extension of the shoulder joint
		Biceps brachii Brachialis	Flexion of the elbow joint
Median	Palmar aspect of paw	Pronator teres Pronator quadratus	Pronation of the antebrachium
		Flexor carpi radialis	Flexion of the carpal joint
		Superficial digital flexor Deep digital flexor	Flexion of the joints of the digits
Ulnar	Caudal antebrachium and palmar aspect of paw	Flexor carpi ulnaris	Flexion of the carpal joint
		Deep digital flexor Interosseous muscles	Flexion of the joints of the digits

cranially directed apex being the tibial tuberosity to which the patellar ligament attaches.

The tarsus, or hock joint, consists of seven bones. The talus (tibial tarsal bone) bears a prominent trochlea which articulates with the tibia and fibula. The calcaneus (fibular tarsal bone) is an elongated bone projecting proximocaudally as the tuber calcis, to which the Achilles tendon is attached. A central and four distal tarsal bones complete the tarsus.

The metatarsals are longer than the metacarpals but otherwise the bones of the four main hindpaw digits resemble those of the forepaw. A reduced first metatarsus may be present but the phalanges of the first digit are absent.

The Cardiovascular System

Oxygen, nutrients and excretory products of metabolism are all carried by the blood between the organs of the body. The blood is circulated in a system of vessels under the influence of the pumping action of the heart.

The normal constituents of feline blood are shown in the anaemia discussion in the Cardiovascular System chapter.

The Heart

The heart is a cone-shaped muscular organ located in the thorax between the second and sixth ribs. The apex of the heart is directed caudoventrally and to the left of the midline.

Table III
HINDLIMB

NERVE	SOMATIC AFFERENT COMPONENT	SOMATIC EFFERENT COMPONENT	
		MUSCLE	MAIN ACTION
Obturator	None	Gracilis Pectineus Adductors	Adduction of the hindlimb
Gluteal	None	Superficial gluteal Middle gluteal Deep gluteal	Extension of the hip joint
Sciatic	Sensory to lateral and caudal aspects of crus	Caudofemoralis Internal obturator Quadratus femoris	Outwards rotation of hindlimb
		Gemellus	
Femoral	Sensory to medial aspect of thigh, crus and hindpaw	Capsularis coxae Sartorius Rectus femoris Quadriceps femoris	Flexion of the hip joint Extension of the stifle joint
Peroneal	Sensory to cranial aspect of crus and dorsal hindpaw	Tibialis cranialis	Lateral rotation of hindpaw
Tibial	Sensory to plantar aspect of paw.	Long digital extensor Lateral digital extensor Short digital extensor	Extension of the joints of the digits
		Peroneus longus	Medial rotation of hindpaw
		Peroneus brevis	Flexion of the tarsal joint
		Biceps femoris Semitendinosus Semimembranosus	Extension of the hip joint and stifle joint
		Popliteus	Flexion of the stifle joint
		Gastrocnemius Soleus Tibialis caudalis	Extension of the tarsal joint
		Superficial digital flexor Deep digital flexor Interosseous muscles	Flexion of the joints of the digits

The heart is enclosed by the pericardium. The shiny outer surface of the heart is the visceral pericardium. This is separated from the parietal pericardium by the pericardial cavity which normally contains a small amount of serous fluid.

The myocardium represents the great majority of the heart wall and is lined on its inner aspect by the thin endocardium.

The lumen of the heart is divided into four chambers and normally there is no connection between the two chambers on the left side and those on the right side of the heart. Towards the apex of the heart the two thick-walled compartments are the left and right ventricles. The thinner walled and smaller chambers at the wide dorsocranial end of the heart are the left and right atria. Before birth the septum between the atria is perforated by the foramen ovale; persistence of the foramen post-natally is the condition of hole-in-the-heart.

Blood can pass from atrium to ventricle on the same side but is prevented from flowing in the reverse direction by the presence of an atrioventricular valve (A-V valve). In the cat both A-V valves consist of two cusps, or flaps, controlled by the delicate chordae tendinae and papillary muscles.

Blood leaves the left ventricle via the aorta and the right ventricle via the pulmonary trunk. The semi-lunar aortic and pulmonary valves prevent reverse flow of blood.

The Arteries

Blood is conducted away from the heart by the arteries. These are vessels with thick walls consisting mainly of elastic tissue with some muscle fibres. This construction allows the arteries to expand and recoil according to the pumping action of the heart.

The Veins

The veins are the thin-walled vessels that return blood to the heart. The blood pressure is lower than the arterial pressure and so possible backflow in the larger veins is prevented by valves.

The Capillaries

The smallest branches of arteries are called arterioles. These are continuous with the smallest veins, or venules, via a network of microscopic vessels called capillaries. It is through the walls of the capillaries that oxygen and nutrients must diffuse to reach the tissues. Waste products of metabolism diffuse in the reverse direction to be transported by the venous blood.

The Circulation of Blood

Blood is returned to the right atrium of the heart by the cranial and caudal venae cavae. During ventricular contraction (systole) blood accumulates in the atria, being prevented from entering the ventricles by the increased pressure within them. During ventricular relaxation (diastole) the pressure gradient allows blood to flow from the atria into the ventricles through the A-V valves.

As right ventricular systole proceeds the increase in ventricular pressure results in closure of the right A-V valve. Once the pressure in the ventricle exceeds that in the pulmonary artery, the pulmonary valve opens and blood enters the pulmonary artery. At the end of ventricular systole, blood tends to flow back into the ventricle but is prevented by closure of the pulmonary valve.

The left and right pulmonary arteries conduct blood to the lungs for oxygenation in the pulmonary capillary bed. The oxygenated blood is then transported to the left atrium of the heart by the pulmonary veins. A cycle of events similar to that described on the right side of the heart occurs. The two sides of the heart function simultaneously and the heart sounds are caused by blood turbulence during (1) ventricular systole (first sound or 'lub') and (2) closure of the artery valves (second sound or 'dup').

Oxygenated blood leaves the left ventricle via the aorta to be distributed to the tissues of the body. In the foetus blood can pass directly from the pulmonary artery to the aorta through the ductus arteriosus, thereby by-passing the non-active lungs; shortly after birth the ductus arteriosus becomes occluded.

The first major artery to arise from the aortic arch is the brachiocephalic trunk (fig. 8) which in turn gives origin to the right and left common carotid arteries and the right subclavian artery; the left subclavian artery arises directly from the aorta.

The two common carotid arteries supply most of the blood supply to the head; they bifurcate just caudal to the angle of the jaw to give rise to the internal and external carotid arteries.

The internal carotid arteries of the cat are usually fibrous and non-patent; it is the external carotid arteries which give origin to the major arteries of the head.

The subclavian arteries pass cranial to the first ribs and cross the axillary spaces as the axillary arteries to provide the arterial supply to the forelimbs.

The aortic arch turns caudally to become the dorsal aorta. The dorsal aorta gives off numerous arteries as it passes through the thorax and abdomen towards the tail. The most important arteries arising from the dorsal aorta are:

(1) coeliac artery to stomach, liver, spleen, pancreas and duodenum.
(2) cranial mesenteric artery to small intestine and pancreas.
(3) renal arteries (paired) to kidneys.
(4) gonadal arteries (paired) to testes or ovaries.

(5) caudal mesenteric artery to descending colon.

At the level of first sacral vertebra the aorta gives rise to the paired external iliac arteries. These continue on the medial aspect of the thighs as the femoral arteries and are the major blood supply to the hind limbs. Subcutaneously situated, the femoral arteries are easily palpable for pulse-taking.

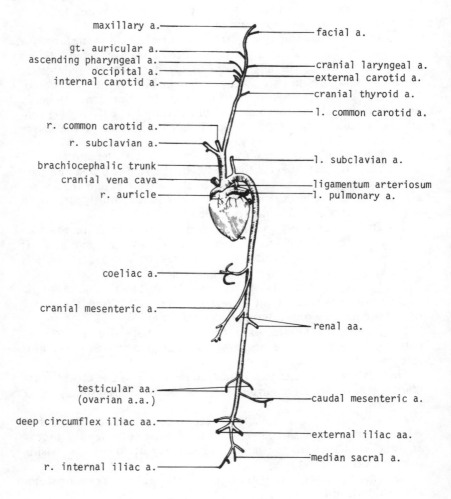

FIG. 8 Heart and major arteries of the cat

The Venous Drainage

The names and positions of the veins closely resemble those of the arteries. Clinically, probably the most important vein in the cat is the cephalic vein lying subcutaneously on the cranial aspect of the antebrachium; it is a frequent site for venepuncture.

The caudal vena cava returns blood to the heart from the tissues of the hindlimbs, pelvis and abdomen.

The paired external jugular veins drain blood from the head and their subcutaneous position in the neck makes them a suitable site for blood collection. The external jugular veins empty into the cranial vena cava via the brachiocephalic veins.

The two venae cavae empty blood into the right atrium.

The Lymphatic System

Tissue fluid is the product of diffusion from the blood through the capillary walls. Tissue fluid can also diffuse into capillaries, transferring crystalloids, gases and some colloids into the blood.

Tissue fluid may also drain into the capillary network of the lymphatic system. Lymphatic capillaries are very similar to blood capillaries but allow much easier diffusion of colloidal protein and also allow passage of particulate matter and phagocytes.

In addition to the lymphatic capillaries the lymphatic system consists of large calibre, thin-walled lymphatic vessels and compact discrete aggregations of lymphoid tissue, called lymph nodes.

The tissue fluid within the lymphatic system is called lymph. Afferent vessels conduct lymph from the tissue to a lymph node. The lymph node filters the lymph both mechanically and by phagocytosis, thereby removing bacteria and other particles.

Lymphocytes, produced in the lymph nodes, are added to the lymph which is then conducted away from the nodes in efferent vessels. All lymph eventually enters the thoracic, left tracheal or right tracheal ducts. The thoracic and left tracheal ducts converge before emptying into the left external jugular vein, just as it becomes the left brachiocephalic vein. The right tracheal duct empties lymph into the right external jugular vein.

The lymph nodes are of considerable clinical importance as they may become enlarged when infection or neoplasia is present in the tissues drained by their afferent vessels. The following lymph nodes are usually palpable in the cat, even when normal:

a) Mandibular; located just ventral to the angle of the jaw.
b) Superficial cervical; just cranial to the cranial edge of the scapula.
c) Popliteal; in the popliteal fossa between the biceps femoris and semitendinosus muscles just caudal to the stifle joint.

The following lymph nodes are palpable in the cat, when enlarged:
a) Superficial inguinal; embedded in fat just ventral to the pubis.

These nodes receive afferents from the three caudal pairs of mammary glands in the female.

b) Axillary; lying within the caudal part of the axillary space. These nodes receive afferents from the cranial three pairs of mammary glands and the forelimbs.

c) Mesenteric; located within the mesentery of the small intestine.

The Spleen (fig. 12)

The largest lymphoid organ in the body is the spleen. It differs from the lymph nodes in that its afferent and efferent vessels are blood vessels, not lymphatics. The spleen of the cat is a relatively large, elongated and flattened organ, lying around the greater curvature of the stomach in the left flank.

In addition to the production of lymphocytes and the destruction of erythrocytes, the spleen functions as a blood reservoir.

The Thymus

In the young cat the thymus is present as a lobulated mass of lymphoid tissue situated between the lungs and just cranial to the heart. As the cat grows older the thymus involutes until it is hardly discernible. The full functional significance of the thymus is not clear although its ability to produce lymphocytes indicates an immunological involvement.

The thymus is of clinical importance in the condition of thymic lymphosarcoma.

The Tonsils

The tonsils are lymphoid masses located in the walls of the pharynx. The paired palatine tonsils lie in the lateral walls of the pharynx just caudal to the glossopalatine arch, a fold of tissue between the soft palate and the base of the tongue.

The pharyngeal tonsil is dorsally situated in the nasopharynx and the lingual tonsil lies at the root of the tongue.

The Respiratory System

Oxygen is essential for the metabolic processes of all the tissues of the body. Carbon dioxide is a waste product of those processes. The respiratory system is responsible for the exchange of these two gases between the atmosphere and the blood. Transport of the gases by the blood is either by chemical combination with haemoglobin in the red cells or in solution in the plasma.

During resting respiration air is inspired through the nostrils and passes through the nasal cavity (fig. 9) where it is warmed and humidified. From the nasal cavity it passes through the nasal pharynx, the chamber dorsal to the soft palate. In order to enter the larynx the air must cross the common pharynx, a region through which food passes during swallowing. The inhalation of food or fluid is prevented by the combined movements of the soft palate and epiglottis.

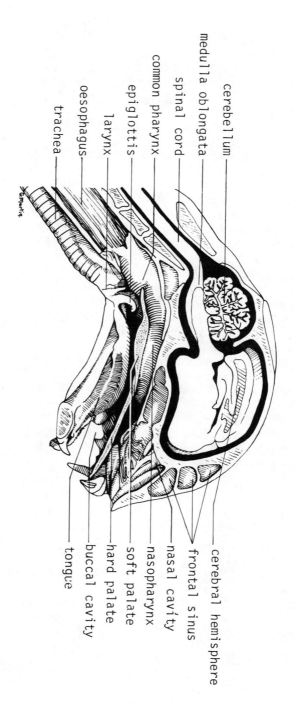

cerebellum
medulla oblongata
spinal cord
common pharynx
epiglottis
larynx
oesophagus
trachea

cerebral hemisphere
frontal sinus
nasal cavity
nasopharynx
soft palate
hard palate
buccal cavity
tongue

FIG. 9   Sagittal section through the head

37

The larynx (fig. 9) is an incompressible cylindrical structure consisting essentially of the unpaired epiglottis, thyroid, cricoid and interarytenoid cartilages and the paired arytenoid cartilage. The epiglottis is the spade-like structure seen when the pharynx is viewed through the open mouth. The thyroid cartilage is the largest of the laryngeal cartilages and the cricoid cartilage is the most caudal. There are two folds in the mucous membrane lining the lateral walls of laryngeal vestibule; the more cranial of these is the vestibular fold and the more caudal is the vocal fold.

Beyond the larynx air passes into the trachea. This is a flexible, incompressible tube which consists, in the cat, of about 40 C-shaped cartilages arranged in series. The gaps in the cartilages are on the dorsal aspect adjacent to the oesophagus; the deficiency in each cartilage is filled with muscle.

Within the thorax the trachea bifurcates into two primary bronchi which enter the lungs and further divide. The bronchi also contain cartilaginous plates and, like the trachea, are lined by a ciliated, mucus-secreting epithelium. The ultimate sub-divisions of the bronchial tree are the respiratory bronchioles and it is from these that the alveolar ducts lead. Alveoli open on all sides of the alveolar ducts; they are the areas of gaseous exchange. The air in an alveolus is separated from the blood only by a single layer of flattened epithelial cells and the capillary endothelium.

The right lung consists of cranial, middle, caudal and accessory lobes; the left lung has only cranial and caudal lobes. The lungs are covered by a thin, transparent membrane, the visceral pleura. The thoracic wall is lined on its inner aspect by the parietal pleura and the space between the pleura, in which the lungs are free to move, is called the pleural cavity. There is normally a small amount of fluid in the pleural cavity which acts as a lubricant between the two pleura.

The Mechanism of Breathing

The surface tension of the thin film of fluid lining the alveoli together with the elastic fibres distributed throughout the lungs, result in a tendency of the lungs to collapse. This, in turn, promotes a slight negative pressure in the pleural cavities. When the thorax is expanded the pleural cavities increase in volume and the lungs expand to fill the increased space, the negative pressure overcoming the tendency of the lung tissue to collapse. The pressure inside the lungs drops below atmospheric pressure and so air rushes into the expanded lungs.

Expansion of the thorax is brought about by contraction of the muscle of the diaphragm, which flattens and moves caudally, and contraction of the intercostal muscles so that the ribs swing outwards and ventrally.

During expiration the diaphragmatic and intercostal muscles relax and, aided by the elasticity of the lungs, the thorax, pleural cavities and lungs return to their pre-inspiratory volume.

If the chest wall is perforated the equalisation of pressure between the pleural cavity and the atmosphere results in collapse of the lung.

The Digestive System

The digestive system comprises the mouth, oesophagus and gastro-intestinal tract together with the liver and pancreas (fig. 10, 11 and 12).

The mouth of the cat is a short and wide cavity in all breeds. The upper lip has a central bare area with a midline groove, the philtrum, extending to the muzzle.

The Teeth

The teeth of the cat are adapted to the carnivorous habits of the species. The canine teeth are long and pointed with a curved crown; they are used to catch and hold prey. The premolar and molar teeth are adapted for the cutting and crushing of meat. The third upper premolar and the lower molar are large teeth specially modified and apposed to have a scissor-like action; they are called carnassial teeth.

The dental formulae of the cat are as follows:

<table>
<tr><td>Deciduous</td><td>Permanent</td></tr>
<tr><td>$I\frac{3}{3} \quad C\frac{1}{1} \quad M\frac{3}{2} = \frac{7}{6} \times 2 = 26$</td><td>$I\frac{3}{3} \quad C\frac{1}{1} \quad PM\frac{3}{2} \quad M\frac{1}{1} = \frac{8}{7} \times 2 = 30$</td></tr>
</table>

The eruption times of the permanent dentition and the number of roots of the individual teeth are given in Table IV.

The Tongue

The tongue is a mobile, muscular structure overlying the floor of the oral cavity. The dorsal surface of the tongue is covered by papillae of various shapes and sizes; the numerous filiform papillae are cornified giving the tongue a roughened surface. On the ventral aspect the midline lingual frenulum attaches the body of the tongue to the floor of the oral cavity.

The Salivary Glands (fig. 10)

There are four pairs of salivary glands in the cat.

The parotid gland is a lobulated, oval shaped structure lying just ventral to the ear. The parotid duct crosses the masseter muscle of the cheek to open into the oral cavity opposite the second upper premolar tooth.

The mandibular gland is a large, oval, well-encapsulated structure found just caudal to the angle of the jaw. The small sublingual gland has a monostomatic portion just rostral to the mandibular gland and a polystomatic portion adjacent to the oral mucous membrane. The ducts of the sublingual and mandibular glands, either separately or conjoined, open on a papilla adjacent to the lingual frenulum.

The zygomatic gland lies ventral to the orbit. Its four or five ducts open into the oral cavity opposite the upper third premolar.

The Oesophagus

During the act of swallowing, food is directed over the laryngeal aditus by the epiglottis. It enters the oesophagus and passes caudally to the stomach under the influence of waves of contraction of the muscular tissues in the wall of the oesophagus.

The mucous membrane lining the oesophagus is arranged in longitudinal folds, aiding its ability to dilate. There are three regions in which there is some limitation on the expansibility of the oesophagus and, hence a danger of obstruction. The first is at its origin, where the oesophagus passes dorsally to the larynx. Secondly, as the oesophagus crosses the dorsal aspect of the base of the heart and thirdly, as the oesophagus passes through the diaphragm.

The Stomach (fig. 12)

The stomach is a large, pouch-like organ lying largely to the left of the midline and caudal to the liver. The stomach is very distensible and its position depends on its fullness; the full stomach protrudes caudally to the costal arch. Various glands are present in the lining mucous membrane and secrete mucus, dilute hydrochloric acid or digestive enzymes into the lumen of the stomach.

The convex side of the stomach is the greater curvature and provides attachment for the great omentum, a two layered membranous sac which extends caudally to cover the whole of the ventral aspect of the abdominal organs. The lesser omentum attaches to the portal fissure of the liver and the concave lesser curvature of the stomach.

The distal exit from the stomach is constricted by a thickened annulus of muscle, the pyloric sphincter.

The Duodenum (fig. 11)

The first part of the small intestine is called the duodenum. It extends cranially from the pylorus for 2 cm before bending caudally as the descending limb; it lies dorsally on the right of the abdomen. At the caudal flexure the duodenum bends towards the midline, and then cranially, as the ascending limb.

Both the common bile duct and the main pancreatic duct open into the descending duodenum. The duodenum is relatively immobile owing to its attachment to the dorsal body wall, the mesoduodenum, and the common bile duct.

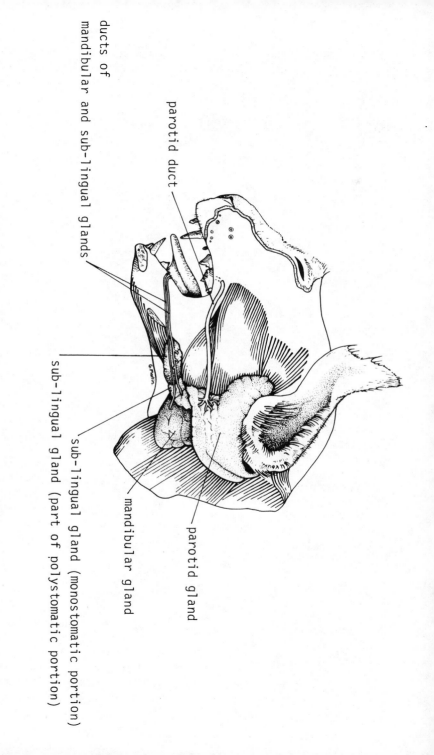

parotid duct

ducts of
mandibular and sub-lingual glands

sub-lingual gland (monostomatic portion)

sub-lingual gland (part of polystomatic portion)

mandibular gland

parotid gland

FIG. 10 Superficial dissection of the face to show the salivary glands

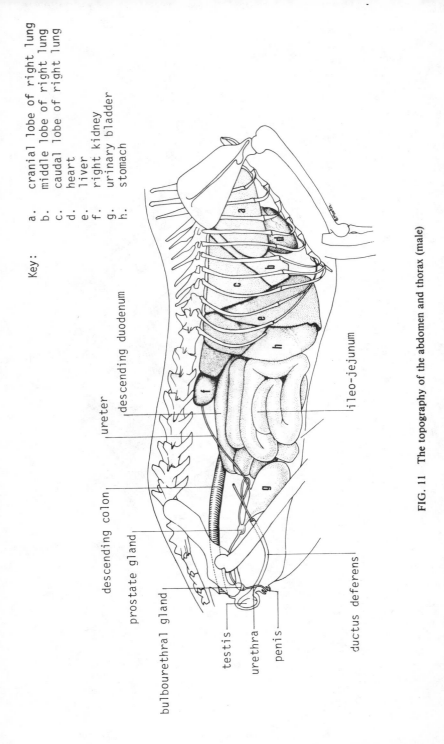

Key:

a. cranial lobe of right lung
b. middle lobe of right lung
c. caudal lobe of right lung
d. heart
e. liver
f. right kidney
g. urinary bladder
h. stomach

ureter

descending duodenum

ileo-jejunum

descending colon

prostate gland

bulbourethral gland

testis

urethra

penis

ductus deferens

FIG. 11 The topography of the abdomen and thorax (male)

Key:
a. cranial lobe of left lung
b. middle lobe of left lung
c. caudal lobe of left lung
d. heart
e. liver
f. left kidney
g. urinary bladder
h. stomach
j. spleen

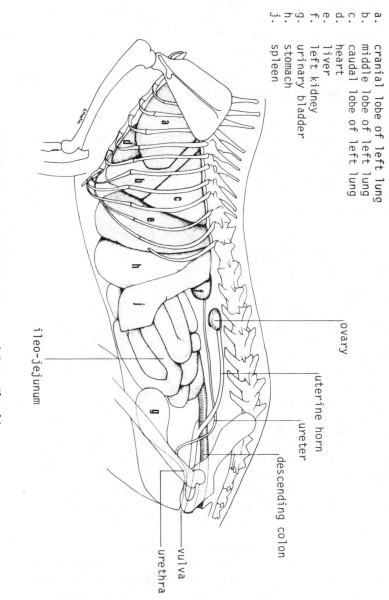

FIG. 12 The topography of the abdomen and thorax (female)

ileo-jejunum

ovary

uterine horn

ureter

descending colon

vulva

urethra

43

The Ileo-Jejunum (figs. 11 and 12)

The duodenum is continuous with the jejunum and, in the cat, there is no gross difference between jejunum and ileum.

The ileo-jejunum is arranged in numerous coils, all linked by the fan-shaped great mesentery containing radiating blood vessels.

The mucous membrane of the small intestine bears many finger-like projections called villi, which increase the surface area for the absorption of the products of digestion.

Oval-shaped aggregations of lymphoid tissue in the wall of the small intestine are called Peyer's patches.

The Large Intestine (figs. 11 and 12)

The ileum opens into the colon at the ileo-colic sphincter. The short ascending colon is in the middle of the right flank and turns to the left as the transverse colon close to the pyloric end of the stomach. The descending colon passes caudally in a dorsal position on the left side. Within the pelvis the colon inclines to the midline where it continues as the rectum to open to the exterior at the anus.

The caecum is a small, blind-ending comma-shaped diverticulum of the ascending colon.

The colon and rectum are attached to the body wall by the mesocolon and mesorectum respectively.

The Liver

The liver lies almost entirely within the rib cage. It is a large organ comprising left and right medial lobes, left and right lateral lobes, a caudate lobe and a quadrate lobe. The gall bladder is located between the right medial and quadrate lobes. The falciform ligament extends from the umbilicus, in the midline, between the left medial and quadrate lobes, to the diaphragm.

The liver receives blood from the gastro-intestinal tract via the hepatic portal vein. This blood contains products of digestion absorbed through the wall of the intestine. The cells of the liver are capable of initiating and controlling various complex biochemical processes. The liver plays a role in the metabolism and storage of carbohydrate, the metabolism of lipids and in the metabolism of protein. In addition to these important functions, the liver converts unwanted nitrogenous compounds into urea for excretion by the kidneys and is the chief organ for the detoxification of harmful chemical compounds or drugs.

Red blood cells, or erythrocytes, have a life span of from two to six weeks. Old erythrocytes are removed by phagocytosis either in the spleen or liver. In the liver the products of breakdown of haemoglobin contribute to the formation of bile. Bile is a green fluid, continuously secreted by the liver and accumulated in the gall bladder. During periods of digestion bile is released from the gall bladder to enter the duodenum via the common bile duct.

The Pancreas

The pancreas is an elongated, lobulated organ contained largely between the two limbs of the duodenum. The main pancreatic duct enters the duodenum close to the orifice of the common bile duct. In the cat the accessory pancreatic duct is often absent.

The pancreas is a complex aggregation of glandular tissue, having both exocrine and endocrine elements. The exocrine function of the pancreas is concerned with the production of pancreatic juice, a particularly potent mixture of digestive enzymes with actions on proteins, lipids and carbohydrates. The secretion of pancreatic juice and its release into the duodenum is under both neural and hormonal control.

The endocrine part of the pancreas comprises numerous isolated collections of cells, called the islets of Langerhans. Two types of islet cells are distinguishable; the beta cells produce insulin and the alpha cells secrete glucagon. These two hormones are concerned with carbohydrate metabolism, though their actual action and control are most complex. Insulin promotes the utilisation of blood glucose by the tissues, either for oxidation (energy release) or glycogen synthesis. Glucagon, on the other hand, promotes the release of stored carbohydrate (glycogen) from the tissues and hence an elevation of blood glucose.

The Urogenital System

The organs of urination and reproduction (figs. 11 and 12) are grouped together because of their morphological and developmental association. Postnatally, however, only the most distal parts of the two duct systems share a common tract.

The Kidneys

The kidneys are the organs of urinary excretion. The production of urine is a complex process involving an initial filtration of blood followed by selective reabsorption mechanisms. In addition the kidneys preserve water and electrolytes and maintain the acid-base balance of the body.

The structural and functional unit of the kidney is the nephron. The proximal part of a nephron is the double-walled Bowman's capsule which envelops a tuft of blood capillaries, called a glomerulus. The initial filtrate accumulates in the capsule lumen and then flows through the elongated renal tubule. The proximal and distal parts of the tubule are convoluted but the middle section, the loop of Henle is a U-shape with straight limbs. It is in the tubule that the various reabsorption processes act to restore required substances (e.g. glucose) to the blood. Some urea returns to the blood by simple diffusion but creatinine is actively and totally excreted. Certain drugs are also actively excreted by the nephrons.

The distal convoluted tubules empty urine into collecting ducts which, in turn, discharge into the renal pelvis, the enlarged proximal end of the ureter.

There are two kidneys; they are bean-shaped organs located against the dorsal body wall within the abdominal cavity. Both kidneys are palpable in the normal cat. The left kidney is at the level of the third and fourth lumbar vertebrae and the right kidney is level with lumbar vertebrae two and three. The kidneys of the cat are unique in the possession of the prominent sub-capsular stellate veins which radiate over the surface from the hilus, the medially-facing concavity of the kidney.

In section the kidney is seen to consist of an outer cortex and inner medulla; the Bowman's capsules are in the cortex and the loops of Henle extend into the medulla. The renal artery is a short direct branch of the aorta and enters the kidney at the hilus; the renal vein and the ureter both leave the kidney at the hilus.

The Ureters
The two ureters are muscular tubes lying against the dorsal body wall; they open into the dorsolateral aspect of the caudal part of the urinary bladder.

The Urinary Bladder
The bladder is a piriform sac situated ventral to the rectum and just cranial to the pubis. The size and position of the bladder vary greatly according to its fullness. The empty bladder of the cat may contract to a diameter of only 2-3 cm but can distend to a diameter 8-9 cm if the urethra is obstructed. The wall of the bladder is strongly muscular, containing three layers of muscle tissue. The bladder is easily palpable through the ventral body wall, when full.

The Urethra
The caudally situated neck of the bladder leads into the urethra. In the female the urethra is a straight musculomembranous tube extending to the external urethral orifice at the boundary between the vagina and vestibule. In the female the lumen of the urethra is 1-2 mm and is easily dilated.

In the male the urethra has a smaller lumen than in the female and is further constricted as it bends ventrally over the ischial arch. The urethra of the male cat is joined at its origin from the neck of the bladder by the two ducti deferentes. The urethra is thus the common tract to the exterior for either sperm or urine. The early, or pelvic part of the urethra is enclosed by the prostate gland.

The Female Genital Organs (fig. 12)
The Ovaries

The two ovaries are oval-shaped and about 1 cm long; they are located just caudal to the kidneys. A pouch of peritoneum, the ovarian bursa, almost completely surrounds the ovary. Cranially a fold of peritoneum anchors the ovary to the body wall near the last rib; this is the suspensory ligament of the ovary. Caudally the proper ligament of the ovary attaches the ovary to the cranial end of the uterus.

Small, fluid-filled protuberances from the ovary surface are Graafian follicles. Following coitus, ripe follicles rupture and release ova (one ovum from each follicle). This process is known as ovulation and is followed by the formation of a corpus luteum, a solid mass of cells at the site of the follicle.

The Vagina

The vagina is long and narrow; it extends from the external orifice of the cervix to the external urethral opening. The mucous membrane of the vagina is arranged in longitudinal folds and includes a prominent dorsal ridge extending caudally from the cervix.

The Vestibule, Clitoris and Vulva

The vestibule extends from the external urethral orifice to the vulva, the opening to the exterior. The longitudinal folds of the vestibular mucous membrane contrast with the smooth lining of the vulva.

The vestibule is encircled by the strong constrictor vestibuli muscle. In the ventral floor of the vestibule near the vulva, lies a small papilla, the clitoris.

The Male Genital Organs (fig. 11)
The Testes

The male gonads are oval-shaped and lie with their long axes in a craniocaudal direction; they are enclosed by the scrotum and located just ventral to the anus. The highly convoluted duct system arising from the testis is the epididymis. Leading from the epididymis, on the ventral aspect of the testis, is the ductus deferens, a long, narrow tube passing cranially through the inguinal canal to loop around the ureter of the same side and finally empty into the prostatic urethra. Just cranial to the epididymis the testicular artery is surrounded by a network of veins called the pampiniform plexus.

The Accessory Sex Organs

The prostate is a large bi-lobed gland surrounding the proximal urethra.

The paired bulbourethral glands are pea-sized structures lying either side of the urethra, just caudal to the ischial arch.

The secretions of both the prostate and bulbourethral glands are added to the semen during ejaculation.

The Penis

The penis of the cat is directed caudally and lies, enclosed in its preputial sheath, just ventral to the scrotum. The presence of a small bone, the os penis (often cartilaginous in young cats), can predispose obstruction of the urethra by calculi. The distal extremity, the glans penis, is covered by small cranially-directed spines.

The Central Nervous System (CNS)

A peripheral and a central division of the nervous system are distinguished. The central nervous system comprises the brain and spinal cord and the peripheral nervous system consists of all the nerve trunks and ganglia outside the C.N.S. The peripheral nerves are either afferent or efferent in function, depending on whether an impulse travels from the periphery to the C.N.S. or vice versa. Afferent impulses arise by stimulation of receptor endings of nerves. Efferent impulses travel from the C.N.S. to target tissues, e.g. muscles or glands.

The nervous system is also considered to consist of autonomic and somatic divisions. The somatic nervous system is responsible for voluntary activity and the autonomic nervous system exerts visceral control. However, such a division is not as clear as it would seem and in fact a marked characteristic of the nervous system is its highly integrated nature.

The Brain (figs. 13 and 14)

The dominant feature of the brain is the cerebrum, comprising two large hemispheres crossed by ridges (gyri) and depressions (sulci).

The olfactory bulbs project rostrally beyond the cerebrum and caudally, on the dorsal aspect, the multi-fissured structure is the cerebellum.

On the ventral aspect, in the midline, the pituitary gland is located as a small projection from the area known as the hypothalamus. Just rostral to the pituitary gland the optic nerves arise from a cross of neural tissue, the optic chiasma. Caudal to the pituitary gland the region ventral to the cerebellum is the pons and this is continued caudally as the medulla oblongata.

It is beyond the scope of this book to describe the very complex internal structure of the brain other than to mention that the thalamus is located in a central position dorsal to the hypothalamus. The cavities

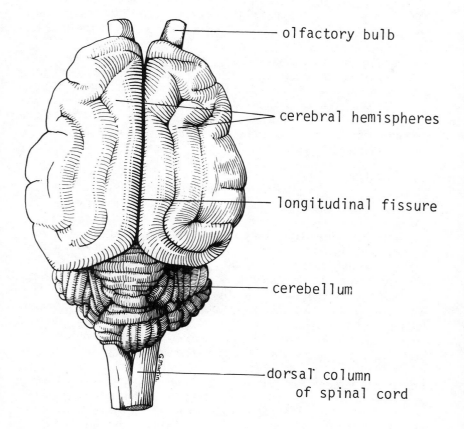

olfactory bulb

cerebral hemispheres

longitudinal fissure

cerebellum

dorsal column
of spinal cord

FIG. 13   Dorsal view of the brain

of the brain are called ventricles; there are two lateral ventricles connected to the midline third ventricle. The cerebral aqueduct connects the third with the fourth ventricle, located between the cerebellum and the pons. The fourth ventricle is continuous with the central canal of the spinal cord and also opens through a pair of lateral apertures into the subarachnoid space.

The meninges are three membranous layers that completely surround the brain and spinal cord; they are called the pia mater, arachnoid mater and dura mater. The pia mater is the innermost layer and the dura mater the outermost layer. The subarachnoid space lies between the pia mater and the arachnoid mater and is expanded at the following two locations; (i) on the caudal aspect of the cerebellum, the cisterna magna may be entered with a needle via the atlanto-occipital space, (ii) the lumbar cistern is at the level of the first sacral vertebra.

The ventricles of the brain, the central canal of the spinal cord and the subarachnoid space all contain cerebrospinal fluid, a dialysate of blood, similar to tissue fluid.

The Spinal Cord (fig. 15)

The medulla oblongata is continued caudally by the spinal cord which extends in the vertebral canal to the level of the seventh lumbar vertebra.

When seen in transverse section, the spinal cord consists of a central area of 'grey' matter, around the central canal, and an outer annulus of 'white' matter. The grey and white matter are not as easily distinguished as their names suggest, the terms deriving rather from the fact that grey matter contains the cell bodies of nerve cells and the white matter comprises the pale-coloured processes, or axons, of the cells.

Many of the axons in the white matter are either ascending or descending in the spinal cord, according to whether they carry afferent or efferent impulses. Nerve fibres carrying the same modalities (e.g. touch, pressure, pain, heat or cold) travel together in collective pathways or tracts. Similarly efferent fibres are disposed in specific tracts in the white matter. Furthermore, nerve fibres carrying a specific modality or modalities from a particular region of the body, travel together.

Whereas, in principle, these concepts of somatotopic localisation and association of nerve fibres within spinal tracts are correct, it should be appreciated that the tracts are not well defined bundles and the existence of certain tracts (e.g. spinothalamic, carrying pain and temperature modalities) may only be partial in the cat.

The central part of the grey matter, around the central canal, and continuing rostrally into the brain, is called the ascending reticular formation; it comprises a network of interconnecting nerve cells. The ascending reticular formation arouses the whole of the cerebral cortex

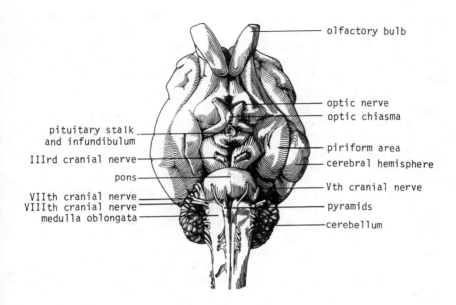

FIG. 14   Ventral view of the brain

so that conscious registration of specific stimuli may occur. General anesthetics probably act by blocking the connections between the nerve cells of the ascending reticular formation.

The Peripheral Nervous System (PNS)

Twelve pairs of nerves arise from the brainstem and are designated cranial nerves I—XII; the names and functions of the cranial nerves are given in Table 5.

Pairs of spinal nerves arise at regular intervals along the spinal cord, corresponding with the vertebrae; it is only at the level of the fourth lumbar vertebra that the spinal cord segments begin to be shorter than the vertebral bodies.

The somatic efferent nerve cells have their cell bodies in the ventral horn of the spinal cord; the autonomic efferent nerve cell bodies are in the lateral horn.

Each spinal nerve (fig. 15) arises by union of dorsal and ventral roots, the ventral root consists of the efferent nerve fibres. Just before the two roots unite a ganglion is situated on the dorsal root; the dorsal root ganglion is the location of the afferent nerve cell bodies. After union of the two roots the spinal nerve divides into dorsal and ventral rami, each containing both afferent and efferent fibres. The spinal nerves innervate the muscles of the body wall and the limbs and also

51

conduct impulses from receptors in e.g. skin, parietal peritoneum, parietal pleura, joints and muscles.

The ventral rami of spinal cord segments C6, C7, C8, T1 and T2 combine as the brachial plexus from which the nerve trunks of the forelimb are derived. The ventral rami of spinal cord segments L4, L5, L6, L7, S1 and S2 comprise the lumbosacral plexus from which the nerve trunks of the hindlimb are derived.

The motor components of the autonomic part of the P.N.S. consist of neurons innervating the glands and smooth (involuntary) muscle of the viscera. In the somatic system a single motor neuron conducts an impulse direct to the target tissue; in the autonomic system it is a relay of two neurons that conduct an impulse from the C.N.S. to a target organ. Motor neurons of the autonomic nervous system are designated either preganglionic or postganglionic.

The outflow of the sympathetic system is restricted to the lateral horn of the thoraco-lumbar spinal cord segments. The cell bodies of many sympathetic postganglionic neurons are located in the vertebral ganglia which are segmentally arranged in a chain outside the vertebral canal. Some sympathetic preganglionic nerve cells by-pass the vertebral ganglia and synapse with postganglionic neurons in the prevertebral ganglia, located within the abdominal cavity, e.g. coeliac and cranial mesenteric ganglia. The postganglionic neurons are distributed to the viscera.

The outflow of the parasympathetic system is restricted to the brain and sacral spinal cord. Parasympathetic preganglionic neurons extend all the way to the target organ before making a synapse with the very short postganglionic neuron.

The Functions of the Nervous System

Through a variety of receptors the central nervous system receives information. Some of this information reaches the conscious level at the cerebral cortex. Some stimuli initiate a reflex response through interconnections between afferent and efferent neurons in the spinal cord e.g. sudden stretching of the patellar ligament results in reflex contraction of the quadriceps femoris muscle (knee jerk reflex).

Voluntary activity can be initiated in the cerebral cortex (e.g. locomotion) but is carefully regulated according to results. This automatic control is achieved largely through feedback circuits and the cerebellum plays a particularly important role in assuring the precision of motor activity.

The Special Senses

The special senses are the specialised abilities to receive and recognise the stimuli of vision, hearing, balance, taste and smell. The receptors of each of the special senses are assembled in specific locations. The olfactory organs consist of groups of olfactory neuroepithelial cells in the lining of the nasal cavity. The taste buds are located in the tongue.

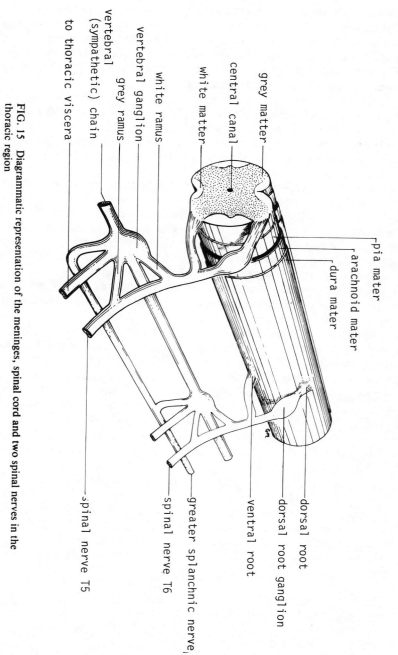

grey matter

central canal

white matter

white ramus

vertebral ganglion

grey ramus

vertebral
(sympathetic) chain

to thoracic viscera

pia mater

arachnoid mater

dura mater

dorsal root

dorsal root ganglion

ventral root

greater splanchnic nerve

spinal nerve T6

spinal nerve T5

FIG. 15 Diagrammatic representation of the meninges, spinal cord and two spinal nerves in the thoracic region

The Eye (fig. 16)

The special receptor cells of vision are the rods and cones of the retina. The ability of the cat to distinguish colours is probably very limited but its vision in darkness seems to rival its ability in daylight. The eyesight of the cat is undoubtedly well-developed and is helped by the relatively large size of the eyes and the possession of stereoscopic vision (both eyes can focus on the same object).

Light enters the eye through the transparent cornea and passes through the fluid aqueous humour. The degree of light reaching the retina is controlled by the iris, a muscular diaphragm, perforated by the pupil. Light passes through the pupil and is refracted by the lens, which is suspended by the ciliary body. Between the lens and the retina is the jelly-like vitreous humour.

The view of the back of the eye via the pupil is known as the fundus. The optic disc, the point of entry of the optic nerve to the eye, is ventrally situated in the fundus. Arising from the central retinal artery in the optic disc, the retinal arteries radiate across the retina. Around the optic disc and extending dorsally is a yellowish-green area; this is the tapetum lucidum of the choroid, the middle tunic of the eyeball. The white, outer, fibrous layer of the eyeball is the sclera.

The pink mucous membrane lining the eyelids and continuous with the outer layer of the cornea is the conjunctiva. In the medial corner of the eye the fold of tissue covered by conjunctiva is the third eyelid, or membrana nictitans. Protrusion of the third eyelid is a common symptom of many feline diseases and is thought to be due to resorption of periorbital fat. Tear fluid is produced by the lacrimal gland just dorsal to the lateral corner of the eye. Drainage of the tear fluid is through two tiny orifices in the medial corner of the eye into a duct system that leads to the nasal cavity. The drainage apparatus is rendered inefficient in some individuals of the long-haired breeds where the face is excessively flattened.

The eyes of kittens do not normally open until 8-10 days after birth.

The Ear (fig. 17)

The ear has the dual function of detecting sound and registering disturbance of balance.

The external ear is supported by cartilage and surrounds the vertical part of the ear canal, or external auditory meatus. The ear canal turns medially to end at the tympanic membrane (ear drum).

The middle ear cavity lies within the tympanic bulla and is connected to the nasopharynx by the auditory (or eustachian) tube. The middle ear cavity is crossed by a chain of three tiny bones, the auditory ossicles; the malleus bone attaches to the tympanic membrane and articulates with the incus. The third bone, the stapes, completes the chain and attaches to the membranous window of the vestibule (oval window) on the opposite side of the middle ear cavity to the ear drum.

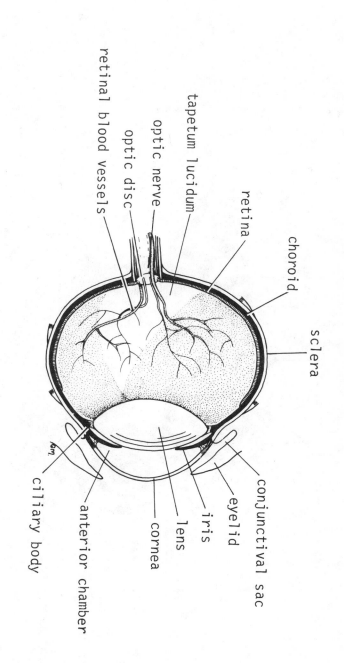

retinal blood vessels

optic disc

optic nerve

tapetum lucidum

retina

choroid

sclera

conjunctival sac

eyelid

iris

lens

cornea

anterior chamber

ciliary body

cm.

FIG. 16   Sagittal section through the eye

55

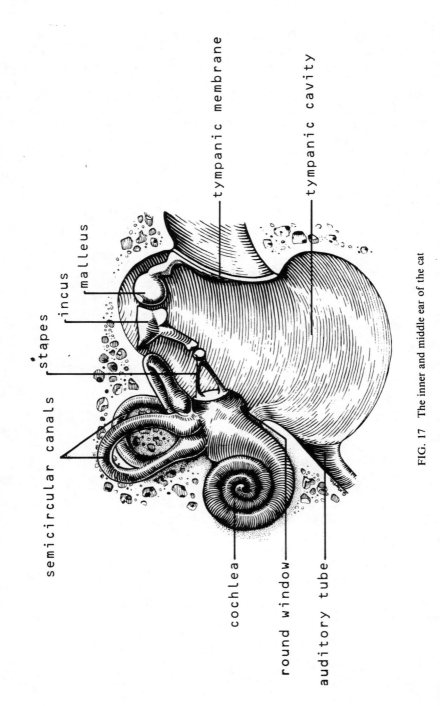

FIG. 17 The inner and middle ear of the cat

tympanic membrane

tympanic cavity

malleus

incus

stapes

semicircular canals

cochlea

round window

auditory tube

The inner ear cavity lies on the other side of the window of the vestibule. The inner ear cavity is contained in a complex excavation of bone, known as the osseous labyrinth. A completely separate connective tissue sac, the membranous labyrinth lies within the osseous labyrinth and is separated from it by a fluid, the perilymph. The membranous labyrinth contains another fluid, the endolymph.

Sound vibrations are transmitted from the ear drum to the window of the vestibule via the auditory ossicles, thus setting up movement in the perilymph; this movement is compensated for by movement of the membranous cochlear window (round window). The shock waves in the perilymph are detected by special receptor cells in the organ of Corti of the membranous labyrinth. The receptor cells begin the transmission of an impulse to the auditory area of the cerebral cortex.

The membranous labyrinth also includes three semicircular canals contained in osseous semicircular canals; the canals are each arranged in a different plane. Special receptor organs in each semicircular canal detect movements of the contained endolymph. Similar balance organs are located in the utricle and saccule, which are also sac-like parts of the membranous labyrinth. The receptor cells of the utricle and saccule, however, respond to the movement of crystals of calcium carbonate, called otoliths.

REFERENCES

King, A.S., Smith, R.N., & Kon, V.M. (1958). Protrusion of the intervertebral disc in the cat. *Vet. Rec.* **70**, 509-512.

McClure, R.C., Dallman, M.J., and Garrett, P.G. (1973). *Cat Anatomy: An atlas, text and dissection guide.* Lea and Febiger, Philadelphia.

Nomina Anatomica Veterinaria (1973). 2nd Ed., International Committee on Veterinary Anatomical Nomenclature of the World Association of Veterinary Anatomists, Vienna.

Sisson, S. and Grossman, J.D. *The Anatomy of the Domestic Animals,* Vol. 2. 5th ed. revised by Getty, R. (1975). W.B. Saunders & Co. Philadelphia.

Skerritt, G.C. and McLelland, J. (1973). *A Guide to the Functional Anatomy of the Limbs of the Domestic Animals.* Department of Veterinary Anatomy, University of Liverpool.

Smith, R.N. (1969). Fusion of ossification centres in the cat. *J. Small Anim. Pract.* **10**, 523-530.

Taylor, W.T. and Weber, R.J. (1958). *Functional Mammalian Anatomy.* D. Van Nostrand Co. Inc., Princeton.

Walker, W.F. (1967) *A Study of the Cat.* W.B. Saunders & Co., Philadelphia.

Table IV
Eruption Times of the Permanent Dentition

TEETH	AGE	NUMBER OF ROOTS
Incisors	3½ - 5½ months	One
Upper first premolar	4 - 5 months	One
Upper third premolar	4 - 5 months	Three
Upper and lower molars	4½ - 5½ months	Two
Upper second and lower premolars	5 - 6 months	Two
Canines	5½ - 6½ months	One

This table was prepared from data given by McClure et al. (1973)

Table V
The Cranial Nerves of the Cat

CRANIAL NERVE	COMPONENTS	FUNCTION
I Olfactory Nerve	Special senses afferent	Afferent pathway of smell
II Optic Nerve	Special senses afferent	Afferent pathway of vision
III Oculomotor Nerve	Somatic efferent	Muscles responsible for movement of eyeball (except lateral rectus and dorsal oblique muscles)
	Parasympathetic efferent	Constriction of pupil
IV Trochlear Nerve	Somatic efferent	Dorsal oblique muscle of eyeball
V Trigeminal nerve	Somatic afferent	Sensory to skin of head, mucous membrane of mouth and nasal cavity, rostral two thirds of tongue, the teeth, the cornea of the eye.
	Special visceral motor	Muscles responsible for opening and closing the jaws
VI Abducens Nerve	Somatic efferent	Lateral rectus muscle of eyeball
VII Facial Nerve	Somatic afferent	Shared sensation from integument of external ear
	Autonomic afferent	Taste from rostral two thirds of tongue and palate

	Parasympathetic	Sub-mandibular and sub-lingual salivary glands Lacrimal gland and glands of nasal cavity
	Special visceral motor	Muscles of face responsible for movements of eyelids, lips, ears, cheeks and nostrils
VIII Vestibulo- cochlear nerve	Special senses afferent	Vestibular division: pathway of balance sensation from inner ear. Cochlear division: sensation of hearing from inner ear
IX Glossopharyngeal Nerve	Somatic afferent	Shared sensation from integument of external ear
	Autonomic afferent	General sensation from mucous membrane of pharynx and caudal third of tongue Taste from caudal third of tongue Sensory receptors in carotid body, detecting changes in the oxygen concentration in the blood Sensory receptors in the carotid sinus, detecting changes in arterial blood pressure
	Parasympathetic efferent	Parotid salivary gland
	Special visceral motor	Stylopharyngeus muscle: this is a dilator of the pharynx
X Vagus Nerve	Somatic afferent	Shared sensation from integument of external ear
	Autonomic afferent	General sensation from the epithelia of the cervical oesophagus, larynx and the gastro-intestinal tract as far caudally as the transverse colon. Sensory receptors in the aortic arch detecting changes in oxygen concentration in blood and changes in arterial blood pressure
	Parasympathetic efferent	Smooth muscle and glands of the gastro-intestinal tract as far caudally as the transverse colon

XI Accessory Nerve (cranial division)	Special visceral motor	Muscles of the pharynx and larynx
XI (spinal division)	Somatic efferent	The sternocephalicus mus- cle turns the head: the brachiocephalicus and trapezius muscles are both protractors of the forelimb
XII Hypoglossal Nerve	Somatic efferent	The musculature of the tongue

Table VI
The Endocrine System

Below is a brief summary of the *major* endocrine glands of the cat together with the hormone that they produce and the *major* physiological effects of those hormones.

ENDOCRINE GLAND	HORMONE	ACTION
Pituitary Gland Anterior lobe	Follicle stimulating hormone (FSH)	Stimulates development of ovarian follicles in the female and production of sperm in the male
	Luteinising hormone (LH)	Stimulates formation of cor- pora lutea in female and secretion of sex hormones by interstitial cells of testes
	Luteotrophin (LTH, prolactin)	Maintains corpora lutea and stimulates lactation
	Adrenocorticotrophin (ACTH)	Stimulates secretion by the adrenal cortex
	Thyrotrophin	Stimulates secretion by the thyroid gland
	Somatotrophin	Stimulates body growth
Posterior lobe	Oxytocin	Stimulates contraction of the uterus and initiates milk ·let-down

	Antidiuretic hormone (ADH, vasopressin)	Controls water resorption in the kidneys and raises blood pressure by causing constriction of smooth muscle of arterioles
Thyroid Gland	Thyroxin	Increases metabolic rate
	Calcitonin	Lowers the concentration of blood calcium
Parathyroid Glands	Parathormone	Increases the concentration of blood calcium
Pancreas Islets of Langerhans	Insulin	Promotes carbohydrate metabolism and storage
	Glucagon	Increases blood-glucose concentration
Adrenal Gland Cortex	Glucocorticoids	Controls conversion of protein to carbohydrate for energy source
	Mineralocorticoids	Controls water and electrolyte balance
Medulla	Adrenalin and Nonadrenalin	Action similar to sympathetic nervous system; prepares body for fight or flight
Ovaries Follicles	Oestrogen	Controls secondary sexual characteristics of female
Corpora lutea	Progesterone	Prepares uterus for pregnancy and mammary glands for lactation. Inhibits ovulation
Testes	Testosterone	Controls secondary sexual characteristics of male

Chapter 3

RESTRAINT, SEDATION AND ANAESTHESIA

The handling and restraint of cats calls for a careful approach to the problem whether the restraint to be applied is physical or pharmacological. It might reasonably be said that idiosyncrasy to both is a feature of the species. All materials used must be selected in the light of our knowledge of cat temperament and drug responses.

Handling

The handling of cats is an art which is inherent in some people but which can be developed by all. Unlike the dog, cats are not usually amenable to physical restraint thus the basic principle of handling is to use as little physical force as necessary but to be always watchful and ready to apply full forcible restraint instantly when the reaction of the cat demands it. Cats are seldom co-operative patients but some degree of co-operation can be obtained by a sympathetic approach and use of fondling techniques known to elicit pleasure responses, e.g. firm but gentle stroking of the back from neck to croup, tickling beside the base of the ear or under the chin; this will often ensure a quiet and reassured patient while preliminary history-taking or other preparations are under way.

Nervousness in cats is often shown by the rapid onset of quite copious sweating via the pads, damp or even wet footmarks being visible on surfaces such as linoleum; rapid panting with slight protrusion of the tongue from which drops of moisture also fall is likewise seen. In some cats copious salivation with incredibly quick production of long strings of tacky saliva indicates nervous tension, e.g. before anticipated injections or during dressing of ears.

Although restraint often necessitates holding the loose skin of the scruff of the neck this is often resented and should be applied only when full restraint is necessary and not automatically for any type of examination.

Cats are far more apprehensive of and therefore more likely to resist approach from in front rather than above; thus baskets or boxes with a lid rather than a door at the front are to be preferred. Similarly any cat which is to be admitted for a short time and which seems nervous or bad tempered is better put into a basket rather than a cat cage, from which it can be lifted out with little resistance. Baskets or boxes containing cats should not be placed on the floor of a surgery or waiting room where they can be sniffed at by dogs. Attention to just this sort of small point may make all the difference between a handleable cat and a raging tiger.

Restraint

A superficial clinical examination of most cats can be carried out with comparatively little control; it is wise to ask the owner to hold and make a fuss of the cat's head but a warning must also be given as to the dangers from a bite and the method of holding advisable.

The simple process of temperature taking may evoke much resentment on the part of the cat. A small stubby-ended thermometer is best used and lubricated with vaseline to facilitate insertion. In over 50 per cent of cases the thermometer will meet an obstruction some $\frac{1}{2}$ inch inside the anus, pressure on which causes discomfort and annoyance; this is the internal sphincter of the anus which can be kept constricted voluntarily. It is essential that the thermometer be inserted beyond this point or rectal temperature will not be registered. Steady but firm pressure results in relaxation of the sphincter within 30 seconds in most cases; it is well to warn the owner that the cat's vocal reaction is mainly one of resentment and that discomfort only, not pain, is being felt.

Unlike the dog, cats seldom show a rise of body temperature due to apprehension or excitement; any rise may usually be accepted as a true bill.

The mouth and throat may be examined by placing the palm of the hand over the cat's skull with fingers on one side and thumb on the other grasping gently just anterior to the temporo-mandibular joint; tilting the head backwards results in the mouth opening $\frac{1}{4}$–$\frac{1}{2}$ inch and the jaws can be fully opened by a finger of the other hand being pressed on the lower incisor teeth. During the examination it is a reflex action on the part of many cats to raise one or both fore feet in an endeavour to remove the examining hand; the owner or surgery assistant should be asked to watch for this movement and apply the necessary restraint. If violent resentment is evinced it may be necessary to drape a blanket or large towel around the animal or even to roll it in it. A useful tip to owners to prevent their being scratched when administering drugs at home is to put the cat's head through the slit pocket of an old raincoat and allow the coat to envelop the body lightly. This often facilitates single-handed dosing.

Abdominal palpation can be carried out in most cats without resistance, one hand being used gently to restrain the head and neck while the other is palpating.

It is appropriate at this point to discuss the collection of a urine specimen. Owing to the cat's modesty over natural functions it may be difficult for an owner to get the required specimen and in such cases it is possible to produce the urine by manual pressure in at least 90 per cent of cases, always provided the owner is given instructions that will obviate the cat being presented with an empty bladder! Considerable patience is required and steady pressure must be maintained on the bladder, preferably at the trigonal end but keeping the fundus under pressure also in the palm of the hand, for some 30 seconds to 2 minutes. Not only has the physical reflex to be overcome but also the cat's voluntary resistance to the artificially induced desire to urinate; relaxation of the sphincter is often accompanied by a cry from the cat that sounds like a wail of despair and owners should be warned that this may occur. By this means it is regularly possible to obtain adequate samples of urine from cats, which is especially useful in cases of diabetes mellitus. The only drawback to this method is that in a small proportion of cases a small blood-vessel is ruptured during the application of pressure and thus allowance must be made for blood in urine which may be of no clinical significance. Adverse effects do not occur even when haemorrhage is quite marked.

Restraint for injections

Subcutaneous, intramuscular and intravenous routes are all used. A careful choice of needles is desirable and the best for injections other than intravenous is a moderately stout, fairly short needle with a short point; suitable needles are a $\frac{9}{10} \times 10$ mm. with short dental cut or the Agla V.R.3. For intravenous use a $\frac{8}{10} \times 13$ mm. needle with short dental cut is ideal but only needles with a first-class point should be used. The $\frac{6}{10}$ mm. needle advocated by some is so liable to get blocked with a blood clot during the course of an injection that it is usually unsatisfactory.

Subcutaneous injections

Opinion as to the ideal site varies widely. Anywhere where there is sufficient loose subcutaneous tissue is suitable but it seems logical to avoid sites which may be handled subsequently, e.g. the back of the neck or the mid-lumbar region; sites over the lateral aspects of chest wall or lumbar region are usually satisfactory.

Intramuscular injections

The best site is the muscle mass at the posterior aspect of the thigh, the semi-membranosus and semi-tendinosus. Needles should not exceed $\frac{3}{4}$ inch in length and during injection should be directed obliquely upwards into the main muscle belly. This obviates the risk of injecting an irritant or slowly absorbed solution around the sciatic nerve. Cases have occurred in which the intramuscular injection of a suspension of procaine penicillin has resulted in paralysis of the limb.

Restraint for subcutaneous and intramuscular injections is similar; the owner or assistant holds the cat's scruff in one hand and with the other presses gently but firmly over the cat's scapulae keeping the forehand of the animal firmly in contact with the table.

Intravenous injections

Four veins are available, the two radials and the two femorals, the former being far more readily accessible but the latter useable in case of difficulty.[1]

For intravenous injections the assistant must be clearly and precisely instructed in the method of restraint. With the hindquarters of the cat towards the assistant the scruff of the neck is grasped firmly in the left hand *immediately behind the occiput*; the commonest fault is for assistants to hold the loose skin of the neck much too far down thus allowing too free downward and lateral flexion of head and neck. Some difficulty may be found in adult entire males and occasional females in which the skin behind the head is thick and taut. The right hand is used to extend the right foreleg by complete extension of the elbow, and the thumb is brought over the anterior aspect of the elbow flexure to press on and raise the vein. Thumb pressure is relaxed as soon as the anaesthetist indicates that the vein is entered but the hand behind the elbow should not be moved as even in the stage of deep narcosis or light anaesthesia flexion and withdrawal of the limb can occur. The hands are naturally reversed for using the left radial vein.

Whilst most cats remain reasonably quiescent during these procedures some raise the unrestrained forelimb in an attempt to dislodge the approaching syringe; use may here be made of the cat's natural—almost reflex—action in clutching the far edge of the table when the head is being pulled backwards.

Various methods for restraint have been devised from time to time and may be used at the discretion of the clinician, but whenever possible anaesthesia should be induced to afford restraint except in the most minor and speedy, procedures. For minor quick interferences about the head the cat may be rolled tightly in a blanket enclosing all four limbs, the head being restrained by holding the blanket immediately behind the occiput. For the hindquarters the cat may similarly (and safely) be rolled in a blanket enclosing head and forelegs and enveloping the trunk as far as the pelvic girdle but the interference should not exceed 1–2 minutes.

Intrathoracic and intraperitoneal injections are used in the cat and both have some advocates as methods of inducing anaesthesia with pentobarbitone sodium. In both cases dosage has to be computed on a weight basis and results are irregular. In the author's opinion the former route should never be used and the latter only in exceptional circumstances for any purpose other than euthanasia.

Premedication and Sedation

By R.S. Jones, M.V.Sc., M.R.C.V.S., D.V.A.

There are a number of groups of drugs which are used for sedation and premedication in the cat.

The phenothiazine derivative or ataractic drugs are used extensively in veterinary anaesthetic practice. These drugs produce sedation and calm the animals, making them less aware of their surroundings. They do not cause drowsiness. Ataractic drugs potentiate the action of anaesthetic agents and hence decrease the total dose, thereby reducing the overall danger of toxicity. Their sedative action facilitates the handling of bad tempered cats; it ensures a quiet cat for venepuncture and reduces the resistance which often occurs during the induction of inhalational anaesthesia. There are a number of drugs in this group but the most common one is acepromazine which is usually administered by intramuscular injection at the rate of 0.11-0.2 mg/kg (0.05-0.1 mg/lb). Occasionally these drugs may be given by the oral route, but their action is often irregular and undesirable side effects may be seen. Ataractics may sometimes be combined with pethidine to produce sedation and analgesia; it is usual to use approximately half of the recommended dose of each drug.

The analgesic drug pethidine, which is used primarily to relieve pain, also has a sedative action in the cat. It is a synthetic drug which is used at a dose rate of 1 mg/kg (0.5 mg/lb), administered by the subcutaneous route. Overdosage rarely occurs, but if it does the signs include hyperaesthesia, disorientation and incoordination; convulsions are seen only occasionally.

Xylazine is a synthetic non-narcotic sedative with mild analgesic properties. It produces muscular relaxation and emesis in a large proportion of cats. It is used at dose rates of 1.0-4.0 mg/kg (0.5-2.0 mg/lb) and the degree of sedation would appear to be dose related; a variety of routes of administration have been recommended but the one of choice is by intramuscular injection.

Atropine sulphate is used for premedication in the cat mainly for its blocking action on the parasympathetic nervous system. Its main action is on the heart rate, which it increases and hence offsets the deleterious slowing of the rate which may be produced by some anaesthetic agents (e.g. halothane). Atropine reduces the flow of saliva and respiratory tract secretions, which can be a problem during anaesthesia when irritant agents such as diethyl ether are being used. The recommended dose for the average cat is 0.3 mg and it is given for preference by intramuscular injection but may also be given intravenously or subcutaneously.

Analgesia

The requirement for analgesia in the cat is not great, but it can be useful in the postoperative period; operations on the thorax and limbs can produce postoperative pain. The analgesic agent of choice for this purpose is pethidine.

Regional anaesthesia by lumbar injection of a local anaesthetic agent is not recommended in the cat. Apart from the risk of sepsis, the problems of restraint of an active animal make the technique inhumane and hence it is not recommended.

Local analgesia produced by infiltration with a local anaesthetic solution such as 1% lignocaine is limited in its application in cats mainly due to their temperament. It may be used for the removal of small skin neoplasms but should not be used for opening abscesses; it is bad surgery to infiltrate the region of an infected focus.

Anaesthesia

Veterinary surgeons have a wide range of anaesthetic agents and techniques available to them for use in the feline species. It is important, however, to relate the choice of technique to the surgery being carried out and to the experience and preference of the person administering anaesthesia.

It is convenient to describe anaesthesia as having four stages. During the induction of anaesthesia with inhalational agents, it is possible to distinguish the separate stages, whereas with intravenous agents it may be difficult due to their rapidity of action.

Stage I is that of voluntary excitement which lasts from the beginning of induction to loss of consciousness. During this period the animal may exhibit signs of apprehension and a rise in pulse and respiratory rates occur. The cat may also hold its breath; urine and faeces may be voided; the pupil is dilated and palpebral and pedal reflexes are still present.

Stage II is the stage of involuntary excitement and lasts from the loss of consciousness to the onset of automatic respiration. Violent and unpredictable movements often occur and the responses to stimuli are often exaggerated; cats may struggle, breath-hold and possibly vomit. The pupil is still dilated and the palpebral and pedal reflexes are present.

Stage III is the stage of surgical anesthesia which lasts from the onset of automatic breathing to the eventual cessation of respiration. For convenience it can be divided into three planes of anaesthesia. Plane I is the plane of light anaesthesia. It is characterised by the onset of automatic respiration which is regular, deep and rapid. This plane is adequate for minor surgical procedures and investigations. The pedal and palpebral reflexes are abolished at the end of Plane I. Plane II is characterised by the onset of slower respiration, the presence of muscular relaxation and constriction of the pupil; this plane is considered to be medium anaesthesia and is adequate for the majority of surgical techniques apart possibly from intraabdominal procedures. Plane III is characterised by an increase in respiratory rate with a decrease in its depth. As anaesthesia deepens, a pause develops between inspiration and expiration (an intercostal lag). This plane is deep anaesthesia and is adequate for all surgical procedures.

Stage IV is the point at which respiratory paralysis occurs. Its onset is characterised by the initiation of diaphragmatic respiration which eventually ceases as anaesthesia deepens. The pulse rate is rapid and pupils dilate; cyanosis occurs, quickly followed by cardiac arrest and death.

For descriptive purposes, anaesthesia can be divided into three sections, premedication, induction and maintenance. It is important to note that one "state" gradually merges into the other and that drugs which are used predominantly for one purpose may also be used for the other (e.g. whilst thiopentone is normally used for the induction of anaesthesia if it is given in repeated doses, it can be used for maintenance).

Premedication has been discussed in an earlier section.

Induction

Induction of anaesthesia in the cat can be carried out using a number of different drugs, mainly barbiturates. Only three barbiturate drugs will be considered. They are all water soluble and normally administered intravenously in cats. They are all primarily hypnotic drugs with little or no analgesic properties.

Thiopentone sodium is one of the most widely used drugs for the induction of anaesthesia in both man and animals. It can be used as a sole agent for procedures of short duration or alternatively it can be given by intermittent injection to produce anaesthesia of prolonged duration; the latter technique is not to be recommended as it may produce complications such as prolonged recovery. Thiopentone sodium is irritant and if the solution is injected extravascularly it can cause tissue necrosis and sloughing. If accidental extravascular injection occurs, the solution deposited under the skin should be diluted at once with normal saline. For the induction of anaesthesia in the cat a 1.25% solution should be used and a dose of 20 mg/kg is computed. Approximately half of this dose (10 mg/kg) is normally given by rapid intravenous injection to induce anaesthesia. The actual amount injected will depend on a number of factors such as the clinical condition of the cat, the skill of the anaesthetist and the rate of injection, plus the effects of premedication.

Methohexitone sodium is similar to thiopentone in its action and is considered to be twice as potent as thiopentone. It is more expensive than thiopentone but its advantage is due to the fact that it is more rapidly redistributed and hence recovery is more rapid.

Pentobarbitone sodium has been used for many years as a sole anaesthetic agent in the cat. Its use has now been largely superseded by modern techniques in view of the number of disadvantages that were associated with its use, not the least of which was the prolonged recovery period. A dose of 30 mg/kg is recommended by the intravenous route, but there is wide variation and the drug should be administered slowly and to effect. A total time of 3-5 minutes should be taken to make the injection and anaesthetic depth should be assessed after each incremental dose. The drug has been administered by the intraperitoneal or even the intrathoracic route but this is not to be recommended.

A combination of the steroid anaesthetic agents alphadolone acetate and alphaxalone have recently been introduced into feline anaesthetic practice. It is a unique combination in that the two drugs are not water soluble and are dissolved in polyoxyethylated castor oil; e.g. "Saffan."* It has been used extensively in cats both for the induction of, and for short duration anaesthesia; it is used at a dose rate of 9 mg/kg (0.75 ml). It is non-irritant if given extravenously and can also be used for sedation and possibly anaesthesia by the intramuscular route. The injection should be made deep into the quadriceps mass and up to 18 mg/kg can be used by this route but results may be variable. The administration of "Saffan" in cats can sometimes produce histamine release with mild anaphylactoid reaction. The common signs are hyperaemia of the ears, nose and paws with occasional oedema of the ears and interdigital areas. Such reactions are usually of little consequence.

*Saffan (Glaxo Laboratories Ltd.)

Maintenance

Maintenance of anaesthesia in the cat is usually carried out with either a gas or volatile liquid or a combination of these.

Nitrous oxide is a colourless gas with a faint smell which is available as a compressed liquid in blue cylinders and vaporises on release from the cylinder. It is relatively non-toxic, a good analgesic, but a weak anaesthetic which often requires supplementation with a volatile agent. It should always be administered with at least 30% oxygen. Halothane is widely used for the maintenance of anaesthesia in cats and may occasionally be used also for induction. It is a non-inflammable, non-explosive colourless liquid with a boiling point of 50°C. A concentration of 1-2% is recommended for the maintenance of anaesthesia and up to 4% for induction. It is best administered in a semi-closed circuit, with either oxygen or nitrous oxide and oxygen, utilising an accurate temperature compensated vaporiser.

Diethyl ether is commonly used in feline anaesthesic practice for the maintenance of anaesthesia. It is a colourless liquid and when its vapour is mixed with air or oxygen it is inflammable and explosive therefore extreme care is essential in its use. The vapour has a typical smell and due to its irritant effect increases the flow of saliva and mucus from the respiratory tract, therefore the administration of atropine is essential. It is best administered in semi-closed circuit with either oxygen or nitrous oxide-oxygen as a carrier gas. Its use for the induction of anaesthesia is not recommended due to its low potency and hence the long period of time accompanied by struggling. Methoxyflurane is a colourless liquid with a boiling point of 104°C. It is very similar to ether in its properties although it is non-inflammable and non-explosive. Due to its high boiling point, it is not satisfactory for the induction of anaesthesia. It is used for the maintenance of anaesthesia in a similar manner to ether and halothane.

Methods of Administering
Inhalational Anaesthetic Agents

At the present time, there is one preferred method of administering inhalational anaesthetic agents to cats and that is by the semi-closed method utilising either a Magill circuit or a modified Ayre's T piece. An anaesthetic machine with a source of oxygen, plus or minus nitrous oxide, and fitted with a vaporiser is essential.

In the Magill circuit the gases pass from the machine to a reservoir bag and down a wide bore corrugated tube and are delivered to the patient either from a mask or endotracheal tube. The expired gases pass partly out to the atmosphere through the expiratory valve and partly back up the corrugated tube. During the expiratory pause, the fresh gas flow forces the expired gases out to the atmosphere.

An Ayre's T piece, preferably as modified by Jackson-Rees, with an open ended reservoir bag on the expiratory limb is the method of choice for the administration of inhalational anaesthetic agents to the cat. It is simple, inexpensive and offers little resistance to respiration. It has the advantage that artificial ventilation can be performed either for resuscitation or open chest surgery by occluding the open ended bag and applying pressure to it.

The administration of the anaesthetic agent to the patient can be achieved by using either a malleable rubber mask such as Hall's mask or an endotracheal tube. In view of the restriction of the diameter of the trachea which is produced by an endotracheal tube it is preferable to use a mask as a routine, although for operations on the mouth, face, pharynx, gastro-intestinal tract or within the thorax endotracheal intubation is essential.

Due to the ease with which laryngeal spasm can be provoked in the cat, intubation of the trachea is not as simple as in most other domestic species. It is necessary to suppress the nervous activity of the larynx either by spraying it with a local anaesthetic solution or by the administration of a muscle relaxant such as suxamethonium. The mouth is held open with a gag and it is preferable to use a laryngoscope to enable one to visualise the entrance to the larynx. In small cats, it may not be possible to obtain cuffed endotracheal tubes of sufficiently small diameter, in these cases a pharyngeal pack of bandage moistened with saline is desirable.

Dissociative Anaesthesia

Dissociative anaesthesia is a term borrowed from the human and is described as disconnected unconsciousness combined with profound analgesia. The eyes remain open, laryngeal and pharyngeal reflexes are unimpaired. Catalepsy or muscular rigidity is present. Apneustic respiration is seen commonly in dissociative anaesthesia. Ketamine hydrochloride is the only compound recommended for use in the cat; a dose of 22 mg/kg will produce anaesthesia of short duration. Premedication with acepromazine and xylazine have been recommended and atropine is essential to offset the bradycardia. Xylazine premedication will abolish the apneustic respiratory pattern and will produce muscular relaxation and is, therefore, the drug of choice.

Chapter 4

SIGNS OF HEALTH AND DISEASE, ROUTINE CLINICAL EXAMINATION

Reflexes of Health: Positions of Disease: Temperament

Some indication of a cat's state of health may be obtained from its response to certain stimuli.

It is true that in relatively mild disease conditions some normal responses can still be elicited but their absence in the average cat may be taken as significant evidence of severe abnormality.

1. In response to firm stroking of the back from behind the neck to the base of the tail cats arch their backs against the stroking hand and raise the tail to a perpendicular position with hindquarters slightly elevated, the hind legs being somewhat extended.

Variations from this response may be noted in; (a) cats which are severely ill, in which it is absent, or (b) in some cases of parasitism by fleas when stroking of the posterior dorsum results in exaggerated and abnormal responses, the cat either licking itself violently in any accessible place or attacking by licking and biting either the caressing hand or the affected area of skin; growling sounds are often made.

2. Response to fondling by tickling the chin, cheeks or parotid region by rubbing the head into the caressing hand. This response is apparently under greater voluntary control than the previous one, is not so regularly elicited and is of less help as a guide to health.

PURRING

The mechanism which produces purring is still unknown but it is a sign widely accepted as an indication of pleasure and comfort. Owners often interpret it as evidence of health: this, however, is not true since many cats, especially old ones, will purr during the later stages of fatal illness. It is often necessary to disabuse owners' minds of the idea that because a cat has purred it is either not seriously ill or is convalescent.

WASHING

Cats are usually fastidious as regards personal cleanliness although exceptions do occur, sometimes because of the owner's neglect of the coat and sometimes for no apparent reason.

In cats which normally wash regularly absence of this activity is evidence of a considerable departure from health whereas the reestablishment of a washing routine is reliable evidence of impending recovery. In some cases washing may be inhibited by local factors such as the ulcerated tongue in cases of ulcerative glossitis.

In health normal sleeping positions are either curled up in lateral recumbency, head tucked into chest and abdomen or, less commonly, in extended lateral recumbency with limbs extended in a relaxed manner. A normal resting posture is the sternal position with forelegs flexed under brisket and head drawn slightly back into the neck.

In disease a sternal posture is often adopted but the forelegs are seldom tucked under the body—they are usually extended below the elbow and the cat's head droops over them in an extended position.

Cats dying of, for example, feline enteritis or chronic nephritis may adopt a sternal posture, head hanging over a dish of milk or water, making feeble attempts to lap for hours on end. Adoption of this type of sternal posture is a serious sign.

Cats presented in extremis from any cause are often found to be lying in lateral recumbency with spine arched convexly and limbs drawn towards one another.

SPRAYING

Spraying by male cats, i.e. the emission of small jets of urine against an object, e.g. wall or curtains, with the hind-quarters raised, penis directed backwards and tail held quiveringly erect, is usually taken to be evidence of territory demarcation and is thus assumed to be an activity peculiar to entire males. This does not account for all cases of spraying, however, which can also occur in castrated males and be evidence of any form of resentment, e.g. jealousy over the introduction of another cat.

Territorial spraying by tom cats is a strong reason for castrating male cats kept in urban areas.

In cases of cystitis or urethral obstruction it is necessary carefully to distinguish between spraying and repeated attempts to micturate; in the latter case the more usual posture for urination is usually adopted, i.e. hindquarters directed downwards in a squatting position and tail held horizontally.

TEMPERAMENT

The feline temperament renders it peculiarly liable to various forms of mental trauma such as change of environment or some physical interference which subjects the cat to indignity. Complete loss of appetite, correctly called anorexia nervosa, may result. One particularly graphic example which may be cited is that of a Blue Persian castrated male cat which had been given an enema for relief of a rectal impaction. For one month subsequently the cat refused all food but every clinical investigation proved negative. It was eventually decided that the cause must be psycho somatic and treatment by phenobarbitone and Vitamin B complex was successful.

It is a curious and somewhat contradictory fact, in view of the foregoing, that the author has never seen any evidence of mental trauma
due to restraint for the routine method of kitten castration; it is the
adult cat which is more prone to mental disturbance.

A condition which might loosely be described as shell-shock was seen
far more often in cats than dogs after air-raids in the last war. A curious
'psychosis' has also been described by Mitchell (1953) in which 6 of
10 cats rescued from Canvey Island after the disastrous East Coast
floods developed a syndrome of anorexia associated with signs of mental
disturbance shown by attempts to catch imaginary objects both in the
air and on the ground. There was slight fever. Symptoms resolved in
four days, possibly assisted by sedatives.

It is thus clear that the psyche of the cat cannot be ignored by those
who have to deal with it whether as pet or patient.

Routine Clinical Examination

It is always wise to establish a fixed routine of preliminary clinical
examination. If this routine is rigidly adhered to in every case other
than those confined to a single obvious superficial lesion it is unlikely
that serious error will arise.

The following routine will usually suffice for the first clinical examination.

1. TEMPERATURE

Rectal temperature is recorded, using a lubricated stubby-ended
clinical thermometer which must be inserted beyond the internal
sphincter of the anus. Normal temperature is usually regarded as being
38·6° C. (101·5° F.) but the range 38–39° C. (100·5–102° F.) will cover
most afebrile patients. Rise of temperature due to excitement is not
common.

2. PULSE

This may be checked at the femoral artery during the previous procedure.

The volume of the cat pulse is small and minor variations are therefore more difficult to detect.

Regular intermittence which is so common in the dog and is regarded
as normal in that species does not occur in the cat.

Pulse rate is increased in any form of nervous tension. In some
cardiac conditions the pulse rate is so greatly increased as to be virtually
uncountable. Quality and rate are probably less helpful in the cat than
any other of the veterinary surgeon's usual range of patients.

3. VISIBLE MUCOUS MEMBRANES

Palpebral conjunctiva, gums and tongue should all be examined. The
normal conjunctiva of the cat is somewhat pallid compared with the
dog and is seldom deeper in colour than a pale pink.

Gum colour is likewise somewhat pallid and may even appear faintly bluish in normal subjects.

The tongue is probably the best visible guide to adequacy of blood in anaemia or haemorrhage cases.

The sclerotic is a clear almost bluish-white in normal subjects. Contusions are often present after accidental wounds. Icterus may not be easily detected in the sclera unless it is very intense; it is more easily detected in the mucous membranes of the inside of the lips. Detection is often facilitated by the pressure of a finger to cause local ischaemia and subsequent withdrawal, the colour being observed before blood returns. The integument of the ear flap frequently shows yellow staining which is difficult to detect with certainty elsewhere in cases of mild jaundice.

During this examination of the mucous membranes of the mouth, the presence or absence of gingivitis or, more rarely, ulceration may be observed.

The presence of missing, loose or broken teeth, tartar deposits, parodontal disease, alveolitis or caries and the mouth odour is noted; uraemia in the cat gives rise to a distinctly ammoniacal smell.

4. PHARYNX AND TONSILS

These will be examined by opening the mouth as previously described.

Inflammation of the pharynx of the cat differs from the diffuse reddening of pharyngitis in the dog and is shown by congestion of the network of blood-vessels coursing over the pharyngeal mucosa; these are virtually invisible in the normal cat.

Tonsillitis is rare in the cat; the tonsils are usually tucked well into the crypts. In older subjects they should be examined for evidence of carcinoma, a relatively rare condition.

Ulcers are occasionally seen on the soft palate.

5. THE TONGUE

This should be observed as a guide to anaemia and haemorrhage and for evidence of marginal or dorsal ulceration. The ventro-lateral surfaces should be observed for signs of inflammation, ranula or neoplasia.

6. EYES AND NOSTRILS

Should be observed for presence of aqueous, catarrhal or purulent discharges.

It is not uncommon to find a dark brown mucoid discharge accumulated in the conjunctival sac or exuding from the inner canthus; this is often described by owners as 'blood coming from the eye'.

7. LYMPH NODES

Those at the angle of the jaws are palpated. Any enlargement should lead to palpation of all other superficial nodes.

8. EARS

The flap is examined for signs of wounds or haematomata. The external canal should be examined for parasitic (otodectic) or pyogenic infection.

9. GENERAL BODILY CONDITION

Bodily condition is assessed with particular reference to recent loss of muscle or adipose tissues. The state of hydration is also noted.

At the same time a rough estimate of coat condition can be made in respect of coat change, adequacy of grooming, abnormal scratch reflexes, parasites, scurf and obvious lesions.

10. EXTERNAL GENITALIA

The most important information to be derived from a glance at these is the sex of the cat. Reliance should not be placed on the owner's word as to its sex although this will have to be accepted as to neutering or otherwise since no external evidence of castration or spaying should be obvious. Difficulties arise in the case of stray adults which may be spayed females and males without visible testicles which, rarely, may be cryptorchid.

In the case of entire females vaginal discharge will be looked for.

11. ABDOMINAL PALPATION

Routine abdominal palpation is a highly desirable habit to acquire; surprising and unexpected lesions are often detected.

The state of the large bowel should be ascertained and the bladder palpated to assess fulness and thickness of bladder wall.

Pregnancy may be detected from about 24 days onwards with great ease.

Enlarged liver, kidneys or spleen are also easily detected.

During this palpation lesions such as abscesses, mastitis or neoplasms in mammary glands will usually become obvious, and also abnormal breaks in the abdominal wall such as umbilical or ventral hernia.

Painful areas of any part of the trunk may likewise become evident indicating incipient sepsis which is often a cause of ill-defined malaise.

12. CHEST

Respiratory rhythm should be initially observed during temperature and pulse recording at which time most cats remain reasonably quiet in lightly restrained sternal recumbency.

Auscultation of heart and lungs may be undertaken; it is highly desirable that both sides of the chest should be auscultated.

The bronchial area should receive careful attention.

If preliminary examination leads to suspicion of fluid, abnormal tissue or air in the thoracic cavity, percussion will be helpful. Fluid levels especially can often be accurately delineated by this means.

Fluid in the pleural cavity causes dulling and muffling of the heart sounds; breath sounds are absent below the fluid level but clearly audible above it; on percussion resonance is only present above the fluid line.

In pneumothorax the paradox of co-existence of inaudible breath sounds with extreme resonance on percussion is virtually diagnostic.

13. MOVEMENT

In view of the cat's proneness to escaping, examination of the completely unrestrained cat is best kept to a minimum but it is essential in some cases of lameness and in neurological cases.

Persuading a cat to show its paces needs patience and tact. Most cats when placed on a strange floor make for a space under furniture and remain there; they do not come when called. Whenever possible they should be placed in the middle of the floor and left undisturbed and so far as possible unobserved and not molested. After some time natural curiosity overcomes most cats and they start investigating their surroundings. Those that just stay put in sternal recumbency may be gently stimulated by stroking along the back or by a very gentle push on the rump.

Abnormalities of gait and tail carriage can be detected in this way but often the examination is time and patience consuming.

As a result of the foregoing procedures, of which the last is only used when necessary, it is unlikely that gross abnormality will be overlooked. At best a firm diagnosis can be made, at worst an indication of which systems require detailed investigation. This will be dealt with more fully under the appropriate headings.

REFERENCE

Mitchell, J. R. (1953) *Vet. Rec.* **65**, 254.

SUGGESTED FURTHER READING

Worden, A. N. (1959) *Vet. Rec.* **71**, 966. (Abnormal behaviour in the dog and cat.)

Chapter 5

THE HEAD (EXCLUDING EYES, EARS AND MOUTH)

The head of the cat is subject to a number of traumatic lesions affecting both hard and soft tissues. Accidental injuries are caused by street accidents in which the head is particularly susceptible to damage due to the habit of dashing out from behind hedges and fences and hitting the hub caps of passing cars head first. Cat bite injuries are common, dog bites less so as it is more usually the hind end of the cat damaged in this way; rat bites are often said to be common but the author believes that most punctures attributed to rats are in fact inflicted by other felines. Marauding cats are often said to have been hit by missiles thrown by irate garden enthusiasts but the evidence for this is more circumstantial than factual. However, air-gun injuries do occur, usually involving the eye. Injuries resulting from ordinary falls are common.

Fractures

Fractures of the bones of the cranium are uncommon even after blows on the head caused by impact with cars. One case is on record in which a penetrating wound had resulted in a triangular section of bone being forced through the lateral part of the right cerebral hemisphere coming to rest on the floor of the cranium. The fracture clearly resulted from deep penetration by a long, sharp instrument and it was difficult to visualize how this could have occurred accidentally yet there was nothing to suggest malicious infliction. The clinical picture was of initial depression and inappetence for which routine clinical examination could show no cause; during the eight hours following this examination severe neurological signs developed comprising blindness, alternating periods of hyperaesthesia and profound depression, complete disorientation and loss of placing reflexes. (Joshua 1962).

Fractures of the hard palate and nasal bones are common following street accidents.

Hard Palate

Whenever a cat is presented which shows any evidence of damage to the head at all, particularly with a history of street accident, the palate should be examined.

Not uncommonly it will be found that the posterior part of the hard

78

palate is split for a distance of 0·75–1·5 cm. The fissure is usually narrow, from 2–5 mm.

The prognosis is far better than in congenital cases and frequently spontaneous healing occurs without any intervention; during the healing period fluids should so far as possible be withheld. Should surgical repair be necessary operation should be undertaken as soon as possible after shock has worn off. Anaethesia will be best induced by an intravenous barbiturate, pentobarbitone sodium or continuous thiopentone sodium. If the edges of the fissure are already undergoing resolution they should be freshened and apposed by closely applied non-absorbable sutures of braided nylon, monofilament nylon or silver or steel wire. It is seldom necessary to undertake relaxation techniques by making parallel incisions as in the dog. (Knight 1958). Routine antibiotic cover is desirable for 5–8 days post-operatively and sutures are removed in 12–16 days, again under anaesthesia.

Nasal Bones

These are often damaged in street accidents although obvious depressions are seldom detected. It is probable that the turbinate and ethmoid bones are also involved.

The cat is presented shortly after a street accident and usually looks a sorry sight. Respirations are difficult and noisy; mouth-breathing is often present; there is a varying degree of haemorrhage from one or both nostrils; eyes, muzzle and nostrils are often clogged with dried and clotted blood; the cat is depressed and holds the head low; intermittent snorting and sneezing may occur.

If examination of the patient discloses no signs of severe brain damage it is always worth undertaking treatment no matter how apparently hopeless is the condition. Haemorrhage is usually self-limiting and treatment is confined to careful removal of caked blood and dirt together with routine attention to shock etc. Within 24–36 hours considerable improvement is usually evident and recovery is rapid and complete.

Jaws

Fractures of the jaws are not uncommon, more frequently involving the mandible but occasionally the superior maxilla around the incisor arch and canines.

Fractures of the symphysis of superior and inferior maxillae occur, mainly as the result of street accidents and are usually self-evident. Signs include inability to close the mouth, malocclusions and excessive mobility at the symphysis; the normal direction of the canine teeth may be altered. Cases showing minimal displacement and no soft tissue damage may require no active treatment and will heal well if carefully nursed on a soft, nourishing diet requiring no mastication.

All cases showing displacement or soft tissue damage should be dealt with surgically once initial shock has passed off.

Under general anaesthesia—preferably intravenous barbiturate—lesions in soft tissues are cleaned and débridement undertaken where necessary. The jaws are carefully re-aligned and held in place by silver or stainless steel wire around the base of the canine teeth; a suitable groove to embed the wire is necessary in most cases and can be prepared by using a small triangular file on the lateral aspects of the canines.

A similar method is applicable to the superior maxilla. Antibacterial therapy for 5–7 days is advisable to obviate infection of soft tissues or loosened tooth roots.

Occasionally despite careful alignment of the fractured mandible malocclusion of the premolar teeth persists; this may be corrected by extraction of the lower carnassial on the appropriate side.

Fracture of the horizontal ramus of the mandible also occurs. Displacement and mobility are often so slight that spontaneous recovery occurs in 10–18 days if the patient is fed carefully. Alternatively a small stainless steel intramedullary pin may be inserted from the posterior aspect of the vertical ramus, and passed forwards beneath the tooth roots to beyond the point of fracture so immobilising the lesion effectively. One case of fracture of the vertical ramus (for which treatment was not sought) which resulted in ankylosis of the temporomandibular joint causing complete trismus has been seen.

Luxation of the Temporo Mandibular Joint

Dislocation of the jaw has been seen arising spontaneously, as in man, during over-extension while yawning; it can also be of traumatic origin. The cat is unable to close the mouth and there is lateral displacement of the mandibles. Diagnosis is confirmed by radiography—advisable to eliminate the existence of a fracture—and reduction is easily accomplished under anaesthesia.

Infection of the frontal sinuses: Sinusitis

This is always a sequel to a catarrhal infection, usually of a chronic nature. Two types of chronic nasal catarrh are recognised in cats, viz:

(a) In kittens from 6–14 weeks of age in which no history of acute disease is forthcoming. Vitamin A deficiency may be an aetiological factor, possibly with concurrent Vitamin D deficiency, causing some deformity and thickening of the bones of the nasal cavity, especially the turbinates and some abnormality of the overlying mucous membranes resulting in decreased resistance to infection.

(b) Persistent muco-purulent or purulent nasal discharge following an attack of one of the feline respiratory virus infections. This is mainly in adult cats.

In many cases infection spreads to the frontal sinuses and once established is difficult to eliminate owing to inadequate drainage. The bacteriological picture is varied but is of secondary importance since response to systemic antibacterial therapy is incomplete and temporary; it is, however, helpful to know the bacteriology and drug sensitivity before proceeding to radical measures. According to Smith (1964) both haemolytic *Staphylococci* and *Fusiformis* spp. may be involved. It is also desirable to ascertain that *Cryptococcus neoformans* is not present.

Symptoms. There is always a history of chronic nasal catarrh as shown by sneezing, noisy respirations or nasal discharge for periods varying from a few weeks to several years.

When sinus infection is present the history is usually of a fluctuating severity with periods of severe sneezing and nasal discharge alternating with periods of relative remission of symptoms and signs. As time goes on the discharge, which may at first have been only catarrhal, becomes frankly purulent and often quite large gobbets of semi-inspissated pus are evacuated from the nostrils. Fever is not regularly a marked feature but quite commonly periods of depression and inappetence occur lasting several hours to 3 days to be followed by an episode of frequent sneezing and discharge of considerable quantities of pus. Depression may be accompanied by apparent 'headache', the cat adopting a sternal posture with head drooping and eyes half-closed; gentle tapping of the bone overlying the frontal sinuses may elicit a definite pain response. Following the period of acute sneezing and discharge considerable symptomatic relief is evident for a varying length of time although nasal discharge never entirely ceases.

As time goes on these cats become a serious problem not only on grounds of ill-health but because of the unpleasantness associated with the repeated ejection of purulent nasal material. Owners may well request euthanasia at this stage.

Treatment. In cases of early nasal catarrh every attempt should be made to eliminate the condition by vigorous antibacterial and vitamin therapy. In young kittens Vitamins A and D by injection and a broad spectrum antibiotic systemically may be completely effective.

In adult cats the use of antibacterial drugs during an attack of feline respiratory virus infection is justified in an attempt to prevent persistent infection of the upper respiratory tract. These, however, may do more harm than good unless sensitivity tests are positive. Vitamin C in massive doses has been credited with recoveries in such cases; it is probable that the improvement noted is due to the fact that tenacious tacky discharge is rendered more fluid and is thus better able to drain. The author has been unable to obtain cures by the use of Vitamin C.

Once pyogenic infection is present in the frontal sinuses (and even in the absence of obvious signs this may be assumed in prolonged chronic cases of nasal catarrh in which neoplasia is not a factor) antibacterial therapy will not provide a cure although temporary improvement is common.

It is necessary at this stage to consider directing therapy to the site of infection itself. Laboratory tests for bacteriology and sensitivity are highly desirable before proceeding to surgery as the anti-bacterial agent of choice may then be used; failing this a broad spectrum antibiotic such as chlortetracycline or chloramphenicol should be selected.

The author has adopted a simple technique of trephining the frontal sinuses with a suitable drill or even an intramedullary bone pin, irrigating the cavity thoroughly with saline and then introducing the antibacterial agent of choice. Results have been encouraging and the method is quick and simple.

Recently Startup (1963) has described a more elaborate technique in which the sinuses are entered, free drainage is established via the nasal cavity and an indwelling polythene tube is left for a few days for repeated irrigation and introduction of antibiotics; good results are claimed.

More recently, Winstanley (1974) has reviewed the technique and stressed the very limited accessibility of the sinuses in the young kitten. He also suggests repeated anaesthesia to be necessary for adequately thorough irrigation and this view is supported by Proud (1974) who emphasizes the inadequacy of natural sinus drainage because of anatomical placement of sinus foraminae in the cat. A further development of this technique, claimed to be successful when carefully performed with meticulous removal of sinus mucosa and periosteum, is sinus occlusion by implantation of autogenous (subcutaneous) fat. (Thomlinson & Schenk 1975).

Prognosis is poor in all cases of chronic nasal discharge unless radical methods are adopted.

Recently Colegrave *et al.* have described the investigation of chronic rhinitis endemic in a cattery from which organisms resembling *Mycoplasma* spp. (*PPLO*) were isolated. Treatment with spiramycin at a dose rate of 50 mg. per kg. bodyweight was effective after a single injection. The duration of recovery is not stated.

'Snuffles' endemic in a community rather resembles the similar condition which is so great a problem to rabbit breeders and should probably be regarded as aetiologically different from the previously described syndrome although it may well be related to virus infections.

In outbreaks of this type careful bacteriological investigation is required as well as attention to nutritional standards and general hygiene. Complete closing of an infected cattery for 6–12 weeks or even longer may well be necessary to eliminate infection.

Neoplasia of the Nasal Cavity

Neoplasia of the nasal cavity in older cats is not uncommon and should always be suspected in cases of unilateral nasal discharge in cats over middle life which are not due to a previous attack of a respiratory virus.

Of a series of 119 neoplasms from cats fully investigated in practice two involving the nasal cavities were seen; one a solid carcinoma involving the right nasal chamber in a 10½ years old entire male, the other a mucoid adenocarcinoma involving the nasal cavity of a 13 years old castrated male.

Symptoms. These are usually local. Nasal discharge may be seen, unilateral initially but occasionally becoming bilateral later, often blood-stained and there may be periods of frank epistaxis. Sneezing or noisy respirations frequently co-exist. Swelling of the bridge of the nose may become obvious in some cases at a later stage; ulceration into the buccal cavity is not usual.

General health remains unaffected in the early stages, appetite and body weight being maintained.

Later depression, inappetence and weight loss may occur.

Metastasis is not usually clinically evident before local signs necessitate euthanasia.

Diagnosis. This is based on clinical signs of which the age group and unilateral character are important differential points. Biopsy involves radical surgery and is thus rarely acceptable to the owner unless improvement can be promised as a result; visual examination of the nasal chambers by rhinoscopy is, in the author's experience, not practical owing to the small size of the cavity to be explored.

Treatment. This is not feasible. Euthanasia should be undertaken as soon as general ill-health is evident.

Neoplasia of the Bony Structures of the Head

Under this heading are included tumours apparently associated with the bony structures even if on pathological examination the tumour is derived from soft tissues.

Tumours of the head are not uncommon and are usually visually obvious, often not giving rise to clinical symptoms unless they involve the buccal cavity and so interfere with eating, or until metastasis has occurred.

Of the series of 199 tumours the following six were apparently associated with the hard tissues of the head.

	Age	Sex	Site(s)	Histology
1	14 year	♂	Left mandible	Squamous cell carcinoma
2	12 year	♂	Gum, hard palate, cheek	Spindle-cell and cartilaginous sarcoma
3	16 year	♂	Lower jaw	Carcinoma arising from gum epithelium
4	15 year	♀	Left side gum	Fibrosarcoma
5	8 year	♀	Zygomatic ridge	Osteosarcoma: Lung metastases
6	—	—	Palate	Osteogenic tumour of low malignancy

Key to sex symbols: Male = ♂; Castrated Male = ♂; Female = ♀; Spayed Female = ♀.

With the exception of the case of osteosarcoma of the zygomatic ridge all tumours of the head occurred in aged subjects. This fits into the general picture of osteosarcoma in the cat which occurs mainly in late middle life, viz. from 6–10 years of age.

Diagnosis is based on clinical evidence, possibly biopsy. Treatment is usually not feasible, surgical excision being rarely possible. X-ray therapy is not a humane proposition in the age group concerned.

Soft Tissues of the Head

Labial Ulcers

'Rodent Ulcer'. The name is a misnomer as the condition is not analogous with the neoplastic lesions seen in man but it has unfortunately become recognised as a clinical entity under this title.

The lesion is an infective granuloma with erosive properties; the site is the anterior part of the lip at the muco-cutaneous junction. There is no specific age incidence but it is usually found in adults.

Symptoms. These are often absent, the lesion being noticed by the owner.

Signs. The lesion commences almost invariably in the upper lip just lateral to the midline; it comprises a shallow concave ulcerated area sometimes with raised proliferative edges. If untreated the erosion spreads involving a larger area of the lip with a tendency to deepen. Spread to the opposite side or to the contiguous area of the lower lip is common. There is no tendency for spontaneous resolution.

Treatment. At one time local treatment was the rule. Curettage and cautery and painting with a 1 per cent aqueous solution of gentian violet have been successful (Patchett 1944); the latter treatment must be used with discretion, as over free application of the dressing by the owner has been known to cause a severe chemical pharyngitis.

Modern treatment is on antibacterial lines with broad spectrum antibiotics, e.g. chlortetracycline 100–500 mg. daily in divided doses, combined with corticosteroids (betamethasone 0·125 mg. daily in divided doses) the latter being introduced after a few days on antibiotics.

Steroid therapy in the form of "Ovarid" (Glaxo-megoestrolacetate) tablets by mouth has been claimed successful, also a good response is claimed for irradiation therapy (Baker 1972) and application of cryosurgical techniques.

Resolution is slow being complete in average cases in 14–28 days. Recurrence is not common.

Cranium

Concussion

Concussion is sometimes seen in cats after accidents involving the head, especially street accidents of the type previously mentioned. In mild cases there may be no loss of balance or disorientation but slight nystagmus is observed which usually passes off within a few hours. In more severe cases nystagmus is more marked, the cat appears blind and there is often loss of righting reflexes so that the animal remains in lateral recumbency. In really severe cases limb spasticity may be shown. Nausea does not seem to be a feature of concussion in the cat. With the exception of severe cases most cats make a rapid recovery if kept warm and quiet; pethidine in moderate dosage may be given if other painful lesions are present but ataractic drugs of the phenothiazine group are best avoided.

Intracranial Abscess

This is occasionally met unassociated with otitis media. It is not usually possible to incriminate a previous pyogenic infection in these cases as distinct from pus in the neural canal in which a previous lesion can usually be found.

Symptoms will vary with the location of the lesion but profound depression and anorexia usually exist; vomiting or rise of temperature occasionally occur. The cat tends to sit in sternal recumbency with head hanging as it does in frontal sinusitis or panophthalmitis. Neurological signs related to the site of the lesion will occur, e.g. ataxia, vestibular signs etc.

Diagnosis. This is virtually impossible in life.

Differential diagnosis includes frontal sinusitis (when nasal discharge is suggestive), panophthalmitis (usually with pain on pressure of eyeball) and otitis media.

Treatment. None is feasible. Euthanasia is usually requested by the owner owing to the profound misery of the patient.

Otitis Media

This is an important condition which will be dealt with under the heading of 'Ears'.

Nasal Polyp

Polyps are reputed to be the occasional cause of sneezing and nasal discharge. The author has never been able to confirm the presence of such a lesion.

Skin

Notoedric Mange

Localized lesions of Notoedric mange are fairly common, the typical site being the forehead anterior to the ears, running forwards and downwards to the upper margins of the orbit.

Early cases merely show a thinning of hair at this site possibly associated with pigmentation of the affected area; irritation is relatively mild in such cases and is shown by rather frequent washing of the head.

More severe cases cause intense pruritus and lesions spread to involve the integument of the pinna and later the top of the head. Advanced neglected cases spread backwards along the neck and shoulders. The skin becomes dry, flaky, scabby, thickened and rugose with superficial epidermal damage due to self-inflicted trauma.

Spread to the inner aspect of the forelegs in the metacarpal area is common in older cases owing to excessive washing and rubbing.

Diagnosis. May be based with some confidence on the distribution of lesions and confirmed by finding of mites in skin scrapings.

Prognosis. This is good in all except advanced cases where considerable skin thickening has occurred.

Treatment. This consists of local application of suitable acaricides, care being taken over their selection, bearing in mind that ingestion of some of the dressing is inevitable when the forelegs are washed after rubbing of the affected areas.

Sulphur ointment well rubbed in every second or third day for 3–4 weeks is simple and effective in mild cases and is relatively non-toxic if sensibly applied. Alternatives are emulsion of benzyl benzoate or suspension of gamma benzene hexachloride applied similarly remembering that the active principle of these is more toxic than sulphur.

Sepsis

General considerations of cat sepsis will be found in a later chapter.

Sepsis about the cat's head is frequent and may occur in almost any site, the commoner of which include:

Temporal Region

Abscesses due to fighting with other cats are common over the whole parieto-temporal area.

Symptoms. These are minimal when the lesions are small. The discharge of pus usually causes the owner to seek advice. In other cases general malaise, anorexia and possibly a rise of temperature occur; sometimes swelling is obvious especially immediately over the eye. In very early cases careful examination of the head may reveal a pin-head scab over a sensitive spot; in such cases expectant treatment is justified.

Diagnosis is easy if pus is already present; in older cats consideration must be given to neoplasia. Haematomata do not occur in these sites.

Treatment. This is by antibacterial therapy, usually antibiotics, generally or locally. Routine treatment for any ordinary sepsis lesion should be 600,000 units procaine penicillin suspension intramuscularly every 48 hours for 4–8 days and expression of pus if a puncture is patent or incision of the abscess if spontaneous rupture does not rapidly occur. A cruciate incision may be needed for abscesses on top of the skull. After expression of pus antibiotic in the form of the appropriate intra-mammary cerate introduced into the cavity via the puncture may obviate surgical incision in many cases when drainage is inadequate.

In such cases it is essential that the puncture be kept open twice daily if too early healing with trapping of residual infection is to be avoided.

Cheeks. The sides of the face are common sites of abscess formation and the skin at this part in the adult entire male is so thickened—this is a secondary sex character—that spontaneous rupture of the abscess may not occur, necessitating surgical incision. Infection in this region is usually due to cat bites but may be due to dental disease. In any case when an abscess of the side of the face recurs more than once careful examination of the mouth, under anaesthesia, is necessary with extraction of any suspect teeth.

Discharging sinuses below the eyes, usually nearer the inner canthus, are more often than not associated with dental infection. The lesion in some respects resembles the malar abscess (dental sinus) of the dog but the site is not identical. Treatment which does not include attention to the mouth will fail.

Chin

A curious form of infection occurs which is not always associated with infected teeth; when unassociated with dental disease the aetiology is unknown.

The lesion comprises painful, firm swelling of the chin often with some drooping of the lower lip away from the lower incisor arch.

General malaise and pain are often present in a degree not consonant with a comparatively small lesion often without fever. Pressure on the chin causes severe pain.

Some cases respond to systemic antibiotic and steroid therapy but some require local injection of these agents into the substance of the chin itself, when anaesthesia is usually necessary. Recurrence is not uncommon. Frank pus formation is rare, probably owing to the density of the tissue at this site.

Bridge of Nose

Infection of the soft tissues overlying the bridge of the nose occasionally occurs and is of a relatively chronic nature with the production of considerable amounts of fibrous tissue.

There is rarely generalised malaise in the early stages, the lesions being obvious and sometimes painful on pressure. Ulceration or sinus formation may occur with a scanty discharge of pus. Bacteriological examination is desirable as the infecting organism may not be one of the usual cat pathogens.

Treatment will be dictated by the bacteriological findings.

Differential diagnosis must exclude neoplasia. Biopsy may occasionally be required. It is also desirable to eliminate cryptococci as a possible cause.

REFERENCES

Baker, G.J. (1972) *J.S.A.P.* **13**, 373.

Colegrave *et al.* (1964) *Vet. Rec.* **76**, 67.

Joshua, J.O. (1962) *Mod. Vet. Pract.* **43**, 40.

Knight, G.C. (1958) *Vet. Rec.* **70**, 680.

Patchett, E.H. (1944) *Vet. Rec.* **56**, 164.

Proud, A.J. (1974) *Vet. Rec.* **95**, 426.

Smith, J.E. (1964) *J. Small An. Pract.* **5**, 517.

Startup, C.M. (1963) *Vet. Rec.* **75**, 752.

Thomlinson, M.J. & Schenk, N.L. (1975) *J.A.V.M.A.* **167**, 927.

Winstanley, E.W. (1974) *Vet. Rec.* **95**, 289.

Chapter 6

THE EYES

Certain conditions of the eye and associated structures which are commonplace in the dog are rare or absent in the cat. The author has never seen luxation of the Harderian gland in the cat, papillomata of the eyelids or distichiasis. Entropion is not common, neither is hordeolum. Although superficial abrasions of the cornea may occur, corneal ulceration comparable to the common canine lesion is virtually nonexistent. Luxation of the lens occurs but is uncommon, dermoids are not common.

Congenital Abnormalities

Ablepharon (*absence of lids*), usually partial and more commonly occurring towards the outer canthus, is often associated with microphthalmus.

Kittens of all types may be affected. Although in the author's experience it is rather more common in the Siamese this difference is probably more apparent than real. In the present state of knowledge it is fairer to regard this as a congenital abnormality rather than an inherited defect; none the less the pros and cons of breeding from affected stock should always be fully discussed.

In many cases kittens are born with their eyes open and this is sometimes evidence of prematurity. Sheppard (1951) states that such kittens often die within a few days of birth but that, in less severe cases that survive, keratitis and conjunctivitis develop. She suggests treatment of these kittens by excision of a triangular piece of skin above the affected area as for entropion, the conjunctiva being stripped from the corneo-scleral junction.

Even if a normal eye is present the condition is virtually inoperable as a great part of the lid, tarsal border and palpebral conjunctiva are absent, the remaining conjunctiva being confluent with the ordinary skin above the eye. This results in inability completely to close the eye with resulting pathological changes in the cornea due to drying and increased susceptibility to infection. Severe cases, especially if associated with microphthalmus, merit euthanasia.

Entropion. Is uncommon in the cat and when it occurs it does so in the central portion of the lid rather than at the corners; both these findings are probably due to the comparatively spherical palpebral aperture.

Smyth (1947) records one case (age and breed not stated) corrected by surgery and one case in a 5-week-old kitten, partly of White Long-haired ancestry, which was destroyed owing to the co-existence of microphthalmus.

Sheppard (1951) considered that entropion was becoming commoner especially in the Blue Long-hair (Blue Persian). It is interesting to speculate whether the large round eye desired by breeders may force the lids, when the eye is open, into an abnormally stretched position causing compensatory rolling in of the tarsal rim and subsequent spasm.

Symptoms are those of corneal irritation with lachrymation and a tendency to blepharospasm.

Treatment by the classical operation of removing a crescent-shaped piece of skin from the affected lid or lids gives satisfactory results. General anaesthesia is essential and care should be taken that the incision nearer to the lid should be as close as possible to the tarsal rim and that a portion of the orbicularis muscle should be excised with the skin to be removed.

Accidental wounds of the lids may occur and are treated on routine lines.

Protrusion of the Membrana Nictitans

This is a common occurrence in the cat and may be associated with local lesions of the eye or conjunctiva or be evidence of sub-normal health. In the latter context its protrusion is believed due to rapid disappearance of the retro-orbital fat during any debilitating condition. Cats are often presented with the history that they have gone blind or have a film across the eye; a careful clinical examination is always called for to establish or eliminate the presence of systemic disease or local abnormality. In the former case a common finding is that the cat is convalescent following a very mild virus infection for which the owner has not sought advice. It is not unusual to find that certain cats lose condition in the late spring and summer months, possibly because of a heavy coat change; anorexia and protrusion of the nictitating membrane sometimes co-exist. This summer decline in some cats is an odd but definite condition. It may be reasonable to postulate hormonal factors following an active breeding season in the entire male but a similar if milder syndrome occurs in some neutered males despite the absence of gonads; the author does not recall the condition in entire or neutered females.

Signs. The condition is obvious, the membrane covering from $\frac{1}{4}$–$\frac{2}{3}$ of the eye surface.

Treatment. Will be according to aetiology. Foreign bodies, trauma or inflammation will be dealt with appropriately and poor condition following infection or other causes may be improved by diet and vitamin additions.

Prognosis. Recovery occurs in 7–28 days. Persistence, associated with progressive weight loss, indicates the need to seek a serious underlying disease process.

Contusions of the Sclera

These are common in street accidents and after cat or dog bites. Usually adjacent tissues are also involved; puncture wounds or small tears may be found in the adjoining lid. There is variable haemorrhage into the normally very white sclerotic. Symptoms may be negligible. Resolution without specific treatment to this lesion occurs rapidly, within 48 hours–7 days.

Conjunctivitis

Is a common eye condition in the cat which may be associated with virus infections, traumatic lesions of the periorbital structures, hypersensitivity or be an entity caused by bacterial invasion.

Intense oedema is a somewhat frequent tissue reaction to inflammation of the conjunctiva peculiar to the cat, which may be persistent and cause mechanical obstruction to vision as well as difficulty in examination of the globe and application of treatment. This oedema is not confined to any one type of conjunctivitis and may occur in all the groups mentioned.

Bacterial Conjunctivitis

Various types of conjunctivitis as a sole clinical lesion may occur. These are varied in manifestation including diffuse reddening and injection, oedema and vesicular, granular or follicular conjunctivitis; the latter group are usually of a somewhat chronic nature and liable to recurrence. Bacteriological findings in these cases are varied and the author is unaware of the incrimination of any specific organism common to this type of case. Since several cats housed together may be affected it is clear that an infective and transmissible organism is involved.

Symptoms are usually of lachrymation, the presence of a brownish mucus at the inner canthus or protrusion of the membrana nictitans. Evidence of photophobia, blepharospasm or irritation causing rubbing is not as common as might be expected.

In vesicular or follicular conjunctivitis the lesions may be numerous or few; in the former as translucent blebs about 1 mm. in diameter, in the latter as raised, red solid granules of similar size.

Treatment. Drops are usually more easily and effectively applied since the space in the conjunctival sac is small for the introduction of ointments or creams; the latter, unless very rapidly melted, are extruded by the tightly fitting globe.

Sulphacetamide or Collosol Argentum drops or ointments of broad spectrum antibiotics may be used. Of the latter oxytetracycline is probably the best.

Failing response to routine methods a swab should be taken for bacteriological examination and sensitivity tests (*not* immediately after a course of antibacterial therapy!). Based on this the appropriate drug may be used systemically or locally by sub-conjunctival injection if it is available in a suitable soluble form; combination with a cortico-steroid is permissible if chronic inflammation is present, e.g. prednisolone disodium phosphate.

Surface cauterisation with 2 per cent solution of silver nitrate, con-trolled by saline, may be effective in chronic cases of vesicular or follicular conjunctivitis.

A specific conjunctivitis due to infection by an organism resembling *Moraxella lacunatus* occurring as an outbreak in a cattery has been described by Withers and Davies (1961) characterised by inflammation, oedema and purulent discharge. The importance of this finding lies in the fact that *Moraxella* is often isolated in human conjunctivitis, a factor to be considered when the history is met—as occasionally happens—that both members of a family and the cat are suffering from conjunctivitis at the same time. The author has investigated a very limited number of such cases, so far with negative results. It is suggested, however, that whenever coincidental cases of human and feline con-junctivitis arise the possibility of *Moraxella* infection be borne in mind.

Conjunctivitis associated with virus infection

Usually a sign of secondary bacterial involvement superimposed on the catarrhal inflammation caused by the virus. In the first 3–4 days of a virus infection the conjunctiva is slightly injected with a variable amount of aqueous discharge; this changes during the early period to a mucoid or muco-purulent discharge, often very copious. Conjunctival oedema may be present but usually in comparatively slight degree.

Diagnosis will be based on the associated evidence of virus infection, viz: raised temperature, malaise, sneezing and nasal discharge.

Treatment will probably be non-specific. It is possible that antibiotic therapy will be used to deal with the general problem of secondary bacterial infection; in the author's experience antibacterial eye oint-ments or drops are of little avail in these cases; far more important is regular cleaning away of discharge (often necessary at 2 hourly intervals) and the lubrication of eyelids with petroleum jelly or liquid paraffin to minimise caking. Astringent eye-lotions such as 0·1–0·5 per cent zinc sulphate (with or without boric acid) and Collosol Argentum drops are more useful than antibacterial ointments. If oedema is a persistent pro-blem the use of Collosol Argentum drops with 1/500,000 adrenalin is well tolerated and effective in reducing the swelling. The conjunctivitis will clear coincidentally with recovery but protrusion of the nictitating membrane may persist well into convalescence.

Conjunctivitis associated with injuries

Accidental wounds of the periorbital structures often cause coincidental inflammation of the conjunctiva, localised or general. Foreign bodies such as grass awns in the conjunctival sac cause severe inflammation often with marked oedema; examination in such cases may be impossible without general anaesthesia and then it is often difficult, owing to the ballooning of the tissue, to satisfy oneself that no damage to the globe exists. In most cases treatment of the injury or removal of the foreign body will result in improvement of the conjunctiva; in protracted cases where oedema persists astringent lotions or drops may be helpful. In extreme cases resort to saline diuretics may be considered in order to dehydrate the tissue. Irritation does not appear to be so intense as in similar conditions in the dog but if it is marked a suitable eye ointment containing local anaesthetic may be used.

Allergic Conjunctivitis

Is only occasionally seen in the cat and in most cases seems to be related to exposure to pollens during the summer months.

Symptoms are lachrymation and some sneezing; whether the latter is due to a related allergic rhinitis or to the increased flow of tears down the naso-lachrymal duct is impossible to say. There is no progress to a catarrhal or purulent condition nor any evidence of ill-health, thus differentiating it from virus infections. The conjunctiva is seen to be bright pink to red, not oedematous but watery.

Treatment is better by suitable corticosteroids (betamethasone or dexamethasone) systemically and locally than by antihistamine drugs which are often not well tolerated in the cat.

Keratitis

Lesions of the cornea are seldom a serious problem in the cat. Abrasions associated with injuries are usually superficial; they heal rapidly with little inflammatory reaction other than transient leucocytic infiltration with the consequent slight opacity. Problems of vascularisation and pigmentation of the cornea are remarkably rare. Slight marginal keratitis may accompany conjunctivitis very occasionally and there will possibly be slight reaction following penetration by a foreign body; the word possibly is used advisedly as several cases of penetration of the cornea by thorns and air-gun pellets can be recalled in which local reaction by the cornea was totally absent or merely part of a generalised inflammation of the whole globe. Occasional opacity of the whole depth of the cornea has been seen resembling an interstitial keratitis—treatment has been of no avail.

Panophthalmitis

This term is chosen to indicate inflammatory reaction involving many or all of the structures in the eye. The author recognises two types of panophthalmitis, traumatic and idiopathic.

Traumatic

May result from injuries sustained in street accidents but more commonly from animal bites; it is also the inevitable result of penetration by a foreign body such as an air-gun slug which reaches the posterior chamber; this point needs emphasising since foreign bodies such as thorns which enter the anterior chamber and even the lens may not result in generalised inflammation or infection.

The signs are usually obvious and vary according to the stage at which the animal is presented; haemorrhage, contusion, suppuration, and even complete devitalisation may be noted.

Treatment should be surgical, by enucleation as soon as operation can be tolerated; attempts at medical treatment to preserve the remnants of an eye are not, in the author's view, justified in this species.

Idiopathic

It is appreciated that this heading may well be a controversial one but the condition can be recognised as a clinical entity.

The condition occurs in adult cats, usually in middle life or early old age ($\rightarrow$ 12 years).

Symptoms. The cat is profoundly dull, unwilling to move from a position of sternal recumbency with head drooping, complete or partial anorexia exists and a desire to seek a dull light. Lachrymation and blepharospasm are remarkable for their absence.

Examination of the cat reveals little; temperature may be slightly raised but otherwise clinical findings are negative apart from the affected eye. The condition has always, in the author's experience, been unilateral. No inflammatory changes of globe or periorbital structures are evident but palpation over the upper part of the globe (as in testing for intra-ocular tension) elicits a marked pain reaction; very occasionally slightly increased intra-ocular pressure may be detected digitally. Ophthalmoscopic examination of the conscious cat is very difficult owing to the intense photophobia provoked by the light and has in the author's hands revealed nothing of significance when carried out under anaesthesia.

Diagnosis. Is based on the profound dullness coupled with pain on pressure of the eyeball in the absence of all other clinical findings.

Treatment. Medical treatment has failed completely in the author's hands and analgesics are unavailing.

Enucleation is the only answer and response is dramatic and permanent with no subsequent involvement of the second eye in any case which can be recalled.

Technique of Enucleation

The closed lids extra-conjunctival method is advocated even in infected cases. The cosmetic effect is acceptable and the absence of secretion after operation is advantageous.

Anaesthesia. By intravenous pentobarbitone or, if volatile anaesthetics are used, intubation is essential to avoid the presence of a face mask.

Whatever method is employed it is essential that depth should be assessed prior to surgery and should not be increased during operation because of apparent pain reaction when the inner canthus is being incised. The skin at the inner canthus of the eye is intensely sensitive—abolition of all sensation at this site implies dangerously deep anaesthesia.

The cat is restrained in lateral recumbency the head being raised on a small sandbag according to the surgeon's preference. Routine clipping and shaving of an area of some ½ inch around the eye is carried out. Cloths are applied. The lids are sutured together using any suture material (preferably pliable) with interrupted or continuous sutures applied as close as possible to the tarsal borders. The skin is then incised about ⅛ inch from the sutured lids following the outline of the orbit. The globe is freed by 'nibbling' around the orbital rim using 5 inch curved on flat scissors, the convexity following the outline of the orbital cavity; it is necessary to ensure that division of tissues is made distal to the conjunctiva at all points. The tissues, including the four rectus and two oblique muscles and retro-orbital fat are all severed thus freeing the globe from its attachments; this can be ascertained by lifting the eyeball slightly out of the socket and ensuring that the only attachment is now the optic nerve and associated structures. Curved 5 inch artery forceps may now be applied behind the globe which is then severed from its remaining attachment. It is sometimes possible to apply a catgut ligature below the artery forceps but this form of haemostasis is by no means always achieved.

The socket should be packed with gauze while the lids are sutured; there is no need to instil antibacterial dressings into the cavity. The cut edges of the lids are then sutured with interrupted sutures of a suitable non-capillary material such as monofilament nylon, the gauze packing being removed before the final sutures are laid. Finally a pad is sutured over the incisional line.

After care. Routine antibiotics for 4–5 days. The pad is removed in 4–7 days—it is usually surprisingly well tolerated—and the lid sutures in 14 days.

Complications. Haemorrhage; usually the application of the pad is sufficient to limit bleeding and pressure by the clot does the rest. One case has been met in which fatal and completely uncontrollable haemorrhage occurred, death occurring some 12 hours post-operatively. On the evidence available it would appear that this was a case of haemophilia. Post-operative infection of the socket has never been met.

Prognosis. Results are excellent with immediate relief of symptoms. In no case has there been any evidence of the cat being subsequently at a disadvantage and a normal expectation of life can be confidently predicted.

Anterior Chamber

Haemorrhage into the anterior chamber of the eye is not uncommon, usually associated with trauma but occasionally there is no evidence whatsoever of such injury, the owner merely noticing the discolouration of the eye.

Symptoms are negligible:

The lesion is obvious. The anterior chamber being filled with bright red blood to a variable extent, sometimes almost completely.

Treatment. By the use of coagulants or Vitamin K or its analogues. Recovery is usually rapid, within 10 days resolution has occurred in most cases.

Accumulation of pus or leucocytes in the anterior chamber is rare in the cat but is seen occasionally. It is difficult to differentiate positively from neoplasia unless associated symptoms of pyrexia and infection co-exist. Persistence of the foreign material in the eye is another indication for enucleation.

Foreign Bodies

Have already been referred to in connection with conjunctivitis and panophthalmitis but occasionally are found in the absence of these conditions.

Thorns not infrequently become embedded in the cornea and are dealt with routinely.

In one case an adult castrated male cat was presented by the owner who said she 'could see a black speck on the eye'. Examination revealed a pin-head size black spot apparently confluent with the corneal surface. The cat showed no sign whatever of being aware of any abnormality.

Under general anaesthesia a thorn $\frac{1}{2}$ inch long, which had penetrated the cornea virtually at right angles, was removed. It was clear that the lens must have been involved owing to the length of the thorn but the only evidence of this was a very small pigmented spot in the lens which could be clearly seen on opthalmoscopic examination and which persisted for some 6 months. No local reaction occurred before or after removal.

Neoplasia.

Neoplasms of the eye and periorbital structures are not common, papillomata of the lids, for example, being remarkable for their absence.

The author has seen deposits of lymphosarcoma in the eyes, including the iris itself, as part of a generalised visceral lymphosarcomatosis. Two cases have also been seen in which histological diagnosis of malignant tumour has been made after enucleation. Lesions are usually visually obvious but seldom cause subjective symptoms. Enucleation is the only treatment.

Luxation of the Lens

Not a common condition but does occur. In the author's experience cases have been seen in non-pedigree cats hence it seems improbable that it is analogous to the condition seen in certain breeds of dog as a hereditary predisposition.

Symptoms are once again remarkable for their insignificance. Slight lachrymation and conjunctival congestion may occur. Usually the owner notices that reflection from the tapetum lucidum has become both more noticeable and more frequent.

Luxation has been into the anterior chamber, the lens usually being clearly visible lying tilted against the posterior corneal surface. The author has not seen a case at the stage when an aphakic crescent or iridodonesis were present.

Secondary glaucoma eventually occurs but is slower in onset than in the dog; local corneal opacity due to pressure usually results. The author has had no opportunity of performing lens extraction in the few cases seen and necessity for enucleation due to secondary changes has not been so urgently required as in the dog.

The Retina

Cases of retinal haemorrhage, detachment and degeneration have all been seen on rare occasions. No aetiological factors have been incriminated.

Signs noted are of pupillary dilation or blindness and on ophthalmoscopic examination the lesions are usually easily visible.

Haemorrhage may resorb in time; coagulant treatment is warranted. There is no treatment for retinal detachment or degeneration.

In the author's experience blind cats are far less able to adapt than dogs and since they are not amenable to physical control by their owners in the same way they are in greatly increased danger of accident; many become miserably depressed and it is usually inhumane to keep blind cats alive.

REFERENCES

Sheppard, M. (1951) *Vet. Rec.* **63**, 685.
Smyth, R. S. (1947) *Vet. Rec.* **59**, 148.
Withers, A. R. & Davies, M. E. (1961) *Vet. Rec.* **73**, 856.

SUGGESTED FURTHER READING

Smythe. R. H. (1958) *Veterinary Ophthalmology*, London, Bailliere Tindall & Cox.
Coop, M. C. & Thomas, J. R. (1958) *J. Amer. Vet. Medical Association* **133**, 369. (Bilateral glaucoma in the cat.)
Uberreiter, O. (1959) *Adv. Vet. Sci.* **5**, 1. (Examination of the eye and eye operations in animals.)
Michel, G. (1955) *Dtsch. Tierärztl. Wschr.* **62**, 347. (Anatomy of the lacrimal glands and ducts in the dog and cat.)
Morris, Mark L. Jr., (1965) *Cornell Vet.*, **lv**, 295. (Feline degenerative retinopathy).

Chapter 7

THE MOUTH
(INCLUDING TEETH AND TONGUE)

Foreign Bodies in the Mouth

Fish bones are not uncommonly found lodged in the mouth, particularly the smaller vertebrae of fish such as haddock and whiting which may become impacted on the crowns of the premolar or first molar teeth during mastication. The long single bones may wedge between two teeth or a small fragment become lodged at gum level in the interstices between teeth; the latter require great care in examination to detect.

In all cases the cat will show great distress pawing at the mouth repeatedly and often clawing the gums quite severely. In the case of a vertebra on the crown of a tooth there will additionally be inability to close the mouth; in older cats a similar picture will occur with a displaced loose tooth.

The history is usually that the symptoms have arisen suddenly during or after a meal or after the cat has come in from outside where it may have been scavenging.

It is usually possible to remove these types of foreign bodies without inducing anaesthesia; incisor dental or artery forceps are useful instruments and should be ready to hand so that examination and treatment can be carried out during one opening of the mouth. General anaesthesia is occasionally necessary for thorough investigation.

Needles, especially threaded, are often swallowed by cats but more usually lodge in the pharynx (see p. 67). It is rare to find a needle transfixing the tongue as often happens in the dog, probably due to the lack of space in the cat's mouth for the needle to attain any other position than with its long axis parallel to that of the cat until it reaches the pharynx where it may become oblique or transverse.

The Teeth and Gums

Dental attention to cats is very necessary and in some parts of the country is a much neglected subject. In the author's experience dental interferences on cats were required nearly as frequently as in dogs.

Dental Formula: $\dfrac{3131}{3130}$

Change from temporary to permanent dentition: eruption of the permanent teeth commences between 15 and 17 weeks of age; all permanent teeth are through by 6 months and fully developed by 7 months at which time the cat can be said to have a full mouth.

Owing to the greater uniformity of conformation some problems are virtually non-existent in the cat, e.g. abnormalities of the bite and malocclusion due to crowding of teeth as in brachicephalic dogs; persistence of deciduous teeth is also exceedingly rare if it occurs at all. Hypoplastic conditions are likewise no problem. Cat teeth are particularly brittle, the crown being relatively thin-walled and thus present some problems in extraction; the use of dental forceps for this purpose usually results in breaking off the crown unless the roots are exceptionally loose. Dental elevators are very valuable in this connection.

Gingivitis

Occurs in kittens and adults; in the former is apparently a clinical entity the aetiology of which is not established; Builder (1955) refers to this condition as an ulceration.

A. In kittens. Is first noticed at the time of eruption of the permanent teeth, i.e. between $3\frac{1}{2}$ and 7 months.

Symptoms (which may be minimal) include reluctance to eat, difficulty in masticating, increase in salivation and sometimes halitosis. The general health is not obviously affected.

The predilection site is the gum adjacent to the last 2 premolars and first molar but often the entire gingival margin, including the incisor arch, is involved. The lesion is seen as a fiery red line at the junction of tooth and gum. In many cases this line is very fine but in severe ones may involve a depth of 1–2 mm. of gum tissue with frank ulceration; suppuration is not evident.

Aetiology. Not known. No specific bacteria have been incriminated to the best of the author's knowledge. Pasteurellas may be found but as they are present in 94% of cat naso-pharynxes, their significance is doubtful.

The condition seems markedly to resemble the so-called "puberty gingivitis" of adolescent humans which is due to hormonal imbalance at this time of life, i.e. in the girl increase in progesterone and oestrogen and in the boy increasing androgen. Although some cases progress to periodontitis--as do some kittens--cases are virtually self-limiting and spontaneous resolution is usual. (Pèter Mikulski, L.D.S., R.C.S., (Eng.) Personal Communication).

It is tempting to postulate that the persistence of some feline cases may be iatrogenic in that neutering of both sexes is common in this age group and that this may contribute to a lasting hormonal imbalance with failure of gingival lesions to resolve.

Treatment. By no means always satisfactory. Vitamin and antibacterial therapy should be adopted, the former including A, C and D. Whenever possible oral hygiene should be assisted by appropriate bathing of the gums. In many cases clinical improvement results, the kitten showing decreased evidence of discomfort but the inflammation persists. In many cases these cats are candidates for early and multiple tooth extraction. It is desirable to arrange regular (3–6 monthly) re-inspections of these patients in order that further treatments may be instituted as necessary and eventual extraction timed to take place before serious lesions develop.

In adults. Gingivitis may be found in association with conditions such as dental calculus, parodontal disease and alveolitis, but may be seen as an apparently uncomplicated lesion when it not uncommonly spreads to the mucosa where it is reflected at the angle of the jaw in which site it causes severe lesions which may be vesicular, papular or ulcerative.

The evidence of gingivitis in the adult is usually more marked than in kittens with obvious inflammation at the gingival margins. Symptoms are variable in severity but may include difficulty in mastication, salivation (occasionally blood-tinged) and pain on opening the mouth or handling the gums. When severe ulceration in the angle of the jaw is present pain on opening the mouth for examination is often severe.

Bacteriological findings are again non-specific and often disappointing in that antibacterial therapy based on them is often ineffective *in vivo*.

Treatment. Any associated condition should be dealt with appropriately and vigorously when the inflammation of the gums will usually resolve.

As an entity it is tackled by thorough antibacterial therapy systemically and locally, the latter by applying concentrated preparations such as intramammary cerates to the gums. Corticosteroids may be incorporated *after* several days on antibacterial drugs, to reduce inflammatory thickening. Involvement of the angle of the jaw may require attention under general anaesthesia with curettage and cautery using 2–5 per cent silver nitrate solution, controlled by saline.

Prognosis in these latter cases must be guarded; some cases resist treatment and may eventually necessitate euthanasia.

Dental Calculus

Deposits of calculus (tartar) are common; the tendency is for dental calculus to be more frequent in older cats but age is not necessarily a factor.

The deposit is usually fairly hard and brittle varying in colour from cream to orange/brown; it is deposited in layers and frequently the mass exceeds the buried tooth in size. All teeth may be sites for tartar formation but the canines, premolars, and first upper molars, are usually worst affected; the upper carnassials may be carrying a deposit five or six times the volume of the tooth; removal will often reveal a healthy tooth beneath.

Occasionally the calculus is soft, furry and pale; in such cases care should be taken to eliminate the existence of nephritis and diabetes as predisposing factors before proceeding to drastic dental surgery.

The significance of tartar formation lies mainly in the fact that it usually results in the development of parodontal disease or mechanical ulceration of contiguous areas of buccal mucosa; its early and regular removal is a valuable prophylactic measure in maintaining dental health.

Symptoms are not usually present in early uncomplicated cases but will occur when either of the above conditions supervenes; in parodontal disease foul breath will be the predominant sign, in ulceration unwillingness and difficulty in eating possibly with salivation.

The owners may present the cat having noticed the discolouration.

Treatment. Should be carried out under general anaesthesia except in cases where a single tooth is involved (unusually one carnassial only will be the site of heavy tartar deposit) when it may be possible to crack off the calculus with incisor forceps in the conscious patient. In nearly all cases several teeth are involved and anaesthesia is desirable not only on humanitarian grounds but for efficiency of examining the buccal as well as the labial aspects of the teeth and for doing any necessary work on the former surface; also if severe parodontal disease is found after removal of tartar the patient is immediately ready for extractions.

Intravenous thiopentone sodium is the agent of choice for dental work, the syringe being held *in situ* and augmenting doses being given as required by an assistant.

For simple scaling three instruments are particularly satisfactory, incisor forceps to crack off large deposits, a flat scaler to deal with lateral tooth surfaces and a pointed scaler for the interstices of the teeth.

Scaling should be carried out thoroughly and carefully, all macroscopic deposits on all surfaces being removed. Following this a suitable intramammary penicillin cerate should be lightly applied to all gingival margins.

Even when only simple scaling is envisaged permission should always be sought for extractions at the veterinary surgeon's discretion. It cannot be too strongly emphasised that removal of any tissue or organ or performance of any surgical procedure not covered by consent of the owner constitutes surgical trespass for which the veterinary surgeon can be held liable in law.

Caries

A condition of cavitation of the crowns of certain teeth, notably the carnassials, on the lateral, not occlusal, surfaces of the crowns is recognised. Builder (1955) described these as lesions of erosion rather than true caries, and this is supported by the histological studies of Schneck & Osborn (1976) who have termed the condition "Progressive, subgingival osteoclastic resorption."

The lesion is seen as a semi-circular black area adjoining the gingiva, in the author's experience most commonly on the lingual surface of the lower carnassial, about 2–3 mm. in diameter. At this stage symptoms are not usually noted but as the lesion progresses it undermines the crown which eventually separates leaving highly sensitive roots *in situ* which often become infected and covered by friable, vascular tissue which is painful on pressure. At this stage difficulty in eating and other evidence of mouth pain becomes apparent. Not infrequently the lesion is first noted during other dental attention.

Treatment is by extraction which should be carried out with the aid of elevators as the crown is particularly fragile in these circumstances, sometimes only a thin shell, but the roots are fairly sound.

Paradontal Disease

Is common in the cat almost invariably as a consequence of dental calculus.

Aetiologically it is possible to postulate lack of dental work as in the analogous condition in the dog since the food of most domestic cats is provided in a finely divided state thus minimising mastication.

Symptoms. The disease may be well advanced before symptoms or signs are noticed. Foul breath odour is often the first sign. Later owing to loosening of teeth difficulty in eating supervenes. Not infrequently a cat may be presented with the history that it has a bone in its mouth owing to the fact that it cannot close its jaw; examination often reveals a displaced carnassial or molar tooth which is held by the tips of one or two roots only and is acting as a foreign body preventing occlusion; the tooth is often embedded in a large mass of tartar.

On clinical examination a variable amount of calculus is present on the teeth which may effectively conceal more advanced lesions. In severe cases pus can be seen oozing between the tartar and the gum.

As the disease progresses erosion of periodontal tissues occurs resulting in increasing exposure of roots and gum recession; the roots become variably atrophic. Smaller teeth often drop out spontaneously.

Treatment. If active inflammation is present a short course of anti-bacterial therapy pre-operatively is wise.

Surgical treatment comprises extraction of all loosened teeth or those which, while remaining firm, show a marked degree of gum recession. Careful and thorough scaling of all remaining teeth is essential, attention being paid to the immediately sub-gingival areas. Local and parenteral antibiotics are advisable.

Wholesale tooth removal is well tolerated and no difficulty in eating is to be anticipated subsequently. If possible the canine teeth should be preserved to assist prehension of food and retain the tongue. Exposure of more than a few millimetres of the root, however, is an indication for extraction of canines as well.

Tooth Extraction

Owing to the very brittle nature of even healthy feline teeth extraction presents some problems and is seldom satisfactorily achieved by the use of forceps. Gentle manipulation with appropriate elevators is extremely effective. A short length of intramedullary bone pin, $\frac{3}{32}$ inch diameter, may be used as a substitute for a proper elevator. Teeth to which elevators are not applicable (some premolars, canines and incisors), should be gripped very lightly in forceps, the jaws of which do not meet too closely and with edges which are not too sharp. It is essential that broken roots should not be left in the gum when they are liable to cause severe symptoms.

An occasional complication of extraction, even in cases where roots have been positively removed, is a persistent gingivitis/alveolitis which causes severe pain shown by refusal to eat and grinding, champing movements of the jaws; on examination there is often a fine frothy appearance of the gums as though hydrogen peroxide has recently been used. In the absence of infection corticosteroids are very effective in reducing this inflammation.

Alveolitis

Inflammation of the osseous tissues associated with tooth roots is not uncommon. It is usually a consequence of some previous condition such as parodontal disease with gum recession (especially canines) or tooth roots left in the jaw following spontaneous separation of the crown as in caries or incomplete extraction.

Symptoms comprise pain as evidenced by reluctance to eat or difficulty in mastication. The overlying gum is seen to be reddened and swollen; the tissue over buried roots may bleed easily when touched; all affected tissues are painful on pressure. Although malaise is present there is seldom temperature rise.

Treatment will comprise extraction of affected teeth or residual roots but surgery may need to be preceded by antibacterial therapy in severe cases. Medical treatment alone may give transient relief but will not be permanent unless diseased teeth and roots are completely removed.

Infected tooth roots with abscess or sinus development

Occasional cases of infection of tooth roots occurs in the absence of other obvious dental disease. It may be difficult in such cases to locate the affected tooth which is causing symptoms (pain and difficulty in eating) until an obvious abscess or sinus develops.

A condition not dissimilar from dental sinus (malar abscess) in the dog occasionally occurs, the discharging point being subjacent to the inner canthus of the eye and is thus both higher and more medial than the corresponding lesion in the dog. The condition is often initially thought to be the usual cat bite sepsis but failure to heal or rapid recurrence soon cause suspicion of tooth involvement. The lesion may be associated with the last premolar (carnassial) or first molar; extraction results in drainage and rapid resolution.

In the lower jaw a similar condition results in localized abscess formation which eventually discharges on the ventral aspect of the horizontal ramus of the mandible.

Extraction of the lower carnassial should be carried out with the greatest care since the tooth is often firm and the surrounding bone, after pyogenic infection is more fragile and liable to fracture. Elevators should always be used.

In all cases antibacterial therapy should follow surgery for a period of 3–7 days.

Tongue and Buccal Mucosa

Ulceration of the Tongue

May occur as a specific or non-specific lesion. In the former case it involves the anterior and antero-lateral tongue edges in cases of viral ulcerative glossitis (see page 190).

As a non-specific lesion it may occur as chemical burning due to the cat licking therapeutic dressings or attempting to remove accidentally acquired agents on the skin such as lime, paraffin, etc. Severe tongue and pharyngeal ulceration has been seen following too lavish application of 1 per cent methyl violet in the treatment of labial ulcers. Treatment is on routine lines.

Ulcers have been seen on the posterior dorsum of the tongue, occasionally in association with similar lesions on the hard palate, for which no aetiological factor has been found. They are usually oval in shape and from 0·5–0·75 cm. in length. Symptoms are usually of unwillingness to eat or drink.

It is likely that the aetiological agent in many such cases is a calici virus (Povey 1976). Calici virus infections are discussed in more detail in the chapter on Infectious Diseases and in the section dealing with the 'cat flu' complex.

Empirical treatment which has included high dosage of Vitamin C parenterally (100–200 mg. intramuscularly twice weekly) has apparently been successful in promoting resolution.

Neoplasia and Inflammation Ventro-lateral to the Frenum Linguae

The above heading is deliberately selected as the lesions covered by this wording are indistinguishable on clinical grounds and occasionally not easily definable histologically.

The lesion occurs as a granulating mass on the lateral aspect of the underside of the tongue adjacent to the lower premolar teeth. The lesion has often become secondarily infected and is then foul smelling. Size varies according to duration but it is not usually possible to decide what the latter is.

Symptoms. Difficulty in eating, occasionally being obvious that the cat is trying to chew on one side of the mouth only, unilateral salivation which may or may not be blood or pus tinged, a foul breath odour and in the later stages depression, malaise and loss of weight.

Diagnosis. The lesion is visually obvious but no firm differential between inflammation or neoplasia should be made without biopsy and even then can be wrong.

Because lesions may be only inflammatory treatment is always warranted.

Unless the patient is very toxic—in which case antibacterial therapy should be instituted—the lesion should be examined under general anaesthesia and a representative piece of tissue removed for biopsy. When possible the lesion should be subjected to curettage or débridement and any adjacent tooth lesions dealt with (e.g. calculus, parodontal disease); light cautery with 2 per cent silver nitrate is occasionally indicated.

Medical treatment comprises combined antibiotic/corticosteroid therapy which should be continued over a period of 7–14 days. Vitamin therapy is a useful adjuvant, preferably combined A, B, C and D.

Prognosis must always be extremely guarded in view of the possibility of neoplasia; likewise some lesions which have proved to be only inflammatory have not responded to treatment and have necessitated euthanasia.

Of seven cases showing this lesion four proved to be inflammatory only, two definitely carcinomata and the seventh, a 9-year-old spayed female, was reported on biopsy to be squamous cell carcinoma but following euthanasia carried out on the basis of this report post-mortem examination and further histo-pathology showed the lesion to be purely inflammatory; this last case high-lights the difficulty of diagnosis and prognosis. None the less in any case where biopsy provides a diagnosis of malignancy euthanasia should be carried out. Corticosteroids should not be incorporated in treatment until histo-pathology has ruled out neoplasia.

In cases of carcinoma metastasis is usually late in the clinical course and usually destruction is necessitated by the condition of the animal before secondary spread is clinically obvious.

Granulomatous lesions on the dorsum of the tongue, having the appearance of advanced neoplasia, but responsive to antibiotic therapy, have been described by Baker (1972).

Stomatitis

A form of stomatitis occurs in the cat which has already been briefly mentioned under the heading 'Gingivitis' but which occasionally occurs without apparent involvement of the gingivae. It comprises an inflammatory lesion of the buccal mucosa where it is reflected in the angle of the jaws and may be vesicular, papular or ulcerative. It is usually an exceedingly painful condition; there is no particular age group, cases having been seen in adults of all ages possibly with a slight increase after middle life.

An ulcerative stomatitis with necrotic lesions, often associated with spirochaetes, was found to be common in Fe LV positive cats (Cotter, Hardy & Essex 1975--see also chapter on infectious diseases) and suggested to be a manifestation of the immuno-suppressive effects of the disease.

Symptoms comprise difficulty in eating usually followed by refusal to attempt to eat; a foul breath odour is often present; occasionally gagging movements are made by the cat.

Opening of the mouth is attended by a variable degree of pain, often intense.

The lesion is easily seen usually involving a rather square area of tissue up to 1 cm. in diameter or even slightly more.

Treatment should be vigorous from the outset as there is no tendency to spontaneous healing but only to spread.

Antibacterial treatment is often disappointing even when based on bacteriological and sensitivity findings but must be adopted. Attention to general health and particularly oral hygiene is necessary. Local treatment comprises cauterising vigorously with silver nitrate (under general anaesthesia) with 5 or 10 per cent solution or even the silver stick. Previous curettage is often helpful. The action of the caustic is controlled by sodium chloride.

A good response in otherwise refractory cases has been achieved by the combination of radical cryosurgery and dental extraction.

Prognosis: Guarded as about 25 per cent cases are resistant to treatment.

REFERENCES
Baker, G.J. (1972) *J.S.A.P.* **13** 373.
Builder, P.L. (1955) *Vet. Rec.* **67**, 386.
Cotter, S.M.; Hardy, W.D. & Essex M. (1975) *J.A.V.M.A.* **166**,
Mikulski, P. (1978) Personal Communication
Povey, R.C., (1976) *Vet. Rec.* **98** 293.
Schneck, G.W.; Osborn, J.W. (1976) *Vet. Rec.* **99**, 100.

SUGGESTED FURTHER READING

Wakuri, H. *et al.* (1962) *Bull. Azabu Vet. Coll.* No. 10, 99. (Eruption after birth of the teeth in the Japanese domestic cat.)

Chapter 8

THE EARS

1. **Otacariasis.** Infestation with *Otodectes cynotis*.

This is an extremely common condition and may be seen at all ages although the disease is less acute in older cats. The parasite is often acquired by kittens during the suckling period from a dam who may not be obviously infected.

Symptoms comprise evidence of irritation shown by scratching and shaking of the ears but exceedingly heavy infestations may cause only minimal signs.

The parasite causes excessive production of cerumen and the exfoliation of scales and scab; the whole external auditory canal may be filled with a hard mass of this material; usually parasites can be seen macroscopically as small whitish dots moving in or on this accumulation. Very large numbers of mites characterise the feline condition in marked contrast to the dog in which parasites are few but symptoms intense. If parasites cannot be seen by the unaided eye the use of a hand lens is helpful whilst they can be demonstrated in large numbers by microscopic examination of debris macerated in liquor potassae.

It is a useful practice routinely to examine the ears of kittens presented for castration, spaying or vaccination and to recommend and carry out treatment if there is any evidence of infestation.

Complications of a simple infestation can be pyogenic infection or severe ulceration of the integument of the vertical canal; chronic mild infestations may lead to hypertrophy of the integument and eventual occlusion of the canal necessitating aural resection. It does not seem that Otodectes are of any aetiological significance in relation to otitis media.

It is an interesting observation that following fully effective treatment of otacariasis many cats remain resistant to re-infestation which in most cases must be a probability.

Treatment. *Otodectes* is an extremely resistant mite and in one small experiment of a variety of agents applied to live mites on glass slides, (which included ether and Strong Solution of Iodine), only dimethyl-diphenylene disulphide killed the parasites in 5 minutes; this product is now unfortunately discontinued. All acaricidal agents in a suitable vehicle may be used for treating otacariasis, e.g. benzyl benzoate, gamma benzene hexachloride, Pybuthrin, dimethyl trichlorophenyl phosphoro-thionate (fenchlorphos) and various sulphur preparations. All these, used in correct strength and vehicle are non-toxic unless used to excess.

Thorough cleaning of the ears with removal of all debris and parasites is essential and it is therefore recommended that whenever possible treatment should be carried out by or under the supervision of the veterinary surgeon, dressing to be dispensed to the owner only for use in any unavoidably long interval. Although in theory treatments at 10 day intervals should be adequate it is found in practice that more frequent treatments are desirable particularly in severe cases, probably due to the impossibility of being certain that all live mites are removed or killed. In severe uncomplicated cases treatment should be given every fourth or fifth day on three occasions and thereafter once every 7–10 days until all evidence of parasites has gone, usually in 21–28 days. The use of a few drops of liquid paraffin in the ears once weekly subsequently is beneficial in returning the rather dry integument to normal and may have some effect in preventing re-infestation in patients exposed to a high risk.

In cases where secondary infection with pyogenic bacteria has resulted in an acute suppurative otitis externa some degree of malaise is often present and antibacterial therapy must be adopted initially before acaricidal agents are introduced. Suggested therapy is 600,000 units procaine penicillin 48 hourly by intramuscular injection for 4–6 days, together with the introduction into the ear of a penicillin cerate for intramammary use. The accumulated debris should *not* be removed from the ear at the first treatment as it often leaves exposed a large ulcerated area from which the integument has sloughed but at the second treatment the normal routine of cleansing may be undertaken as healing is extremely rapid. Following antibacterial therapy acaricidal dressings should be used for the appropriate period.

In some cases initial treatment and removal of debris discloses a large area of ulcerated, highly vascular integument which bleeds quite freely; in these circumstances the use of acaricidal drugs should be delayed until healing has occurred, bland oily liquids being used for lubrication and softening of deposit prior to removal.

Notoedric Mange

May involve the ear flaps when spread from the temporal region occurs. Alopecia is noticed on the normally hair-bearing surface and the association with the typical lesions as described previously makes the aetiology reasonably evident. Treatment should be extended to cover the ear flaps.

Suppurative Otitis

Occasionally an acute and apparently primary condition of suppurative otitis externa occurs, usually in kittens and young cats and usually bilateral. It is often not possible to incriminate previous ear trouble such as otacariasis.

Symptoms. Acute depression, refusal of food, sometimes a slightly raised temperature. The ears are held outwards giving the cat a somewhat lop-eared appearance. Pus production is copious and purulent discharge is often literally pouring out of the ear canal and soaking and matting the subjacent hair. The pus is usually of a dirty cream or yellow colour, fairly fluid and often containing floccules of sloughed integument.

Treatment. Penicillin as recommended previously (see page 108) by systemic and topical routes is rapidly effective; the ears are usually normal within 7 days of the start of treatment.

This form of otitis may also be accompanied by the formation of a layer in the canal of what looks like a diphtheritic membrane. In such cases care must be taken in removing discharges as large areas may slough at too early a stage. In spite of the presence of large amounts of pus dressing should be minimal until healing is well advanced; for this reason the adoption of systemic therapy is essential.

A less acute suppurative condition of the ears is seen in some cases of chronic hypertrophic otitis which produces small quantities of caseous type pus; this will be dealt with more fully under the appropriate heading.

Sepsis

Both the ear flap and canal are sites of septic infection following cat bites in fights; in the latter case one puncture is found in the skin anterior or posterior to the meatus and the second is found inside the canal. In the ear flap localised abscesses resembling small haematomata may form; the inflammatory reaction in bites involving the ear canal is usually more intense, and often causes the case to resemble a suppurative otitis. Differentiation is by finding tooth marks which are usually reasonably obvious. Abscesses of the flap occasionally require surgical drainage in addition to antibacterial treatment but the lesions involving the ear canal usually respond well to penicillin with which a small dose of betamethasone may be combined to give early symptomatic relief from the pain and irritation of the intense inflammation.

Vigorous and sufficiently prolonged treatment is necessary in septic lesions of the ear in view of the relatively poor healing properties of tissues associated with cartilage.

Chronic Hyperplastic Otitis Externa

In older cats (5 years +) a more chronic inflammatory condition of the external canal is seen which is characterised by thickening of the integument. There may or may not be evidence of bacterial infection. There is usually no evidence of existing otacariasis although it is highly probable that this has previously existed and been an aetiological factor.

Symptoms. Constant irritation is shown by repeated scratching and shaking. Self-inflicted lesions of the skin often appear posterior to the pinna and on the surrounding areas of skin; occasionally the development of a haematoma is the factor which draws attention to the ear canal

On examination the ear canal is seen to be decreased in calibre due to thickening of the integument which is often pigmented; the convolutions of the meatus may be touching one another so creating a vicious circle of increased irritation→scratching→thickening.

If it is possible to introduce the speculum of an auriscope into the canal a careful examination should be made for any ulcerating, bleeding or proliferative lesions in the depth and for evidence of a simple polyp.

Treatment. Medical treatment may be of some avail but surgery is often required.

Medical treatment should include antibacterial and steroid therapy both systemic and local; the canals should be carefully cleaned with a bland preparation such as liquid paraffin or compound salicylic liniment[1]; local anaesthetic ointments such as ung. procaine co. (Hewlett) may be useful in eliminating scratching.

Failure to respond adequately and permanently to medical methods indicates resort to aural resection, an operation which, while carried out less frequently in feline patients, can give results comparing favourably with those achieved in dogs. A simple technique suitable for the cat is described on pages 63 and 64.

Polyps

Occasionally pedunculated benign growths are found arising from the lower vertical or superficial horizontal canal. These may be detected during routine auriscopic examination or may initially appear to be generalised verrucosity of the integument and only on careful examination is it found to be a pedunculated single lesion.

Occasionally extirpation may be satisfactorily accomplished without resection but it is often wise to perform a partial or complete resection to ensure as complete excision as possible.

Neoplasia

Ceruminous adenocarcinoma.

This tumour is virtually peculiar to the cat, its occurrence being rare in all other species (Cotchin 1957).

---

[1] Compound Liniment of Salicylic Acid

        Salicylic Acid   50 g. (1 oz.)
        Industrial Methylated Spirit   200 ml. (4 fl. ozs.)
        Tincture of Cantharides (optional)   25 ml. (½ fl. oz.)
        Castor Oil to 1000 ml. (20 fl. ozs.)

The lesion is seen as a proliferating mass in the depth of the vertical canal. Clinically it is impossible to differentiate from hyperplasia and may even be difficult histologically. Occasionally the tumour behaves like a true carcinoma and metastasises.

Of the series of 119 cat tumours no less than ten were associated with the external auditory canal, details are appended.

1. 4 year ♂   Granuloma.
2. 16 year ♂   Chronic granulomatous polyp.
3. 10 year ♂   Polyp. Infected hyperplastic granuloma.
4. Aged.   Infected ceruminous adenoma.
5. 16 year ♂   Hyperplasia.
6. 10 year ♀   Carcinoma.
7. 13 year ♂   Carcinoma (metastasis +).
8. 8 year ♀   Infected ceruminous gland hyperplasia.
9. 13 year ♂   Ceruminous carcinoma (metastasis +).
10. 9 year ♂   Ceruminous carcinoma.

Apart from evidence of metastasis no prognosis could be based on clinical examination.

Diagnosis and prognosis must be based on histology hence biopsy is necessary; since this usually necessitates resection to reach the lesion it is best to proceed immediately to resection and excision, delaying prognosis.

Haematoma

Ear haematoma is common in cats associated with any condition causing scratching or shaking of the ears viz. otacariasis, other forms of otitis and Notoedric mange. Frequently the development of the obvious lesion is the first thing to draw the attention of the owner to any ear trouble hence a careful examination of the external canal is required in all cases of haematoma.

The haematoma comprises extravasation of blood between the cartilage and skin of the pinna, usually on the inner aspect. The size of the lesion varies from a small bleb at the base of the pinna to a tense swelling occupying the entire flap. The swelling varies in colour from normal to slightly purplish.

Owing to mechanical discomfort from the weight shaking and scratching increase and the ear is held outwards in a lop-eared manner.

Prognosis. Resorption always occurs within 10–42 days but invariably associated with contraction and scarring resulting in a crumpled ear unless surgical treatment is undertaken.

Treatment. In all cases treatment *must* be directed at removing the underlying cause but discretion must be used in choice of dressings to avoid further self-inflicted trauma.

The lesion itself may be dealt with by radical surgery or be left to resolve spontaneously. The latter course is perfectly proper in cases where the cosmetic effect is not important.

Surgical. Minor surgical techniques such as aspiration or the use of small incisions followed by pressure bandaging are usually doomed to failure. If surgery is undertaken it should be drastic. A very wide variety of techniques has been described for haematomata mainly differing in detail of suturing and applying pressure.

The object of surgery is threefold, to evacuate the contents, to eliminate dead space and recurrence of haemorrhage and the avoidance of scarring.

These methods are best achieved by Zepp's technique of making an S shaped incision followed by careful application of multiple wire or other suitable sutures. (Zepp 1949).

The operation must be carefully and thoroughly performed and is thus time consuming necessitating fairly long duration general anaesthesia. The incision must extend to the whole length of the lesion and sutures must be placed in every part of the flap where further exudation could occur. The object of the S shaped incision is to distribute the contractile tensions of scarring in many directions and thus minimise distortion of the pinna.

Conservative treatment must be accompanied by attention to the canal and may need to be assisted in the early stages by bandaging the ear tightly over the head to obviate discomfort and further shaking.

In the case of large haematomata resorption may not commence for some 10 days after the lesion has reached its maximum size and the owner should always be given some indication of the probable duration of resolution when the case is first seen.

In several cases where animals have been on corticosteroid therapy for some other reason it has been noted that resolution has been accelerated and it thus seems not unreasonable to suggest that, unless contra-indicated, betamethasone or other suitable steroid should be given orally for 10–14 days using gradual withdrawal methods of dosage.

Otitis Media

Middle ear disease is not uncommon in the cat and is characterised by neurological signs. It has received some attention in the literature of recent years. Lawson (1957) has discussed a series of eighteen cases in Glasgow, Moltzen (1961) describes otitis media in the dog and cat referring to nine cases in the cat treated by insufflation and drainage via the Eustachian tube, while Wilkinson (1963) briefly describes the condition and says that combined antibiotic/steroid therapy will be effective in most cases.

The disease can occur at any age and may be apparently sudden or insidious in onset. Many cases are not associated with evidence of disease in the external ear. Infection may be via the Eustachian tube and organisms incriminated include *Pasteurella multocida* and haemolytic staphylococci (Smith 1964).

Symptoms. Locomotor ataxia is usually present resulting in an inco-ordinate staggering, swaying or stumbling gait, sometimes with a tendency to circling. Rotation of the head is a common feature and there may be disparity in pupil size and light reflexes. Fever is not a frequent feature of the disease but malaise is often present probably due to distress caused by inability to balance.

Righting reflexes are affected.

Diagnosis. Based largely on the clinical signs plus radiography.

If a purulent discharge is present in the external canal this will be additional supportive evidence but frequently the meatus is macroscopically perfectly normal.

In many cases the osseous bulla on the affected side shows an increased density on radiography, the lateral view is probably preferable but positive results may also be obtained in a ventro-dorsal plane. The radiographic changes are fully described by Lawson and Moltzen but in an X-ray of reasonably good quality the changes are obvious even to the comparatively inexperienced observer. Whilst X-ray diagnosis is helpful in many cases a negative finding does not necessarily indicate absence of otitis media.

Differential diagnosis: Cerebral tumours and 'stroke' (cerebral haemorrhage or thrombosis). Differentiation in the absence of positive radiographic findings may be difficult but tumours of nervous tissue are rare in the cat and the 'stroke' syndrome is met more commonly in aged cats the symptoms being hemiplegic rather than locomotor inco-ordination.

Treatment. Wilkinson considers response is good to systemic broad-spectrum antibiotic/corticosteroid therapy but this view is not shared by Lawson. Moltzen advocates the technique of forced drainage via the Eustachian tube by insufflation via the external ear and obtained 50 per cent success in a small series of cases.

In view of the fact that the pus in the middle ear is often found at post-mortem examination to be inspissated or at best very tenacious in character it seems that drainage techniques cannot be expected to give uniformly good results. In early cases systemic antibacterial therapy may well succeed but in longer standing cases this seems unlikely without associated drainage and topical therapy. In cases with associated external ear discharge improvement has been obtained by performing aural resection followed by irrigation of the middle ear and introduction of suitable antibiotics via the ruptured tympanum. Some degree of head tilt is often left permanently or for long periods after otherwise successful treatment.

One approach to the bulla for surgical drainage using the radical technique of 'Bulla Osteotomy' has been described by Denny (1973) and good results are claimed following careful and repeated cleansing of the bulla by this means.

The spread of pyogenic infection to contiguous cerebral tissues is not uncommon.

Prognosis is obviously, in the light of the difficulty of really satisfactory treatment, very guarded.

Aural Resection

The technique in the cat is similar to Wright's method as for the dog described by Joshua (1958). Anatomically the ear is similar in both species, the vertical canal being less roomy in the cat and shallower. General anaesthesia is essential and since clipping and shaving will have to be carried out in the anaesthetised animal the choice

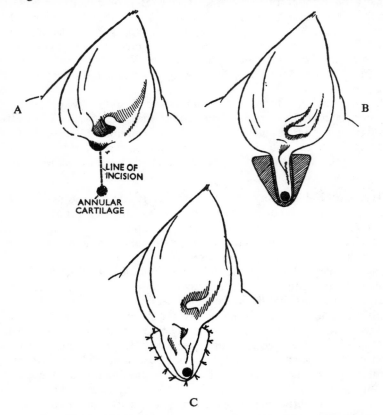

FIG. 18 A. Line of incision must extend to vertical limit of annular cartilage.

              B. Canal exposed. Triangular section of skin removed anterior and posterior to the incision.

              C. Integument and cartilage drawn back and sutured to new skin edge.

of intravenous pentobarbitone sodium is probably best. Use of a face mask is inconvenient. After routine clipping and shaving the vertical canal is vigorously cleaned. Cloths (three are usually sufficient) are applied after the usual skin cleansing processes. A groove director (not probe-ended) is passed into the vertical canal making sure that the lowest limit is reached. An incision is made, if possible through all layers at once, using the groove in the director as a guide. The incision must be continued until the director springs freely out of the canal thus ensuring that the lower limit of the annular cartilage is exposed; this is essential. A triangular area of skin, apex ventral, posterior to the incision is excised, care being taken to remove skin only and to interfere as little as possible with subcutaneous tissues. Haemorrhage may be copious but can be controlled by forci pressure until the tissues are apposed which will serve adequately for haemostasis in most cases. Sutures, preferably of braided nylon (approximately 4 lb. breaking strain) are carefully laid to bring together precisely the edges of integument and cartilage anteriorly and skin posteriorly; Hagedoorns needles are useful for precise penetration of the rather tough lining of the ear canal. Great care must be taken carefully to suture the ventral part of the incision. This procedure is repeated on the anterior aspect of the incision. The amount of skin to be excised must be carefully judged; in most cats the base of the triangle of skin (superiorly) will be some 0·5–0·75 cm.

Bandaging for the immediate post-operative period is advisable in most cases but should be left off as soon as it appears that the cat will not interfere with the ears; alternatively a protective collar can be used in placid cats. Routine antibiotic cover is supplied. Topical dressings will vary with the needs of the case. Sutures are removed gradually from the eighth day. Healing should be complete in 10–14 days. Results are gratifying in most cases.

REFERENCES
Cotchin, E. (1957) *Vet. Rec.* **69**, 425.
Denny, H.R. (1973) *J.S.A.P.* **14**, 585.
Joshua, J.O. (1958) *Vet. Rec.* **70**, 1115.
Lawson, D.D. (1957) *Vet. Rec.* **69**, 645.
Moltzen, H. (1961) *Adv. Small An. Pract. III*, 56.
Smith, J.E. (1964) *J. Small An. Pract.* **5**, 517.
Wilkinson, G.T. (1963) *Vet. Rec.* **75**, 1198. ·
Zepp, C.P. (1949) *Vet. Rec.* **61**, 643.

SUGGESTED FURTHER READING

Cotchin, E. (1956) *B. Vet. J.* **112**, 263.

Chapter 9

THE ALIMENTARY TRACT

Pharynx

Foreign Bodies

Commonly lodge in the pharyngeal region since most are of a sharp and/or irregular shape, e.g. fishbones and needles.

Fishbones

A variety of types of fishbone may become impacted including vertebrae, long straight bones if fairly rigid and flat cartilaginous plates from skate (ray).

If fairly large they may become wedged fairly well forward in the pharynx and can be seen and possibly removed at ordinary visual examination. Many, however, pass into the retropharyngeal area where they are concealed from view by the pillars of the fauces; this type necessitate induction of general anaesthesia for confirmation of diagnosis and removal.

Symptoms. Always arise suddenly after a meal although this significant history is not always available, e.g. if the cat has been out scavenging.

Often exaggerated swallowing movements, gagging and retching are present but sometimes only evident during attempts to eat. The cat is quite unable to swallow and any attempt to do so provokes severe symptoms.

Diagnosis is by visual examination with or without anaesthesia; in the latter case it is often necessary to explore carefully the folds of pharyngeal and retropharyngeal mucosa to locate the bone. There may be localised oedema and inflammation at the site of impaction.

It cannot be too strongly emphasised that any suspicious case should be examined early and thoroughly under anaesthesia and not dismissed with the assumption that the cat has a sore throat. In this respect a meat test may well be unreliable because similar symptoms can occur in cases of pharyngitis and laryngitis as a result of attempted deglutition.

Differential diagnosis will include pharyngitis and laryngitis but must be fully confirmed as above. In pharyngitis the network of engorged blood-vessels will be seen; in laryngitis a history of loss of voice is suggestive.

Handling of the laryngeal area is not helpful since violent gagging may be provoked in both foreign body and laryngitis cases.

Treatment. Removal, if necessary under anaesthesia.

Anaesthesia must be induced with care for two reasons, (a) that the airway may be partially obstructed by the bone, especially skate, (b) in old standing cases (often 5–7 days elapse before treatment is sought) the animal is in a poor nutritional state and less tolerant of anaesthetic agents.

Although it is rare for more than one piece of bone to be involved it is none the less a wise precaution to pass a gum elastic sound into the stomach to ensure that the rest of the oesophagus is free.

Needles

Cats, particularly kittens, love playing with wool and thread from workboxes and thus frequently swallow needles. These rarely impact in the anterior pharynx or become impaled in the dorsum of the tongue as occurs in the dog, but are often held up even if only temporarily, in the retropharyngeal area.

Symptoms may, unfortunately, be minimal and transient. If advice is sought early examination under anaesthesia is essential. If thread is still attached to the needle diagnosis is greatly facilitated but care should be taken in using it to withdraw the needle as the eye may be distal to the examiner and damage could be caused by unwise pulling on the thread. If no thread is attached great care is needed in searching the mucosa; on digital examination the hyoid bones must not be confused with the needle. In the case of a negative examination of a patient with a suggestive history radiography is essential.

If not located and removed from the pharyngeal area two possibilities exist, i.e. that the needle will pass on into the alimentary tract (at any point of which it can cause trouble) and be excreted, or it passes into the deeper retropharyngeal tissues of the neck.

Symptoms will abate temporarily but may recur in a variety of forms, the most common being local abscess formation.

Pharyngitis

Can occur in the absence of intercurrent virus disease but may have some unknown viral or bacterial aetiology as it is not uncommon to meet a number of cases in a locality over a short period of time.

Symptoms. Often mild and indefinite but include exaggerated swallowing movements, 'throat clearing' sounds (not a genuine cough), sometimes gagging on eating although often food is completely refused, occasionally regurgitation shortly after swallowing. Fever is rarely present and the cat remains in good condition although it may appear depressed. The history is not related to a recent meal.

Chemical inflammation of the pharynx due to licking and ingestion of irritant dressings or accidental skin contamination also occurs.

The inflamed pharynx of the cat is rather characteristic, showing a network of fine bright red blood-vessels traversing the mucosa; these are not seen in the normal pharynx.

Care must be taken to eliminate any possibility of foreign body.

Treatment. The condition is usually self-limiting within 4–9 days; in some cases the use of a demulcent such as Glycerin of Borax may be useful. On rare occasions the inflammation persists without change for more than 10 days; provided there is no evidence of infection a suitable corticosteroid in small doses (about half the average) for 2–3 days will cause the inflammation to regress rapidly.

Tonsils

Tonsillitis, if it occurs at all, is very rare or alternatively is not diagnosed, i.e. enlarged inflamed tonsils comparable with the common canine condition are not seen.

Examination of the throat under anaesthesia for other reasons may disclose tonsils which are redder than usual but they rarely protrude beyond their crypts.

Neoplasia of the Tonsil. Much less common than in the dog but does occur. In the series reviewed four tumours involved tonsils:

Age	Site(s)	Histology
1. Not known	Left tonsil,	Polyp.
2. 17 years	Tonsil and cervical nodes,	Lymphosarcoma.
3. 11½ years	Right tonsil and node,	Squamous cell carcinoma.
4. 11 years	Left tonsil, wall of pharynx, root of tongue,	Squamous cell carcinoma.

In case 1, the tonsil polyp was found coincidentally during routine post-mortem examination of a cat with a carcinoma of the subcutis of the shoulder region.

In case 3 the owner noted the enlargement of the lymph node; no other symptoms were present. The tonsil tumour was detected at the first examination but in view of the absence of symptoms no action was taken. The cat lived some 4 months during which time no pain or difficulty in eating occurred but the metastatic growth enlarged and there was eventual loss of condition; at this stage the cat was destroyed.

In contrast case 4 showed a totally different picture, probably due to the invasive nature of the tumour. There was inappetence, pain on opening the mouth and marked depression; there was a foul odour from the mouth. Early euthanasia was necessary.

The clinical syndrome is thus more varied and therefore less typical than in the dog and the condition will only be diagnosed on careful examination of the mouth and pharynx in any case showing difficulty in eating or enlarged submaxillary or first cervical lymph nodes.

The Neck

Is the site of a variety of lesions, usually of a disease process affecting other organs or such non-specific conditions as sepsis.

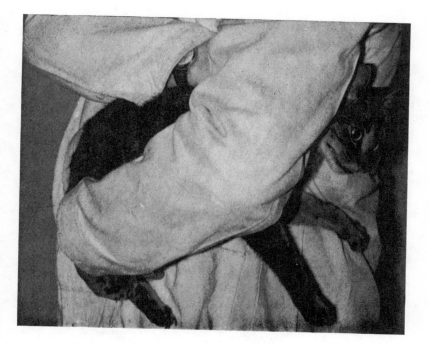

FIG. 19   Method of carrying cat

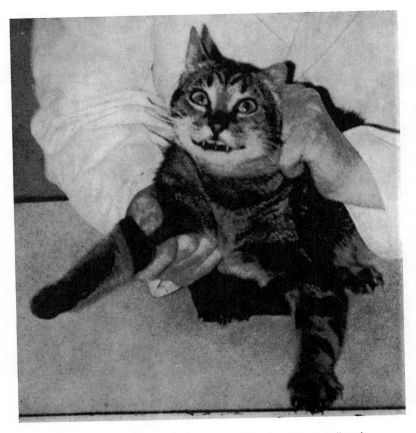

FIG. 20   Cat restrained for intravenous injection into cephalic vein

Lymph Nodes

The submaxillary and cervical lymph nodes may be involved in neoplasia of the tongue and tonsil, lymphosarcomatosis (including the pseudo-Hodgkin type) and tuberculosis. A careful examination of the cat for evidence of an underlying primary condition should be made in any case of cervical lymph node enlargement.

Parotiditis

Inflammation and enlargement of the parotid glands is occasionally seen. It is usually bilateral although swelling may be asymmetrical.

The cat usually remains well and rise of temperature is only slight if present at all.

Resolution is slow, the glands becoming more indurated as they decrease in size but may remain abnormally palpable for several weeks.

Sepsis

The neck region, especially the submaxillary area, is often involved in sepsis due to cat bites. Treatment is routine with antibiotics and surgical drainage when required.

Recurring Abscesses or Sinuses

If a septic focus recurs repeatedly after apparent response to treatment or if a sinus develops two conditions must be considered.

1. TUBERCULOSIS

Tuberculous sinuses of the neck are reputedly common in the cat. The author has, in fact, never been able to confirm this but none the less regards the fullest investigation of any persisting focus of suppuration for the presence of tubercle bacilli as imperative.

2. FOREIGN BODIES

The presence of a needle or other penetrating foreign body.

As previously mentioned needles often penetrate the retropharyngeal mucosa and track into the deeper tissues of the neck where they may cause deep-seated foci of suppuration.

All such cases should be examined radiographically in both ventro-dorsal and lateral planes. Care must be taken not to interpret normal structures as needles, e.g. hyoid bones, clavicle and spine of scapula.

If a needle is positively diagnosed on X-ray a search must be made for it surgically, hence the necessity for several radiographs to attempt to fix the location of the needle. Even so surgery is often like searching the proverbial haystack and failures are often recorded.

Sometimes the needle will make its way to the surface and every time a fresh septic focus bursts or is opened in these cases a careful search should be made for a needle eye or point.

121

Thyroid Tumours

Appear to be of no clinical significance in the cat, the lesions being usually found incidentally at post-mortem.

Two cases occur in this neoplasm series, an unclassified tumour showing a few mitoses in a 13-year-old and an adenoma of the left thyroid in a 15-year-old, both castrated males.

The possibility of such tumours must be borne in mind in the differential diagnosis of neck swellings; they are situated distal to the lower extremity of the larynx and if they attain any size fall to near the point of the sternum.

Oesophagus

Oesophageal obstruction by foreign bodies is not common although needles may occasionally be held up in the thoracic oesophagus and may either pass on to the stomach or, more commonly, penetrate the oesophageal wall, traverse the pleural structures and emerge through the skin of the thoracic wall. Symptoms in such cases are indefinite or even absent, the first indication of trouble being localised sepsis of the thoracic area.

If suspected, radiography will clinch the diagnosis but so far as treatment is concerned it is probably wiser to leave well alone in the hope that the needle will eventually surface rather than indulge in heroic surgery which is usually pre-doomed to failure.

Carcinoma of the oesophagus is a serious and not rare condition of older cats. Cotchin, who has repeatedly drawn attention to the possible significance of carcinoma of the upper alimentary tract of cats, quotes ages of 6–16 for this particular tumour (Cotchin 1956). In the practice series the age of the two confirmed cases was not known.

The history and symptoms are usually characteristic. Occasional vomiting becomes more frequent and is soon recognised as being the prompt regurgitation of solid food. Liquids or very finely divided solids are at first retained. Regurgitation becomes increasingly regular and soon occurs after every intake of solids. Unless kept unusually well nourished on liquid foods the cat becomes ravenous and starts to lose weight. Appetite is usually maintained until an advanced stage of cachexia is reached, as is some degree of brightness and energy.

Diagnosis. The lesion is usually related to the first pair of ribs and is not always of a proliferative type so that diagnosis by palpation is seldom possible; in many cases the entire lesion is within the thorax.

The best method of diagnosis is probably by endoscopy; a tube of suitable dimensions, 30 cm. length × 0·75 cm. diameter may be used for both canine bronchoscopy and feline oesophagoscopy; perspex is a very suitable material, the tube having bevelled edges at its distal end from which the light (which is a proximal source) is thrown forward. The lesion is seen as an irregularity of the oesophageal mucosa which may bleed easily when touched. Diagnosis by passage of a bougie with a brush-like end which will remove and bring away fragments of the abnormal tissue for biopsy has been suggested but the relatively firm nature of some of these tumours militates against its regular success.

In advanced cases when the lesion is either occluding the lumen of the oesophagus or causing stenosis of all layers radiography using a contrast medium can be extremely valuable. Even in cases where stenosis is not marked with resultant hold-up of contrast medium the irregular surface of the tumour may become impregnated with barium and so recognisable.

Prognosis is hopeless and in view of the state of miserable hunger early euthanasia is to be advised as soon as diagnosis is established.

Stomach

Apart from its involvement in other disease states the stomach mainly causes trouble when accumulations of hair cause impaction or when it is involved in lymphosarcomatosis. Freak (1963) records one case of gastric ulcer some details of which are given (see below).

1. Fur Impaction

In the wild state in addition to hair swallowed during grooming the stomach will also contain indigestible remnants of natural prey such as hair and skin hence it is a physiological process for cats to vomit a cylindrical mass of such debris at regular intervals, usually 7–14 days. In domestication this process is not always regular and may result in abnormal accumulations of hair in the stomach and intestine. Affected cats become slightly dull and appetite is lost. Some clinicians claim that the impacted stomach can be felt on palpation; the author cannot confirm this from personal experience.

The condition is most likely to occur during periods of coat change when larger than average quantities of fur are ingested.

Diagnosis is based on absence of other reasons for the inappetence, there is no fever and the large intestine is not impacted.

Treatment by mild aperients, especially oils such as liquid paraffin, is usually effective. In some cases the hair is eventually passed per rectum, in others vomiting is caused and the usual bolus is produced.

In cats prone to fur impactions regular small doses of liquid paraffin (a small teaspoonful 48 hourly) is advisable during coat change; regular assisted grooming should be advised.

Chemical gastritis may result from ingestion of irritant dressings licked off the skin or occur in cases of poisoning, usually indirectly through the eating of poisoned vermin. The fastidious feeding habits of cats make it unlikely that they will often eat the poisoned bait itself.

Freak (1963 personal communication) records a case of gastric ulcer which was confirmed on post-mortem examination. The cat was a

6–7-year-old spayed female with a long (1–1½ years) history of weight loss, debility, anaemia, muscular weakness and pain after eating; the cat would eat a little but leave the food after a few mouthfuls; melaenic faeces were passed. Vomiting was only occasional and slight with no blood. There was some pain on palpation of the anterior abdomen. Radiography without a contrast medium was negative.

Foreign bodies of the type seen in dogs rarely occur and needles are seldom diagnosed at this location.

Bacterial and allergic gastro-enteritis are relatively uncommon although the case described by Noble and Sim might have been the latter.

Neoplasia

The stomach may very occasionally be involved in lymphosarcomatosis when it is not usually the only site. Carcinoma of the stomach has not been recorded in either of two series of cat tumours described by Cotchin, nor in one recorded by Head (1963). In lymphosarcoma cases the syndrome will probably be indefinite and not particularly related to stomach. Vomiting, general wasting and weakness and evidence of neoplasia in other organs may all be present.

Most cases of stomach neoplasia will be found incidentally at post-mortem.

Small Intestine

May be involved in chemical, bacterial or allergic inflammations and reactions as mentioned above under the heading of 'stomach'.

Congestion of an area of the small intestine is usually found in cases of feline enteritis other than hyperacute forms.

Once hair has entered the intestinal tract it usually traverses this without causing trouble but may impact in the colon and rectum. In one case a concretion comprising hair and bone fragments had become impacted proximal to the ileo-colic valve, causing ulceration and perforation of the overlying gut with localised peritonitis.

Diarrhoea

Although diarrhoea is a common symptom in cats it is more commonly due to changes in other organs, e.g. pancreas, than to lesions of the small intestine itself. The exception is diffuse infiltration of large tracts of gut by lymphosarcoma tissue in which case the palpation of a thickened small intestine in any cat showing a progressive wasting syndrome is suggestive. Bacterial gastro-enteritis is not a common condition in cats. Iffey (1964) has recently reported an outbreak of severe enteritis in cats associated with the presence of *Escherichia coli* but the evidence for the pathogenicity of the organism is unconvincing. Langman (1964) has supported the probable pathogenic role of *E. coli* suggested by Iffey but doubt is expressed by Smith (1964) regarding it. The latter author states that, although uncommon, an enteritis of variable severity may occur due to *Salmonella* spp.

In the young kitten a form of diarrhoea occurs which is not associated with intestinal parasites or virus disease. The age group is usually 6–12 weeks, there is no rise of temperature or vomiting but the kitten is usually in rather poor condition despite well maintained appetite and general spirits. Faeces are usually cream to greyish in colour, foul smelling and passed frequently in small quantities often with a good deal of tenesmus. The anus is often excoriated and prominent and moist faecal material contaminates the perineum.

Response to Vitamin A therapy is usually extremely good, often spectacular, which should initially be administered parenterally in the form of an oily solution, 100,000 units Vitamin A per ml., 0·25–0·5 ml. intramuscularly every 48–72 hours at first and subsequently once weekly. Once improvement is obtained vitamin intake should be ensured by oral administration of a suitable multi-vitamin preparation and careful attention to diet.

Antibacterial therapy is seldom needed.

Foreign Bodies

These occur less commonly in the intestinal tract of the cat than that of the dog due both to the more fastidious feeding methods and more thorough mastication of food and to the rarity of retrieving objects thrown in play. Small objects such as plum stones may occasionally be swallowed during play whilst needles and thread are more frequently swallowed by cats than dogs. Textiles are occasionally ingested as some cats develop a habit—occasionally a vice—of eating wool either from garments or carpets which can cause impaction in the small intestine. Rubber toys are seldom chewed by cats hence there is little likelihood of obstruction by pieces of rubber.

Foreign bodies such as fruit stones will cause an obstructive syndrome with symptoms of vomiting, subsequent inappetence and absence of defaecation (not always easily observed). Although palpation of the cat's abdomen is so easy it is not always equally easy to locate the foreign body. Radiography will assist in the case of sufficiently radiopaque objects. Exploratory laparotomy may be necessary.

Although not common intestinal foreign bodies may easily be overlooked in the cat as a possible diagnosis for the very reason that it is not a condition which immediately springs to mind as it would in the case of a vomiting dog. When diagnosed, enterotomy is performed in the usual way but in all cases showing an obstructive syndrome where diagnosis cannot be established exploratory laparotomy should in any event be carried out without waiting too long in further attempts at precise diagnosis. The surgeon should be prepared for the operation of enterectomy in such cases since alternative lesions causing obstructive signs are intussusception and localised constricting neoplasia.

Operation is performed routinely via a flank incision, under general anaesthesia of the surgeon's choice. Great care must be taken in repairing the incision in the bowel in either enterotomy òr enterectomy to avoid stricture at the site post-operatively, a more likely complication in an animal with a bowel of relatively small calibre such as the cat. In enterotomy a single layer of sutures of fine catgut (00–0000 on atraumatic needles) should be used; in enterectomy end-to-end anastamosis is adequate.

Post-operative antibiotic cover should include streptomycin to suppress bacterial activity in the gut. For 24–36 hours nothing should be given by mouth; in dehydrated patients who have been off food or vomiting severely for several days intravenous bovine serum albumen or hydrolysed protein may be given together with subcutaneous administration of glucose saline. After 36 hours glucose water and hydrolysed protein may be given in small quantities frequently, by mouth; milk should not be given because of residual curd. After 3–4 days low residue foods such as lean meat are offered; milk may now be added. A return to normal diet after 7 or 8 days is advisable to ensure reasonable bulk passing through the intestine to minimise contracture at the site of incision.

Needles

The presence of needles in the intestinal tract may cause no symptoms at all or indefinite ones which are not helpful to diagnosis. If suspected, radiography will confirm the presence of a needle but will not indicate whether it is in the bowel lumen or free in the peritoneal cavity having penetrated the bowel wall.

In the case of a 3½-year-old castrated male cat presented with symptoms of inappetence, vomiting and depression which on examination had a temperature of 39·8° C. (103·6° F.) and marked anterior abdominal pain a diagnosis of feline enteritis was confidently made only to be confounded when a week after apparent clinical recovery (which took place in 4–5 days) the patient passed a needle and thread in the faeces.

Even in cases where the presence of a needle in the abdomen is confirmed the wisdom of surgical search is doubtful unless necessitated by the severity of symptoms; such surgery is often fruitless.

Intussusception

Far less common than in the dog, in fact virtually a rarity, and not occurring in similar circumstances, but it does occur.

It is not associated with infant diarrhoea as in the puppy but is more likely to occur in the adult cat due to severely irregular peristalsis caused by foreign bodies such as soft textile material in the bowel.

The history is an obstructive one of medium severity with no previous history of diarrhoea; vomiting and inappetence are usual. Again, despite the ease with which the cat's abdomen can be palpated it is by no means easy to recognise the lesion with certainty and diagnosis may

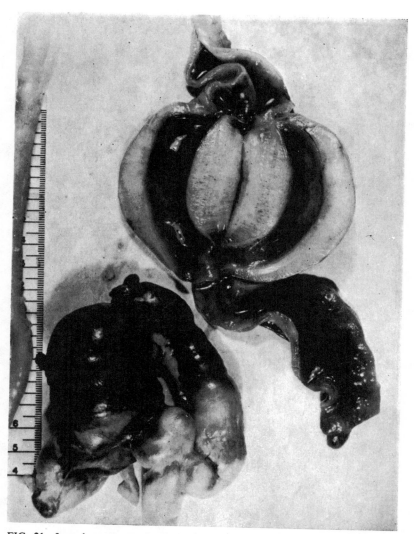

FIG. 21 Lymphosarcomatosis. Lesions in duodenum, caecum, ileo-colic wall and mesenteric node of 9½ year old castrated male cat

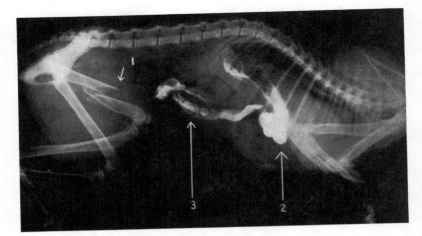

FIG. 22 Four months old kitten. Street accident: 1. Fractured femur. 2. Small intestine (contrast medium) in thorax indicating rupture of diaphragm. 3. An incidental finding. Ascarid worms outlined by contrast medium in small intestine still in abdomen.

have to await exploratory operation. By the time operation is undertaken plastic adhesions will usually have occurred and resection of a few inches of bowel will be necessary. Post-operative treatment is as above.

Neoplasia

The intestine is quite commonly a site of lymphosarcoma deposits, localised or diffuse, single or multiple.

In the neoplasm series quoted, six cases are recorded as having bowel involved, five castrated males ages $9\frac{1}{2}$, 10, 10, 12 and 15 years and one 14-year-old spayed female. No cases of neoplasia other than lymphosarcoma occur in this series.

Localised deposits may cause constriction of the bowel lumen and thus an obstructive syndrome but even when accurately diagnosed it is doubtful if extirpation of the lesion is warranted as it is unlikely to affect the course of the disease for long.

In diffuse or multiple deposits diarrhoea is more likely to be the dominating symptom.

In many cases bowel involvement is but one of many sites in which case the syndrome may not be related to the alimentary tract at all.

Adenocarcinoma also occurs not infrequently in the small intestine as cited by Cotchin (1956 and 1957) and Head (1963). They are mainly mucoid adenocarcinomata and have been recorded from the age of 5 years onwards. Duodenum, jejunum and ileum may all be involved.

The syndrome is an obstructive one and progressive in nature, associated with weight loss. The lesion may be palpable.

Treatment. Surgical excision of a localised lesion is warranted if diagnosis can be made reasonably early while the cat is still in fair condition, and metastasis is not yet apparent.

Large Intestine

Constipation is a condition much beloved of the British public whether in themselves or their animals hence the prosperity of many patent medicine manufacturers. While the term constipation is generally understood it should be the aim of the clinician to decide what is causing delay, infrequency or difficulty of defaecation in each individual and not merely to dispense or prescribe suitable aperients.

It is essential in all cases to obtain a very precise history and to superimpose a careful clinical examination to avoid disastrous errors, such as cases of urethral obstruction being described and treated as constipation or the frequent passage of small amounts of loose faeces accompanied by undue straining being mistaken by the owner for inability to defaecate.

The following conditions may be differentiated in the cat, all causing apparent constipation.

1. LACK OF BULK

The diet of many household pet cats is offered in so refined a form that lack of residue may cause atony of the musculature of the large bowel. In the wild and in those cats that hunt and eat small rodents a quantity of indigestible residue from skin, hair and bones will provide adequate bulk to form a faecal mass which will keep the bowel well exercised. Similarly many modern balanced tinned diets contain cereal designed to provide some roughage.

Lack of bulk may cause one of two syndromes, either infrequent emptying of the bowel with faeces remaining in the colon for unduly long periods from which more water than normal is re-absorbed, resulting in very hard faecal masses of varying calibre which may be mechanically difficult to pass, or the more frequent passage of un-formed rather tacky dark faeces which usually require an abnormal amount of straining to expel owing to their amorphous state; this latter is not, obviously, a true constipation.

The symptoms usually described are infrequency, difficulty or tenesmus in defaecation; in advanced cases of infrequency inappetence or even vomiting may occur.

Diagnosis may be based on abdominal palpation (hard faeces will easily be recognised in the colon) or the nature of faeces in the rectum as determined by insertion of a thermometer; tacky, unformed faeces will adhere to it.

Initial treatment of genuine constipation may be by laxatives or aperients. Useful agents are liquid paraffin, preferably mixed in the food to avoid seepage from the anus of oil which has by-passed the faecal mass; magnesium sulphate in warm water is very useful in softening hard, bulky stools but is not easy to administer. There are also available several proprietary pills containing small doses of a variety of aperient drugs which are easily administered and preferable to a full dose of a single agent.

Subsequent treatment must be aimed at providing increased residue. In cats which are not fussy feeders the addition of prepared cereal, such as bran, to the diet is sufficient. Most cats are difficult as regards diet and will refuse food mixed with alien substances; in these the use of a refined bran preparation with Vitamin B is often possible since the required bulk is smaller and can be mixed with a small quantity of a food readily taken. Similarly bulk laxatives containing agar agar, preferably with Vitamin B, are most valuable, one teaspoonful a day usually providing ample bulk to ensure regular and easy defaecation.

2. FUR

As previously mentioned all cats ingest some hair during self-grooming, especially during the period of coat change, and in most cases this is eliminated by regular regurgitation of a cylinder of matted fur. Some cats, however, do not return fur in this way and in such animals the hair becomes incorporated in the faecal mass causing colonic stasis and/or rectal impaction.

The most regular symptom is loss of appetite; often there is no other abnormality reported. Sometimes dulness is apparent and occasionally infrequent vomiting. The owner may have noticed absence of defaecation.

Examination discloses a normal temperature, the cat usually in good condition but often in the moult and a colon full of faeces of varying calibre and consistency, the latter from doughy to hard.

Initial aperient treatment should be followed by advice to give a small dose (half to one teaspoonful) of liquid paraffin every second or third day throughout the rest of the coat change period and to brush and comb regularly to remove maximum possible dead coat. In these patients this regime should be recommended for each ensuing moult.

Megacolon

A condition of gross dilation and atony of the colon, in some ways analogous to Hirschsprung's disease, is by no means uncommon in the cat and should be recognised as a clinical entity.

The condition may arise at any age from approximately 6 years onwards. The cat is initially presented with a typical history of constipation. On rectal examination with a thermometer or even digitally the rectum is usually found to be empty and may be ballooned but a mass of faeces is usually detected at the pelvic inlet; abdominal palpation confirms the presence of large masses of faeces, often of enormous calibre, in the colon; the whole length of descending and even transverse colon may be impacted.

Diagnosis cannot always be made on one such episode but may be suspected and is confirmed by recurrence of impaction at gradually lessening intervals.

Initial treatment may need to be vigorous including enemata and manual breakdown and removal of the faecal mass. This should always be carried out under general anaesthesia; not only does this assist efficiency but severe cases of anorexia nervosa have been seen due to the restraint and indignity of such a procedure being inflicted on the conscious cat.

Treatment. Usually medical but this has to be maintained for the remainder of the cat's life and even this may only produce infrequent defaecation but will usually avoid complete impaction.

Diet should include laxative foods such as raw liver, adequate Vitamin B and moderate roughage.

The most suitable laxative must be found by trial and error in individual patients. Salines have the advantage of minimising dehydration of the faecal mass but are not easy to administer with the necessary fluid.

One patient in which megacolon was diagnosed at about 9 years of age lived until the age of 14½ on a daily regime of cascara sagrada and Epsom salts which produced evacuation of vast faecal masses on an average once every 14 days.

Resection of the atonic colon has been advocated. The feasibility of lumbar sympathectomy in such patients is a possibility to be explored. Most owners are not prepared to submit cats to drastic surgery when medical treatment will afford some sort of relief and the condition is not usually endangering life.

Sometimes a cat will be presented with a history of constipation or inability to defaecate which on examination is found to have long fibrous grasses or even string coated with faeces protruding from the anus. This should be removed by gentle traction.

Long-haired cats which do not get regular grooming may get faeces matted in the long hair of the back of the thighs which can create a mechanical barrier to the passage of further faeces; it is also a common site of blow-fly strike which may go undetected until maggots are well developed and are already invading living tissues.

Neoplasia

The colon may be involved in spread of lymphosarcoma from the ileum and may rarely be the site of a discrete sarcoma deposit. Carcinoma has not been recorded in either series recorded by Cotchin (1956 and 1957) or by Head (1963), but Rubarth (1934) has recorded a caecal carcinoma.

Symptoms of large bowel involvement in lymphosarcoma are unlikely to be confined to that organ and must be expected to be referable to the overall disease picture.

Anus and Anal Sacs

A condition occurs in cats which is often mistaken for some form of constipation. This is the incarceration of a knob of faeces of normal size and firm but not hard consistence in the anus, between internal and external sphincters.

It usually occurs in cats in middle or older life and causes repeated, distressing and apparently painful attempts to expel the mass.

On examination the faecal knob is detected just within the external sphincter; the size is usually some 1–2 cm. long and 0·75–1 cm. diameter and somewhat oval in shape; it may be incarcerated centrally or to one side of the anal orifice.

The condition is readily differentiated from megacolon by the situation of the impacted knob and the fact that the colon is often empty or at most containing normal quantities and size of faeces.

The cause appears to be atony of the internal sphincter rather than stricture of the external muscle since this is usually found to be manually distensible. There is no evidence of diverticulation.

Treatment is by digital expulsion of the faecal knob by pressure on either side of the anus as for emptying anal sacs; the procedure is usually vocally and vigorously resented by the cat but can be done so quickly that anaesthesia is not warranted. Recurrences are probable in any individual but the normal size and consistence of faeces does not call for general medical treatment. Some owners can be instructed in the method of relieving the situation without seeking veterinary assistance once diagnosis is established.

Anal Sacs

The presence of anal sacs and the possibility of their causing symptoms is often overlooked in the cat. They are situated similarly to those in the dog but the ducts open in the circumanal tissue and are directed in a straight posterior position; the orifice of the duct is usually marked by a small slightly pyramidal elevation.

The only condition seen has been of impaction, the secretion usually being somewhat inspissated. Septic infection of the sac has not been seen.

Symptoms are of irritation usually shown by excessive washing of the anal region but occasionally by the classical 'tobogganing' as in the dog.

Expression of secretion affords relief. This must be undertaken slowly but firmly owing to the dryish nature of the secretion and obviously causes some discomfort. Occasionally the secretion is a drop or two of rich brown fluid material with a pungent odour.

Excoriation of the Anus

May occur in diarrhoea, or impacted anal glands due to constant licking or rubbing

The underlying cause must be dealt with and suitable non-toxic ointments applied. Procaine zinc ointment may be used with discretion and under the supervision of intelligent owners who can prevent ingestion of the dressing.

Intestinal Parasites

Several intestinal parasites occur in cats in the British Isles but are of comparatively little clinical significance. Of the cestodes *Dipylidium caninum* is the most common, *Taenia taeniaeformis* also occurs and the presence of *Diphyllobothrium* in Southern Ireland makes this a parasite to be considered in cats in that area.

Toxocara cati (*mystax*) and *Toxascaris leonina* are the two common nematodes and *Isospora felis* is the species of coccidia which invades cats.

Dipylidium caninum[1] is probably the worm causing most concern to owners because of the presence of motile segments in faeces or in the fur around the anus; there is no evidence that it causes clinical symptoms in the host. Although communicable to man in theory (by children accidentally ingesting infected fleas or lice) in practice it cannot be regarded as a public health hazard.

Infestation is recognized by the presence of mature segments on faeces or on the hair around the anus; fresh segments are white and often motile but soon dry on exposure to air and then resemble rice grains. Although owners sometimes claim that the health of the host cat has improved after expulsion of the worm there is little evidence that it is the cause of clinical disease.

Treatment. Arecoline acetarsol is an effective of the taeniafuge in use. It should not be given to cats under one year of age; dosage 9-18 mg. (½ to 1 tablet) according to the weight of the cat. It should not be administered to an animal which has been starved but preferably given 3 hours after a small meal; a milky diet for 12-24 hours prior to dosing is said to be helpful. Purging with passing of the worm usually occurs in ¾-1 ½ hours after dosing and may occasionally be accompanied by colic. When possible the evacuated parasite should be examined for presence of the scolex.

Dichlorophen. May safely be given to kittens and young cats, dosage 0·5 gm. (1 tablet) per 3 kg. (6 lb.) bodyweight. The action of dichlorophen differs from other taeniafuges in that it causes disintegration of the parasite in the intestine which is expelled as an amorphous unrecognisable mass without obvious purging. This drug may be fully effective in recent infestations, i.e. when the worm is less than 8 weeks old as judged by passage of mature segments for not more than 14 days, but in longer standing infestations segments are usually again shed in some 6 weeks time indicating that the scolex has not been destroyed possibly due to protective tissue reaction at the point of attachment to the mucosa. It is a very useful stand-by for younger animals.

Bunamidine hydrochloride is highly effective against Taenia spp., Dipylidium caninum and adult Echinococcus granulosus. Because the worms are killed and disintegrate, they are not usually seen in the faeces after treatment. The dose of 100 mgm. is orally administered on an empty stomach (*not* before weaning) and may occasionally induce emesis, without loss of efficacy. Feeding is advised three hours after drug administration and in the case of Echinococcus infestation in a second treatment is advisable six weeks after the first.

Tablets should not be broken, crushed, mixed with food or liquid and the irritant particles should be withheld from contact with the eyes. Overdosage can cause severe vomiting and diarrhoea and in extreme cases death from cardiac failure.

Niclosamide is highly effective against all tapeworm species and may safely be administered to pregnant and young animals. A dose of 0.25 to 0.5g. according to size is administered orally after a twelve hour fast and excretion of dead tapeworms occurs from six to forty eight hours later. Initially these may be intact, but later partially digested. In the case of Echinococcus granulosus infection a dose rate increase is recommended.

Available for broad spectrum treatment of tapeworms and roundworms is **Mebendazole** which, having no contra-indications, is available in 100 mgm. tablets for administration orally alone or mixed with food and in a variety of dosage patterns over a period of several days. This drug works by inhibition of the uptake of glucose by stomach and intestinal worms and is extremely safe in use.

In addition to administration of a specific taeniafuge the life cycle of *Dipylidium* must be broken by elimination of the intermediate host, fleas or lice. Infected cats should always be examined for presence of ectoparasites and treated appropriately. Many cats shedding segments are found to be apparently free of fleas and lice; such cats when infested by a single flea may suffer more intense irritation than cats which habitually carry a heavy parasite burden and are thus more assiduous in their grooming efforts and so more likely to ingest the offending visitor.

Infestations of *Taenia taeniaeformis* are dealt with similarly, the difference being that the intermediate host is small rodents such as rats and mice, hence infestation arises from ingestion of the natural prey of cats given to hunting, thus the life cycle is not easily broken.

Round Worms

These appear to cause less trouble in kittens than the corresponding infestation in puppies. *Toxocara cati* (*mystax*) and *Toxascaris leonina* are the two species occurring in the cat and although not specifically incriminated Gibson (1960) feels that the former could be involved in the causation of visceral larva migrans in man. Sprent and English (1958) imply a similar view but conclude as follows: 'It may be stated in conclusion that it is the association between puppies and children wherein lies the greatest danger of "visceral larva migrans". It seems likely that cats are less dangerous in this respect because they become infected later in life, they have more fastidious habits, usually bury their faeces and are relatively aloof from human contact.'

Unthriftiness and diarrhoea can arise due to heavy worm burdens in young kittens but all other causes, including dietary deficiencies should be considered before diagnosing these as due to parasitism or unless there is adequate evidence of a really heavy infestation. Such infestations are more likely to arise in closed communities such as breeding catteries hence it is desirable that breeding queens should be kept as free as possible of nematodes. Ante-natal infection of kittens does not occur.

Diagnosis is based on microscopic examination of faeces for the presence of the characteristic ova either by direct smear or flotation concentration methods, or on evidence of adult worms passed in the faeces.

Treatment has been greatly facilitated by the introduction of piperazine compounds and diethylcarbamazine both of which are effective and well tolerated.

Piperazine compounds are available as tablets of 0·5 gr.; the dose being 0·25 gr. (half tablet) crushed up in milk and given shortly before a light meal.

Diethylcarbamazine citrate is available in tablets of 200 mg., the dose being 50 mg./kg. (25 mg. per lb.) bodyweight, an average of half a tablet for a kitten of 1–2 kg. (4–5 lbs.). A single dose is usually sufficient; vomiting occasionally occurs but does not apparently interfere with the efficiency of treatment. This drug is more expensive than piperazine.

A useful additional anti nematodal drug is the cholinesterase inhibitor **dichlorvos**. Dosed orally at a rate of 10 mgm./Kg. the drug may cause slight emesis without loss of efficacy, and occasionally increased salivation and faecal softening. It is contra-indicated in cases of constipation and should not be used in conjunction with other cholinesterase inhibitors such as organo-phosphorous insecticidal sprays. In cases of overdose atropine is antidotal.

Coccidia

Oocysts of *Isospora felis* (occasionally *bigemina*) are not uncommonly found in the faeces of cats but should not be regarded as of clinical significance unless present in large numbers.

Whilst clinically significant infestations could occur in catteries or other closed communities it is unlikely that individual cats will acquire a pathological burden owing to their method of covering excreta.

Sloan (1964) gives the following figures for incidence of intestinal parasites in cat faeces examined for veterinary surgeons in practice:

Dipylidium caninum		2%
Taenia taeniaeformis		3%
Toxascaris leonina	under	1%
Toxocara cati		20%
Coccidia (usually *I. felis* sometimes *I. bigemina*)		10%

REFERENCES

Cotchin, E. (1956) *B. Vet. J.* **112**, 263.
Cotchin, E. (1957) *Vet. Rec.* **69**, 425.
Freak, M. J. (1963) Personal communication.
Gibson, T. E. (1960) *Vet. Rec.* **72**, 772.
Head, K. (1963) Personal communication.
Iffey, J. (1964) *Vet. Rec.* **76**, 132.
Rubarth, S. (1934) *Skand. Vet. Tidskr.* **24**, 685.
Sloan, J. E. (1964) Personal communication.
Smith, J. E. (1964) *J. Small An. Pract.* **5**, 517.
Sprent, J. F. A. & English, P. B. (1958) *Aust. Vet. J.* **34**, 161.

SUGGESTED FURTHER READING

Seawright, A. A. & Grono, L. R. (1964) *J. Path. Bact.* **87**, 365. (Malignant mast cell tumour in a cat with perforating duodenal ulcer.)
Taylor, J. H. (1964) *Vet. Bull.* **34**, 633. (Toxocara infections in man and animals.)
Sprent, J. F. A. (1956) *Parasitology* **46**, 54. (The life history and development of Toxocara cati in the domestic cat.)
Joshua, J. O. (1960) *Mod. Vet. Pract.* **41**, 36. (Vomiting in the cat.)

Chapter 10

PANCREAS, LIVER, SPLEEN,
PERITONEAL CAVITY

Pancreas

The pancreas is an organ essential to fat digestion and sugar metabolism via its external and internal secretions respectively, deficiencies of both of which occur in the cat.

Exogenous Deficiency

Deficiency of the exogenous secretions of the pancreas, viz. trypsinogen, amylase and lipase, results in inability to digest and absorb fat and impaired digestion of protein. Clinically, cases may present a picture of steatorrhoea or merely intractable diarrhoea. Both types are more likely to occur in cats over 6 years of age.

The classical syndrome is co-existence of a ravenous appetite, loss of weight and passage of large quantities of abnormal faeces. Affected cats remain bright and playful for a considerable time but eventually become cachectic. Stools are typically said to be voluminous, pale in colour, having a foetid or rancid odour and becoming greasy in consistence on cooling; these characteristic changes are not always present however, and the possible diagnosis should not be discarded on this account; neither is the ravenous appetite so marked or regular in occurrence as in the dog.

In milder cases appetite and body weight may be unaffected but a persistent intractable diarrhoea occurs, often of dark coloured faeces with a thick, creamy consistence.

Diagnosis is based on two sets of criteria in conjunction with the clinical picture:

(*a*) Presence of fat globules, undigested meat fibres and starch granules in the faeces on microscopic examination.

(*b*) Relative or complete absence of trypsin in the faeces.

In using this latter test it is important that more than one sample should be investigated since wide variations have been found in normal subjects. It is usually accepted that a titre of 1 : 20 or less—occasionally completely negative—indicates pancreatic deficiency and if this is found on each of two or three examinations of different specimens appropriate therapy is warranted.

Treatment. Is by administration of pancreatin preferably in combination with bile salts, as preparations designed to pass unchanged through gastric digestion.

The feeding of raw pancreas has been advocated and claimed to be effective but the difficulty of ensuring a regular supply of fresh gut-breads, quite apart from doubts as to the effect of gastric digestion, makes this treatment of dubious value.

Various preparations of pancreatin are available either as keratin-coated tablets (which disintegrate only in small intestine) of pancreatin alone or combined with bile salts, or keratin-coated granules of pancreatin single or triple strength. The tablets are medium sized and thus not always easy to administer regularly to feline patients but are less expensive than granules which may, in any case, be rejected by fastidious feeders. Dosage is estimated entirely by clinical response; it is usual to start on a regime of one tablet twice daily or one small teaspoonful of granules daily, increasing or decreasing until a satisfactory maintenance dose is attained. Therapy must be lifelong.

In any case of persistent diarrhoea in a middle aged or older cat for which no cause can be found it is always worthwhile estimating trypsin in faeces as many cases prove to be deficient and respond well to replacement therapy.

Prognosis. The condition is a rewarding one to treat in correctly diagnosed cases and provided regular dosing is possible and easy to maintain the cat may be expected to have a relatively normal expectation of life.

Diabetes Mellitus

This is a condition of the older cat which has received comparatively little attention in the literature and is still regarded as a rarity by many clinicians.

Figures of incidence are not available for the cat but those for the dog vary so widely that it is doubtful whether statistically significant figures for the former could be easily compiled. There is no doubt that it is a condition occurring with some regularity, three cases having been under treatment in one practice simultaneously while other cases were being detected not infrequently by routine urine examination (in many cases confirmed pathologically) of old cats presented purely for euthanasia.

The disease is due to deficient production of insulin by the islet tissue of the pancreas; in the cat, cases have been seen only in older animals (8 years +) thus the condition may reasonably be regarded as being of a degenerative and senile nature. The pituitary-oestrogen mechanism will rarely apply in the cat since the vast majority of cases occurs in neuters, mainly males; neither have cases been found associated with previous stress such as severe shock in accidents, nor is it confined to obese subjects.

Pathologically the picture is typical of diabetes in other species with relative or complete absence of islet tissue from, and evidence of hyaline degeneration in, the pancreas and fatty changes in the liver.

Symptoms. Increased water intake with corresponding polyuria is the earliest and most regular feature. If urine investigation is carried out at this stage no other symptoms may be developed before diagnosis is made. Subsequently weight loss, lack of energy and poor appetite develop. Vomiting is not a regular feature. In advanced cases there is extreme emaciation and often a foul mouth characterised by the rapid deposition of soft tartar and the development of parodontal disease. Slight lens opacity may be noted in some patients but is neither so frequent nor so well developed as in the dog.

Diagnosis. It cannot be too strongly emphasised that any cat, particularly over middle life, showing increased thirst for water should be subjected to urinalysis. Urine specimens are easily obtained by the method outlined on page 10.

Diagnosis is usually based on the presence of glycosuria, confirmed on more than one sample, the greatest care being taken to ensure its collection in clean vessels, together with the clinical picture. Blood sugar estimation although desirable is not always feasible in daily practice; it may not be wise to hospitalise these patients as a routine for diagnosis because changes in food intake due to change of surroundings etc. may mask the picture.

Ketonuria has not been present in most cases diagnosed during life which probably accounts for the absence of vomiting.

It is of interest that in those cases subjected to post-mortem examination which had been diagnosed as diabetes mellitus on the above rather slender criteria all have been confirmed. No case of renal glycosuria, i.e. glycosuria due to a lowered renal threshold in other, possibly kidney, disease has been seen.

Treatment. Diabetes mellitus is a very rewarding disease to treat in the cat. Several patients have lived out what could reasonably be described as a normal expectation of life on insulin therapy. Contrary to what might be anticipated no cat has resented the daily injections and it has been possible easily to train owners in administration.

Treatment is by subcutaneous injection of insulin once daily; Protamine Zinc Insulin or Zinc Suspension Insulin have proved the most suitable forms. Dosage must be estimated on clinical response but usually lies between 5 and 11 units daily. Although it is desirable to maintain urine glucose at below $\frac{1}{4}$ per cent it is not essential to maintain a negative urine; in several patients it has been found that hypoglycaemia is likely if urine sugar is abolished. Dlugach (1953) has drawn attention to this fact and it can certainly be confirmed from experience. It is desirable to achieve a state of clinical balance, i.e. normal appetite, water intake reduced to normal and bodyweight returned to and kept normal.

In one patient which at the time of writing has been on insulin therapy for six years, insulin requirement has progressively but slightly fallen, viz. from 9–7 units; this cat is also given 1 day in 7 off insulin and off food, a regime which appears to prevent hypoglycaemic episodes.

Adjustment of diet cannot be relied upon in cats for two reasons, firstly that in most cats carbohydrate intake is minimal and secondly that a sick cat can often not be persuaded to accept an altered diet, which may seriously jeopardise its chances of surviving.

Oral hypoglycaemic agents have proved useless in the cat, dosage being impossible to get accurately assessed to prevent hypoglycaemic signs; there is also the difficulty in many cats of maintaining regular administration of tablets over a long period of time.

Any diabetic cat which suffers some concomitant illness in which bacterial infection is present or could occur, should receive early and most vigorous antibacterial therapy as resistance to infections is greatly reduced and relatively simple conditions become potentially fatal. Similarly if any surgical interference has to be undertaken extreme care must be taken to avoid infection.

Prognosis. Good in any case diagnosed at a reasonably early stage, i.e. before emaciation is advanced.

It cannot be too strongly recommended that urine examination should be made at once in any older cat showing increased water intake and that owners should be urged to attempt treatment. There is even ground to suggest that regular (3–6 monthly) routine urine checks are well worthwhile in older cats.

In untreated cases it seems that the progress of the disease may be slower than in the dog. In one patient whose owner refused both treatment and euthanasia the time elapsing between diagnosis (known to be early as urine examinations had been made pretty regularly) and eventual destruction was one year. This may not hold good for all cats as several cases diagnosed in cats presented for euthanasia in an advanced state of emaciation were said by owners to have been deteriorating for weeks or a few months only, but this may well be unreliable as to the time of onset.

Other Diseases of the Pancreas

Pancreatitis has not been recognised by the author in any form comparable to the dog, possibly due to a different anatomical arrangement of pancreatic ducts nor has the condition been seen in post-mortem examinations of any patients showing acute abdominal signs. One 6½-year-old castrated male cat which suffered recurring jaundice episodes following an apparent bacterial infection was reported as showing a nodular hyperplasia and focal inflammation of the pancreas.

At the same time it is clear from the literature that occasional cases of acute pancreatitis do occur, e.g. one case is mentioned in a series reported for another condition by Howell and Pickering; this occurred in a 7½ year male cat but no clinical details are given. A case of acute haemorrhagic pancreatic necrosis is reported in a 3-year-old cat in which the main sign was severe abdominal pain. (Recwitch, Bonertz and Carlson). From the limited reports available it seems clear that the condition is equally as difficult to diagnose accurately as in the dog and is equally usually rapidly fatal. The predominant signs are abdominal pain, temperature rise and evidence of shock, i.e. an abdominal catastrophe.

NEOPLASIA

According to Cotchin (1956, 1957) adenocarcinoma of exocrine pancreatic tissue is not uncommon. Clinical symptoms were loss of condition, poor appetite and occasional vomiting. There is a marked tendency to metastasis especially to the liver.

The diagnosis of neoplasia of the pancreas is not easy on clinical grounds alone.

In one case in the neoplasms reviewed, the pancreas was involved in lymphosarcomatosis.

Liver

There is no evidence that virus hepatitis occurs in the cat but there are clinical grounds for believing that a bacterial infection occurs causing both hepatic and renal signs. This is discussed in greater detail on page 197. Jaundice, often of a recurring nature and eventual cirrhosis occur in these cases.

It might be thought probable that *Leptospira icterohaemorrhagiae* infection would occur in cats owing to their contact with rats; a survey of 200 cat sera has demonstrated *L. ictero.* agglutinins in low titre in several cases but in no instance could this be correlated with a suggestive disease picture. The cases mentioned above are clinically strongly reminiscent of leptospiral jaundice but in several fully investigated it has been found completely impossible to incriminate leptospires. Rupture of the liver with rapidly fatal internal haemorrhage is not uncommon in street accidents.

NEOPLASIA

The liver is frequently involved in lymphosarcoma cases but is also a site of neoplasia of other types.

Of the eight cases in which liver is reported as being involved in the neoplasm series one was angiosarcoma, one reticulosarcoma, one lymphosarcoma, two sarcoma (type not stated), two adenocarcinomata and one carcinoma. With the exception of two 6-year-olds (reticulosarcoma and sarcoma) all were 12 years or older. One case of particular interest is that of a 12 year spayed female destroyed for carcinoma of the liver, this cat was examined on arrival in the practice at age 10½, the owner complaining that the cat suffered from chronic constipation. Routine abdominal palpation revealed a grossly enlarged liver but signs specifically related to liver did not arise for a further 12 months and it was 1½ years from the time of first examination to necessary euthanasia, an unusually long survival period for a carcinoma case.

Symptoms of liver neoplasia include dulness, inappetence, variable frequency of vomiting, (usually of bile), loss of weight, (especially musculature of limbs), sometimes jaundice and occasionally ascites.

Liver function tests which may assist in diagnosis include:

1. Serum Alkaline Phosphatase.

2. Transaminase estimations. These two tests considered in conjunction may be helpful in diagnosing liver neoplasia.

3. Electrophoresis may be of assistance in cirrhosis cases.

The work on liver function tests has been carried out mainly in the dog and too ready application of these results to another species could be unreliable.

Toxic Hepatitis

Can arise in many types of poisoning, the most significant probably being that reported by Larson (1963) in a cat given 300 mg. (5 gr.) aspirin daily for 12 days.

Cirrhosis

Is not uncommon in cats. Cotchin referring to a case of cirrhosis with pericapsular accumulation of lymphocytes, remarks 'We do occasionally see cases of rather acute cirrhosis in cats'.

Slight cirrhosis, portal cell infiltration and patchy liver cell degeneration have been seen in patients destroyed following repeated jaundice episodes as a result of the possible infection previously mentioned.

Symptoms are of dulness, inappetence and vomiting; ascites is not infrequent and weight loss is usual in the later stages.

Diagnosis may be assisted by liver function tests.

Treatment is seldom satisfactory as the cause cannot always be determined and it is not possible to reverse pathological changes of this type.

A high carbohydrate, high digestible protein and low fat diet is to be advised; hydrolysed protein solution with glucose is very valuable. Constipation may be an associated feature for which saline purgatives in moderate dosage are preferable.

Chronic Passive Congestion

Passive congestion of abdominal organs occurs in right sided cardiac incompetence or failure. In the cat signs are often not noticed by the owner until the acute development of evidence of failure including pleural and abdominal effusions.

Symptoms will be those referable to liver as above, there may be obvious accumulation of fluid in pleural and/or peritoneal cavities, the liver may be enlarged and palpable. The cardiac dysfunction will be detected on routine examination.

Prognosis is poor and treatment usually unavailing due to the intolerance of most cats for digitalis and its fractions.

Clinico-pathological techniques may well serve to distinguish more accurately between the various liver changes but for purposes of the practitioner recognition of the fact that liver is involved is usually sufficient since this will necessitate a very guarded or poor prognosis, few liver conditions responding well or permanently to therapy.

Spleen

Conditions of clinical significance in the spleen are virtually limited to neoplasia and splenomegaly due to mast cell proliferation. Haematoma of the spleen is not common as it is in the dog, nor is the organ so often ruptured in street accidents.

The spleen is commonly involved in lymphosarcomatosis, lymphatic leukosis and other types of sarcoma but may be the sole site of mast cell proliferation, focal or diffuse.

It is of clinical significance when it is the sole site of the lesion as splenomegaly is easily diagnosed and treated. This type of case usually arises in middle life (6–9 years); symptoms include dulness, weakness, sometimes pallid mucous membranes, inappetence and occasional vomiting; there is usually some loss of weight and the abdomen may be noticeably enlarged.

On examination the much enlarged spleen is easily palpated and recognised; it may fill the greater part of the abdominal cavity extending well into the pelvic area but its edges can usually be accurately identified.

Treatment is surgical, by splenectomy.

General anaesthesia by intravenous pentobarbitone sodium or gaseous agent is induced. An incision 2–3 inches long is made vertically in the left flank about 1 inch behind the last rib. The spleen is invariably immediately below the incision and can usually be manipulated so that one end can be brought through it; if this is impossible due to gross enlargement it may be necessary to enlarge the incision in a cruciate or T-shaped horizontal manner. Once exteriorised, haemostasis is the only remaining problem but is easily achieved by ligating the vessels traversing the omental attachment in small groups, with the exception of the large artery and vein entering at the hilus which must be dealt with carefully, preferably using a double ligature of 0 or 00 catgut. It does not appear in these cases to be necessary to ligate the artery first and subsequently allow blood from the spleen to re-enter the venous circulation since the enlargement is usually due to abnormal cellular elements and not purely retained blood.

The splenic omentum is separated ½ ¾ inch from its attachment to the spleen, distally to the ligatures, and the organ removed. The abdominal incision is repaired routinely; additional transverse incision does not appear to militate against satisfactory and prompt healing.

Recovery is usually rapid and uncomplicated, prognosis being very good.

The idea of splenectomy appears to alarm some surgeons but it is a technique easily and rapidly performed giving gratifying results and is within the scope of any competent small animal surgeon.

Abdominal Lymph Nodes

Are seldom the site of primary disease but are frequently involved in more generalized conditions.

Abdominal lymph nodes are often the site of lymphosarcoma deposits and are usually affected in the lymphatic leukosis picture which causes enlargement of superficial nodes: they may also be sites for metastasis of other types of malignant tumour such as reticulosarcoma and adenocarcinoma.

The local node will often be enlarged in association with any inflammatory lesion of an abdominal organ, especially the ileo-colic group.

Abdominal tuberculosis (becoming rarer since the eradication of bovine tuberculosis) usually involves mesenteric nodes, in fact such a node may be the sole site of a lesion.

Symptoms and signs will be largely related to the underlying disease process although not infrequently an enlarged lymph node is the only palpable abnormality.

Peritoneum, Mesentery and Peritoneal Cavity

Both parietal peritoneum and mesentery may be the site of metastatic tumours, occasionally by implantation spread.

Peritonitis

This is not common as a surgical complication in this antibiotic era but an apparently spontaneous peritonitis has been seen in cats the cause of which could not be established (See Chapter 19, Diseases Due to Infective Agents, Feline Infectious Peritonitis).

Symptoms comprise intense dulness, vomiting, thirst and sometimes restlessness suggestive of abdominal discomfort; defaecation is usually in abeyance. There is fairly rapid loss of weight.

Temperature is usually only slightly raised, the abdomen appears somewhat distended and there is discomfort on palpation but rarely guarding of abdominal muscles. Exudation is not invariable and there is considerable variation in amount when it has occurred.

The condition is usually rather acute but if time permits haematology and examination of exudate, if any, will be helpful in diagnosis. A raised white cell count will be virtually constant and pus cells and possibly bacteria will be present in the exudate.

Treatment. Is rarely successful and unlikely to be so in cases where a primary lesion cannot be found. It must be remembered that superficial lesions of cat sepsis can and do occasionally cause a pyaemia with localised abscess formation in abdominal organs, e.g. liver, kidneys and that in such cases peritonitis is the end result and not the condition at which therapy should have been initially directed. One of the great difficulties of adequately treating peritonitis in cats is the virtual impossibility of leaving *in situ* adequate drainage tubing. Attempted treatment will necessitate anaesthesia (great care is needed and the briefest possible duration advisable), puncture or incision of the abdominal wall—the latter is preferable in order that some examination of the abdominal viscera may be made to determine extent, site and if possible, the cause of the condition. All exudate should be removed, the peritoneal cavity irrigated with normal saline and large doses of anti-biotic introduced; the latter preferably in solution to avoid irritation of already inflamed tissues by suspensions or powders, which limits the choice virtually to crystalline penicillin, streptomycin and chloramphenicol succinate; penicillin and streptomycin may be combined and thus give a fairly broad antibacterial range but chloramphenicol is best left as sole agent. Methicillin is also available in soluble form and can be used. Doses should be massive, e.g. 1 mega unit penicillin, 1 gramme streptomycin or 0·5–1 gramme chloramphenicol.

In the rare case in which early diagnosis is possible and the cause is self-limiting, the above therapy may be successful but the prognosis in peritonitis cases must always be grave.

The question of tuberculosis will be dealt with more fully under another heading but this infection must always be kept in mind as a possible cause and any exploration or treatment carried out with the greatest care and attention to more than usually thorough sterilisation of instruments after use in any suspicious case.

Chylous Ascites and Chylothorax. Are conditions virtually peculiar to the cat and occurring occasionally. They are due to damage, usually of unknown cause, to the cisterna chyli or thoracic duct with escape of chyle into the peritoneal or pleural cavities respectively. The anatomical basis of the condition has been discussed in a detailed review by Lindsay (1974). Symptoms are entirely due to the presence of a large and increasing volume of fluid; the leak in the duct does not heal hence the condition is progressive. In the case of chylous ascites the first sign will be abdominal distension, in the early stages unaccompanied by other symptoms. Subsequently loss of appetite, decrease in energy, progressive wasting and finally respiratory embarrassment due to pressure from the fluid-filled abdomen will occur.

Diagnosis of fluid in the abdomen is relatively easy, a fluid 'thrill' being more easily demonstrated in the cat than the dog, and differential diagnosis is made by paracentesis, the milky homogenous nature of the withdrawn fluid being diagnostic.

There is no practicable treatment. Paracentesis will relieve symptoms temporarily but the continued patency of the cisterna chyli renders this a futile procedure.

Chylothorax will cause earlier and more serious symptoms. Accumulation of chyle in the pleural cavity quickly causes embarassment of respiration, the cat adopting a posture of sternal recumbency with elbows slightly abducted and showing exaggerated and forced respiratory movements. Cyanosis may be present and may be provoked or worsened by forced movement; movement or forcible change in posture can precipitate serious respiratory, and consequently cardiac embarrassment.

The 'fluid line' is easily demonstrable by auscultation, percussion and possibly radiography in the orthodox position (positioning for lateral radiography can provoke fatal respiratory embarrassment in an advanced case and in no circumstances should a ventro-dorsal exposure be attempted) and the exact nature of the fluid determined by exploratory puncture. Treatment is not feasible and early euthanasia is to be advised.

Very recently an article has appeared (Graber 1965) describing the diagnosis and successful surgical treatment of a case of chylothorax due to rupture of the thoracic duct. The duct was ligated just anterior to the diaphragm.

Ascites

Accumulation of serous transudate in the peritoneal cavity occasionally occurs as a sign in cases of cardiac failure or liver disease. In cardiac syndromes transudation is the result of circulatory stasis, a generalised sluggishness of circulation affecting all parts of the body and thus usually causing co-existent pleural transudation, in hepatic cases it is due to back-pressure from a diseased (often cirrhotic) liver causing circulatory stasis particularly of the splanchnic area combined with reduced colloid osmotic pressure resulting from lowered serum albumen.

It is thus clear that the presence of ascitic fluid is not a disease *per se* but the result of primary disease elsewhere which it is essential to locate for proper diagnosis. In many cases the abdominal enlargement is the first sign noticed by the owner and it therefore becomes necessary to make careful enquiry into the health of the cat over the preceding weeks and to carry out a careful clinical examination of the patient.

In primary heart cases there is usually evidence of co-existing pleural fluid and this may make adequate auscultation of the heart difficult since sounds are muffled by fluid not only in the pleural cavity but often pericardium as well. The pulse in these cases will be rapid and thin, it may even be imperceptible. In cases of hepatic origin fluid accumulation will occur only in the abdomen and auscultation of a reasonably normal heart (there will be some abnormality due to splanchnic venous stasis) and the comparatively full pulse provide helpful differential criteria.

Paracentesis shows a fluid serous in nature varying in colour from pale yellow to pinkish; the packed cell volume of the blood will be increased.

Ascites is a late development in heart or liver disease thus prognosis is always grave. Advanced liver changes are irreversible and the virtual impossibility of adequately digitalising feline patients makes treatment of cardiac ascites singularly depressing. In most cases early euthanasia is to be recommended on humane grounds.

REFERENCES

Bloom, F. (1957) *N. Amer. Vet.* **38**, 114.
Cotchin, E. (1957) *Vet. Rec.* **69**, 425.
Cotchin, E. (1956) *B. Vet. J.* **112**, 263.
Cotchin, E. (1960) Personal communication.
Dlugach, J. (1953) *J. Amer. Vet. Medical Association* **123**, 118.
Graber, E. R. (1965) *J. Amer. Vet. Medical Association* **146**, 242.
Howell, J. McC. & Pickering, C. (1964) *J. Comp. Path.* **74**, 280.
Larson, E. J. (1963) *J. Amer. Vet. Medical Association* **143**, 837.
Lindsay F.E.F. (1974) *J.S.A.P.* **15**, 241.
Ruwitch, J., Bonertz, H. E. & Carlson, R. E. (1964) *J. Amer. Vet. Medical Association* **145**, 21.

SUGGESTED FURTHER READING

Kadziolka, A. (1955) *Med. Wet. Warsaw* **11**, 432. (Hyperplasia of spleen and liver in cats.)
Bloom, F. (1960) Gamma Publications, Inc., New York. (The blood chemistry of the dog and cat.)
Zontine, W. J. (1962) *Small An. Clin.* **2**, 136. (Acute pancreatitis in dogs and cats.)
Joshua, J. O. (1963) *J. Small An. Pract.* **4**, 275. (Some clinical aspects of Diabetes Mellitus in the dog and cat.)

Chapter 11

RESPIRATORY SYSTEM INCLUDING DIAPHRAGM

Upper Respiratory Tract

Nasal catarrh
This has been dealt with previously as have other diseases of the nasal cavities.

Laryngitis
Laryngitis occurs as a clinical entity not uncommonly, presumably due to an infective agent although cases tend to arise sporadically and there is little evidence of spread in an average locality. Nothing is known as to incubation period or morbidity. Cases vary considerably in severity from an almost asymptomatic loss of voice to serious and even fatal laryngeal spasm.

Symptoms. The cat is often presented with the history of having a 'sore throat', frequent gulping movements being noticed by the owner. Appetite may or may not be affected. Curiously there is rarely any cough. Gulping and gagging movements are common and the latter may be suggestive of pharyngeal foreign body in which case examination under anaesthesia is often necessary. The cardinal sign is loss of or change in voice. Temperature is rarely raised. Manipulation of the larynx often provokes violent response. Obviously the larynx cannot be seen via the mouth in the conscious cat but none the less this inspection should be made to eliminate pharyngitis as the cause of symptoms.

In the average case spontaneous recovery occurs in 5–10 days and little is needed by way of treatment. Inhalations or administration of Compound Tincture of Benzoin on sugar can give symptomatic relief by provoking increased secretion and thus moistening the irritable larynx.

In severe cases there is no tendency to resolution and the patient becomes increasingly depressed, refuses food and suffers increasingly frequent attacks of a distressing type of dyspnoea during which noisy, gasping respiratory efforts are made, the mouth being kept more or less permanently open. In such cases the use of ataractics such as promazine and chlorpromazine and anti-inflammatory agents (corticosteroids) are warranted and usually give at least temporary relief. Drugs are best administered parenterally owing to the great distress caused to the cat by attempts at forced oral administration; similarly, forced feeding is difficult and even dangerous.

A few cases have been met in which there has been no response to therapy and euthanasia has become necessary on humane grounds, ridiculous though this may seem for so simple a condition. Once again it is a question of species response and the feline tendency to laryngeal spasm creates this unfortunate situation.

Chest

BRONCHITIS

Is a quite common condition, tending to occur seasonally, usually in autumn and winter. The age range is variable and seems insignificant. There is no evidence that the condition is infectious. Affected cats are often subject to annual recurrence.

Coughing is the predominant symptom and is frequent and of variable severity. There is rarely evidence of general ill-health. Temperature is seldom raised nor are respirations markedly abnormal.

On auscultation of the bronchial area exaggerated breath sounds can be heard, often frank bronchial râles, usually dry but occasionally moist. There is no involvement of lung tissue.

Diet should if necessary be adjusted and adequate vitamin intake assured by administration of suitable vitamin supplements. In mild cases annual recurrence can often be avoided or minimised by recommending administration of cod or halibut liver oil during autumn and winter months.

In cases where the cough is sufficiently troublesome to warrant treatment a proprietary pill containing atropine has proved remarkably effective.

Untreated cases often recover spontaneously in the spring. The tendency to spontaneous recovery and seasonal recurrences make it unlikely that *Aleurostrogylus* infestation is of aetiological significance.

PNEUMONIA

Contrary to what might be expected is not a very frequent condition. As mentioned elsewhere, a patchy pneumonia is found in cases of feline pneumonitis but is seldom clinically obvious or significant.

Bacterial invasion of lung tissue can obviously cause pneumonia but bronchopneumonia of the type seen so commonly in canine distemper cases is far less frequent, the lesions of the feline respiratory virus diseases being largely confined to the upper respiratory tract. However, *Escherichia coli* is found in some cases of pneumonia with or without viral involvement. Smith (1964) also names *Pasteurella multocida* as being a common secondary in viral infections of the lung causing a suppurative broncheolitis and bronchopneumonia.

Symptoms include exaggerated respirations, often with mouth breathing, general malaise and a raised temperature.

Auscultation will delineate areas of consolidation. Sneezing and coughing are in abeyance when any widespread consolidation exists.

Treatment. Antibacterial therapy using penicillin, penicillin and streptomycin, broad spectrum agents such as the tetracyclines or chloramphenicol or the broad spectrum penicillins is essential. Administration should be parenteral and a route chosen which necessitates the minimum of restraint, since struggling which increases oxygen requirement, is to be avoided.

Nursing is of the greatest importance. The cat must be kept in an even temperature but with adequate ventilation. It must not be allowed out even for excretory purposes. Windows should be open (avoiding draughts) and covered with wire netting or something similar to prevent the cat escaping. In severe cases with considerable consolidation oxygen therapy is required. For cats nursed at home this is simply achieved by hiring a small cylinder of oxygen from a local chemist and administering the gas via a small funnel of enamel, glass or plastic. Since cylinders are not issued with a reducing value in these circumstances the owner is instructed to turn on until a very faint hissing can be heard; the funnel is held some 6–12 inches from the cat's face and it is allowed to inhale the oxygen enriched air for some 10 minutes in every hour. In small animal hospitals some form of oxygen tent may be available or can be devised.

If forced feeding becomes essential it must be undertaken with the greatest care to avoid distress and inhalation of fluids.

Even in this age of 'wonder drugs' nursing has a great part to play and in no case more than pneumonia. It is the duty of veterinary surgeons carefully to instruct owners in nursing procedure.

Pulmonary Oedema

Is not common in cats but can occur during anaesthesia induced by volatile agents. Respirations become rapidly embarrassed and watery fluid is discharged in variable, often copious amounts, down the nostrils.

The condition is usually rapidly fatal. It is probable that the routine use of atropine for pre-anaesthetic medication would markedly reduce the risk of pulmonary oedema but this is seldom practised for everyday brief procedures such as spaying.

Pleural Fluids. (excluding pyothorax and chylothorax).

In some cases of hyperacute illness associated with calici virus infection a massive accumulation of oedema fluid and neutrophils occur in the chest causing sudden death. (Hoover & Kahn 1975)--See also in chapter on infectious diseases, 'The Cat Flu' complex.

Accumulation of a serous transudate occurs in some cases of heart failure. Once this stage is reached fluid accumulates rapidly not only in the pleural but also in the peritoneal cavity and pericardial sac.

The history is usually of brief duration, up to 3 days. Affected cats are usually in the older age groups (a useful differential from pyothorax which can occur at all ages).

Symptoms. Include exaggerated respirations, a sternal posture with elbows abducted, variable degrees of cyanosis worsened by exertion and extreme reluctance to move. Depending on the fluid level, and quantity of pericardial fluid, heart sounds may be audible and obviously abnormal or may be muffled and even inaudible. Pulse is rapid, weak or imperceptible.

The presence and type of fluid can be determined by exploratory puncture but the advisability of this procedure must be carefully weighed against the disadvantages and dangers to a patient in a precarious condition. It is essential that the cat be allowed to remain in the orthodox position—enforced lateral recumbency can prove quickly fatal.

Prognosis. Is poor since the animal is already in failure. The limitations of treatment of cardiac conditions have already been emphasised. Euthanasia should not be long delayed.

Pyothorax

Synonyms: Exudative pleurisy, empyema thorax, septic pleurisy.

This condition is one of considerable clinical significance in the cat. It occurs regularly but not frequently and is apparently a species tissue response to a wide variety of aetiological factors.

Since the condition is more correctly regarded as a tissue response than a single pathological entity the name pyothorax has been adopted since this merely indicates pus in the thoracic cavity without suggesting specific lesions.

Experience shows that pyothorax is a hyperacute or acute condition occurring in cats of all ages and may be related to a variety of predisposing causes. Pyothorax has been found to follow feline respiratory virus infections, in recovered cases of feline enteritis, during the weeks following apparent recovery from a cat sepsis lesion and in association with infestation of the lungs with *Aleurostrongylus abstrusus*; in some cases no predisposing cause can be incriminated.

Despite the fact that one or both sides of the pleural cavity are filled with what appears to be obviously purulent exudate a proportion of cases is bacteriologically sterile (Wilkinson (1956)) and the remainder associated with bacteria of no specific significance. In some cases the exudate contains large numbers of *Aleurostrongylus* larvae; in others no evidence of this parasite exists. Smith (1964) records the occasional isolation of haemolytic staphylococci from these cases.

From the point of view of the practising veterinary surgeon early recognition of the syndrome is important since despite records of a few successfully treated cases prognosis is usually poor and early euthanasia to be commended.

Symptoms. Hyperacute cases: Symptoms may be in existence for only 12 hours before death. They are of rapidly developing and progressive dyspnoea, profound dulness, complete inappetence, reluctance to move, often pain on handling, greatly increased respiratory distress on forced movement, possibly with cyanosis and mouth breathing.

Temperature is raised in the early stages but is often subnormal by the time advice is obtained.

Auscultation reveals partially or completely muffled heart sounds and absence of breath sounds for a variable level on both sides of the chest. Pulse is rapid, weak, often inapparent. Percussion will often clearly delineate a fluid line with dulness below and resonance above a certain level. Handling of chest and abdomen not only provokes increased dyspnoea but obvious pain due to pressure on parietal pleura of thoracic cavity and diaphragm.

Hyperacute cases are invariably bilateral hence treatment is not feasible and euthanasia to be recommended.

Acute cases: May have been in existence several days to 1 week before advice is sought. Some such cases are unilateral and attempted treatment may be justified; Wilkinson G. T. (1960) records the successful treatment of such a case.

Symptoms are similar to those previously described but being slower in onset their development may be detected in more detail.

Appetite may or may not be lost in the early stages; there is dulness and reluctance to move; a sternal posture is selected and the cat is unable to sleep in a normal position. If forced to move the cat will usually only walk a comparatively short distance and rapidly resumes sternal recumbency. It will not jump onto heights.

Temperature varies from sub-normal to 40·6° C. (105° F.).

Dyspnoea may not be obvious at the outset but becomes progressively more marked and is particularly provoked by exertion. Discomfort on handling the chest or pressing on the anterior abdomen is nearly always apparent. In early cases where little fluid has accumulated auscultation and percussion may reveal little but any suspected case should be re-examined at least 24 hourly with careful auscultation and percussion on each occasion.

In the later stages mouth breathing and cyanosis may occur.

Diagnosis. Is based mainly on the clinical picture since general anaesthesia, especially in bilateral cases, for exploratory puncture is hazardous and the distress occasioned by attempts in the conscious animal even with local infiltration can provoke a fatal respiratory collapse.

None the less in less acute afebrile cases differential diagnosis from serous effusions and chylothorax is desirable and can be established only by withdrawal of fluid. In unilateral cases anaesthesia is obviously less hazardous.

Treatment. Diagnosis is not established until significant exudation has already occurred hence it cannot be too strongly emphasised that treatment which does not include surgical drainage is utterly futile. In cases where bacteriological invasion has occurred systemic anti-bacterial therapy may cause a sufficient temporary remission of symptoms to permit anaesthesia and surgical drainage under better conditions and is therefore justified. Treatment of bilateral cases is seldom successful.

Under light general or local infiltration anaesthesia, a suitable needle is introduced into the pleural cavity of the affected side (usually in the area ribs 5–9) and fluid withdrawn into a sterile syringe (sterile since bacteriological examination is desirable to ensure that subsequent antibacterial therapy is well directed), the process being continued until all fluid is withdrawn, often a considerable volume (in Wilkinson's case 60–70 ml.). In view of the fibrinous deposits usually seen in these cases careful irrigation of the pleural cavity with sterile saline at blood heat is desirable if the condition of the patient warrants prolongation of interference. Subsequently a suitable antibiotic in non-irritant form, e.g. crystalline penicillin in solution, streptomycin in solution, either of the above as intramammary cerates (distribution over the chest cavity is less complete in this form) or solution of chloramphenicol succinate in appropriate dosage and volume is introduced via the same needle which is then withdrawn while maintaining negative pressure. Antibiotics and supportive treatment are given systemically during the next 5–7 days.

Prognosis. Very guarded. Recurrence within a few weeks of apparently successful treatment is very common.

In cases where surgical drainage is not practicable prognosis is hopeless and early euthanasia to be advised.

Infestation with *Aleurostrongylus abstrusus*

Whilst infestation with the lung-worm *Aleurostrongylus abstrusus* is undoubtably more common than is generally believed (Hamilton (1963) records an incidence of 9·6 per cent of 125 cats examined) it is not easy to assess its clinical significance. Lesions caused by this parasite are not infrequently found in the lungs of cats destroyed for reasons totally unconnected with the chest. At the same time Wilkinson has indicated its possible aetiological role in cases of pyothorax and Hamilton attributes the death of one cat with respiratory signs associated with coughing, sneezing and muco-purulent nasal discharge and subsequent hydrothorax to this infestation. The latter author also considers that in five other cats mild clinical disease was probably due to *Aleurostrongylus*.

Diagnosis. If any cat with respiratory signs is suspected of *Aleurostrongylus* infection faeces should be examined for the presence of first-stage larvae. Eosinophilia may be present but is suggestive rather than diagnostic.

Treatment. Various treatments have been reported but there is insufficient evidence to permit strong recommendations being made.

Neoplasms of the Chest

In the neoplasm series quoted nine cases of neoplasia involved the chest and associated organs, mainly as metastatic deposits but occasionally as the primary site.

One 12 year castrated male had an adenocarcinoma of the lung, believed to be of primary bronchial origin.

Two 6-year-old cats, neutered male and female, had mediastinal tumours, one definitely a thymoma the other possibly thymoma or lymphosarcoma.

Two cats had lung metastases from a primary axillary mammary gland carcinoma, one had lung metastases from a ceruminous gland carcinoma of the external auditory canal, two cases of sarcomata are apparently from a primary site near the carpus and the other had sarcomata in various sites including lungs. The ninth cat had lung metastases from a posterior pharyngeal carcinoma.

In most cases symptoms due to the chest lesion will not predominate but in primary cases symptoms will depend on the tissue involved, e.g. if in lung, dyspnoea and cough will prevail; mediastinal tumours will cause pressure symptoms on bronchi and possibly oesophagus.

Any cat having had a tumour removed from another site, especially mammary gland, which develops respiratory signs and weight loss within the few months following surgery should be regarded as possibly having lung metastases. In advanced cases radiography may confirm diagnosis of the presence of tumour tissue.

There is no feasible treatment.

Mediastinal and bronchial lymph nodes may be involved in lymphosarcoma or lymphatic leukosis (pseudo-Hodgkin's type) syndromes and may also become enlarged in other infective conditions, especially the rather uncommon cases of pulmonary tuberculosis. Chest signs are, with the exception of the latter, likely to be secondary to the general disease picture.

As previously mentioned needles which have passed the pharyngeal area may enter other tissues and hence may traverse the pleural cavities giving rise to indefinite chest signs as they do so. Diagnosis can be confirmed by radiography but heroic surgery is not to be advised as such foreign bodies usually emerge at the skin surface in a localised septic focus.

Diaphragm

The diaphragm may be involved in pathological processes as an incidental contiguous structure, e.g. tumour deposits, especially in lymphosarcoma or inflammatory reaction during pyothorax.

By far the most important lesion is rupture of the diaphragm usually with herniation of abdominal viscera into the thoracic cavity.

Rupture of the Diaphragm. Diaphragmatic Hernia

Is a not uncommon lesion in street accident cases when a crushing force is applied to the trunk.

The rent in the diaphragm may be on either side and of variable extent involving muscular and/or tendinous portions.

In extensive tearing the diaphragm may be almost completely separated from the body wall on the affected side.

History. Significant history is not always available but in many cases a street accident is known to have occurred but not necessarily in the immediate past.

Symptoms. Usually of respiratory embarrassment, variable in degree according to the extent of visceral herniation.

The cat tends to remain in sternal recumbency with elbows somewhat abducted. Respirations are exaggerated and obviously requiring voluntary effort. Forced movement increases dyspnoea and may cause cyanosis.

Raising the forehand of the animal may relieve dyspnoea by allowing viscera to drop away from the embarrassed lungs while raising the hindquarters may alarmingly and dangerously increase respiratory distress.

On examination mucous membranes may be pallid or cyanosed. The abdomen may feel and appear unusually empty. If small intestine is herniated peristaltic sounds may be audible on the affected side which is also dull on percussion. Heart and pulse may be rapid and weak and breath sounds can be detected only on the unaffected side of the chest.

Parts of liver and small intestine are usually herniated and spleen and stomach often herniate then or subsequently.

Herniation of the stomach often results in kinking of the oesophagus with the extremely rapid development of severe tympany which can be quickly fatal.

Diagnosis. Based on the history of accident, the clinical findings of a partly empty abdomen and dullness on one side of the chest, the presence of gut sounds in the thorax and the reduced area of functioning lung tissue on auscultation.

Diagnosis is confirmed by radiography, using barium to outline stomach and small intestine which can be seen in the thorax. Care should be taken in positioning for radiography as sudden and fatal dyspnoea can be caused.

Differential Diagnosis. Ordinary post-traumatic shock with bruising of ribs; haemothorax; pneumothorax; pyothorax; chylothorax or pleural effusion due to cardiac insufficiency; the three latter are not associated with a history of accident. Peristaltic sounds in the chest and radiography are the methods of differentiating.

Treatment. Surgical only. Always a hazardous proceeding but repair should always be attempted.

In recent accident cases a delay in order to combat shock is advisable but the hazard of stomach herniation and the consequent need for emergency surgery must be borne in mind.

Whilst it is highly desirable that some means of assisted respiration during anaesthesia should be available successful surgery has been accomplished without, Milnes recording two cases in cats and one in a dog satisfactorily completed without any positive pressure apparatus.

Obviously the best method is that using an endotracheal tube and re-breathing bag which can be manually compressed throughout operation but failing this is a simple expedient using a T or Y piece can be very satisfactory.

The greatest care must be taken in inducing anaesthesia (with an intravenous barbiturate) prior to intubation as this is the time when fatal collapse is most likely to occur.

The surgical approach can be via the abdomen or via the chest; by the latter route two methods are available, entry between the appropriate ribs (rib resection is seldom needed in the cat as satisfactory retraction of the very elastic ribs is usually feasible giving adequate exposure) or less commonly by longitudinal splitting of the sternum. The abdominal and sternal routes do not necessitate accurate diagnosis of the side of the rupture whereas the intercostal approach demands this.

The rent in the diaphragm is sutured using cat-gut, linen thread, braided nylon or even silk.

On completion of the repair as much air as possible must be removed from the pleural cavity. If the abdominal approach is used the anaesthetist fully inflates the lungs while the last suture is drawn tight and tied but in the other two methods this is delayed until the final co-apting suture is tightened round ribs or sternum.

The difficulty of surgical repair is greatly increased in old-standing cases in which retraction and scarring of the torn edges of the diaphragm is advanced, in fact satisfactory suturing may be impossible.

Post-operative treatment is routine.

Prognosis. Always guarded owing to the hazards of anaesthesia but surgically speaking good in recent cases, poor in old cases.

REFERENCES

Hamilton, J. M. (1963) *Vet. Rec.* **75**, 417.
Hoover, E.A.; KAHN, D.E. (1975)*J.A.V.M.A.* **166**,463.
Milnes, J. (1954) *Vet. Rec.* **66**, 13.
Smith, J. E. (1964) *J. Small An. Pract.* **5**, 517.
Wilkinson, G. T. (1956) *Vet. Rec.* **68**, 456.
Wilkinson, G. T. (1960) *Vet. Rec.* **72**, 903.

SUGGESTED FURTHER READING

Blaisdell, K. F. (1952) Thesis. Cornell University.
Sudduth, W. (1955) *J. Amer. Vet. Medical Association* **126**, 211.
Brown, V. K. (1962) *Vet. Rec.* **74**, 829.
(Three articles above on Aleurostrongylus.)
Harbart, W. B. (1964) *J. Amer. Vet. Medical Association* **144**, 46. (Dyspnoea due to cystic thoracic duct in a cat.)
Whitehead, J. E. (1963) *Mod. Vet. Pract.* **44**, 43. (Differential diagnosis of dyspnoea in cats.)
Archibald, J., Clacken, T. & Bishop, E. J. (1955) *N. Amer. Vet.* **36**, 565. (Canine and feline bronchiectasis.)
Holzworth, J. (1958) *J. Amer. Vet. Medical Association* **132**, 124. (Thoracic disorders in the cat.)

Chapter 12

CARDIOVASCULAR SYSTEM

Probably the most important pathological condition of the cardio-vascular system in the cat is arterial thrombosis. Valvular lesions of the heart do occur as do anaemia and lymphatic leukosis but in view of the rather dramatic nature of the signs associated with thrombosis this subject is dealt with first.

Arterial Thrombosis: (Embolism)

The term arterial thrombosis has been deliberately selected to indicate that blockage of vessels other than the aorta by clot can occur; records exist confirming thrombosis of sub-clavian arteries and there seems every probability, as yet unconfirmed, that cerebral thrombosis has also occurred. Holzworth *et al.* (1955) have pointed out that the lesion should more accurately be described as an embolus but that subsequent deposition of material about the embolus renders it eventually a thrombus, hence the usual nomenclature is justified.

Detailed descriptions of cases have been given by Collet (1930), Holzworth *et al.* (1955), Freak (1956) and Joshua (1957); these authors have fully documented nine cases and given brief résumés of the symptoms and findings in eleven other suspected or retrospectively diagnosed cases some of which were confirmed or discovered at post-mortem.

Aetiology. It is usually assumed that the condition is consequent upon primary heart disease but a suggestion has been put forward (un-published) that the suddenness of onset in many cases and relatively large size of the thrombi could indicate primary disease of the blood.

There is no doubt that in many patients there is no evidence of pre-existing abnormality.

Age Incidence. There is no particular age incidence cases having been recorded from 1–15 years but the preponderance occurs in middle life (4–10 years).

Symptoms and Signs. These are variable according to the location of the thrombus, its size and the speed with which it has occluded the vessel. In localised cases (e.g. unilateral iliac or femoral thrombosis) the associated signs give a clear indication of the site of the clot. In all other than very localised lesions there is evidence of considerable circulatory embarrassment and disorganisation the cat being collapsed to a variable degree, temperature usually sub-normal, mucous membranes pallid or cyanotic, showing marked dyspnoea, distress and anxiety with pain in the parts deprived of a blood supply.

If there is posterior aortic or iliac thrombosis femoral pulses are absent but heart sounds may be exaggerated although usually grossly irregular.

The affected limb(s) is cold, withdrawal reflexes are absent and there is no pulse in the associated vessel. There may be pain in muscle bellies; this is particularly marked in cases of iliac thrombosis in which evidence of paralysis and ischaemia is accompanied by a most typical enlargement, spasm and painful cramping of the gastrocnemius muscular bellies. Oedema, necrosis and sloughing have been described in limbs temporarily deprived of a blood supply by thrombosis.

In some cases histories of previous unexplained collapse or shock episodes are elicited; in others following recovery from the initial diagnosed attack further episodes occur often necessitating euthanasia.

In occasional cases where pain is severe (e.g. in cramped gastrocnemius muscles) temperature may be raised, probably purely a pain reaction but it is more usual, as previously mentioned, for temperature to be sub-normal to normal.

Course

In many severe cases death occurs or euthanasia is necessary on humane grounds during the initial period of severe circulatory embarrassment. If this is weathered signs related specifically to the blocked vessel develop, e.g. posterior paralysis, oedema and paralysis of a forelimb, atrophy of individual muscles or groups of muscles, kidney infarction etc.

Spontaneous recovery occurs in many cases, sometimes apparently complete, sometimes with local damage persisting due to ischaemia. Spontaneous recovery is presumably due to two factors, contraction of the clot with increasing ability of blood to flow past it and the establishment of some collateral blood supply. Persisting changes are most commonly renal dysfunction due to infarction and hind limb weakness due to localised muscle necrosis and fibrosis.

Treatment. Initially directed at combatting shock and circulatory stress by warmth, adequate oxygenation and relief of pain. Subsequently anticoagulants such as heparin may be used but the tendency to recurrence and the consequent need for permanent anticoagulant therapy with its attendant risks makes this a procedure to be used only in carefully selected cases.

If bacterial endocarditis is suspected as being of aetiological importance a prolonged (at least 14 days) course of antibiotic, preferably penicillin, is justified.

Prognosis. Always guarded despite the fact that localized cases have apparently made permanent recoveries. The possibility of renal infarction must be borne in mind and signs of renal insufficiency looked for subsequent to apparent recovery.

Anaemia

Anaemia is not uncommon in cats; it occurs specifically as feline infectious anaemia, and frequently in association with Fe LV infection, the latter being established as the cause of both haemolytic and aplastic anaemias as well as anaemias secondary to neoplastic destruction of haemopoietic tissues. See Chapter 19, page 254, Feline Infectious Anaemia.

Non-specific anaemias may accompany bacterial infections, kidney and liver disease, rheumatoid arthritis and mast cell infiltration of the spleen as well as occurring in cats in which no aetiological factor can be established.

In all cases underlying disease processes must be sought. Symptoms related to the anaemia are loss of energy, decreased exercise tolerance, some loss of appetite and loss of bodily condition. In advanced cases dyspnoea may be evident.

The visible mucous membranes in the cat are normally somewhat pallid and although blanching may be seen in advanced cases they are often a comparatively unreliable indicator. Tongue colour is rather more reliable, the dorsum of the tongue in the normal cat being a fairly bright pink but showing variable pallor in anaemias.

The blood picture may or may not be helpful in deciding upon aetiology. The heart rate and pulse are usually increased, differences in the volume of the latter being difficult to detect.

Normal Range of Blood Cellular Elements in The Cat. (Coffin).

R.B.C.	6·2–10 millions.
Hbg.	8–13·8 grams per 100 c.c.
Hemat.	34–46 per cent.
M.C.H.	13–17 micromicrograms.
M.C.V.	51–63 cubic microns.
M.C.H.C.	32–34 per cent.
Platelets.	0·15–0·25 millions.
Reticulocytes.	0–2·5 per cent.

Normal Range For Leukocytes.

Total W.B.C.	8–35 thousands. (Kittens, 8–17·5 thousands.)
Neutrophils.	57 (30–75) per cent.
Eosinophils.	5 (2–10) per cent.
Basophils.	0·1 (0–0·5) per cent.
Lymphocytes.	32 (20–40) per cent.
Monocytes.	6 (1–15) per cent.

Since cardiac incompetence with corresponding peripheral ischaemia is not very common in the cat, likewise spontaneous haemorrhage due to spleen haematoma or angiosarcoma are rare, a pallid tongue is more likely to indicate anaemia. Internal haemorrhage in street accident cases is usually obvious by reason of the history. It is unlikely that thrombosis cases will be confused with anaemia because of the sudden onset and associated severe signs of circulatory embarrassment in the former.

Treatment. In hypochromic anaemia iron therapy is called for. Oral administration of iron is not particularly easy in the cat and it is probably better to use the parenteral route giving twice or thrice weekly injections of a suitable iron preparation such as those used for piglet anaemia.

In microcytic or cytopaenic forms therapy is by injection of liver extracts (refined forms are preferred) or cyancobalamin. Preparations including folic acid and hog stomach are occasionally of value.

Prognosis. Is variable according to aetiology, if known. If associated with hepatic or renal dysfunction it is poor. Removal of enlarged spleen in cases of mast cell infiltration usually results in apparent spontaneous improvement in anaemia. There is usually improvement in general health including the associated anaemia in rheumatoid arthritis cases which respond to corticosteroids.

Heart

Heart disease is not particularly common in cats and when it does occur frequently does not give rise to clinical symptoms until the stage of failure is approaching or reached.

Congenital abnormalities seem surprisingly rare or unrecognised.

Valvular Defects

Murmurs associated with valve incompetence have been noted in adult cats. Clinical signs are minimal, usually some decrease in activity and/or loss of appetite. The murmur is often somewhat sibilant as opposed to the 'blow' heard in the dog; it may resemble a squeak and may be sufficiently loud as to be heard without auscultation. Cases have been seen in which both murmur and symptoms have been comparatively transient especially if treatment with digitalis can be tolerated for even a short time. This suggests that the lesion may be an endocarditis caused by bacterial invasion, e.g. in cat sepsis. For this reason vigorous antibacterial therapy, even in the absence of fever, is warranted in addition to that directed at the heart itself.

In aged cats the so-called 'mitral blow' occasionally occurs but is often not detected until the cat is in failure.

Treatment. The intolerance of many cats for the digitalis glycosides makes treatment of heart disease in this species disappointing. Doses of 15–60 mg. digitalis leaf or 0·1 mg. digitoxin often cause inappetence and vomiting and must be discontinued. Small doses of digitalis leaf or any of the individual glycosides should always be tried as response in the few cats which can tolerate it is very good. Bentley (personal communication) finds that some cats which cannot take conventional preparations can tolerate digitalin granules in a dosage of 0·1 mg. (1/600 gr.). Mild sedation with small doses of phenobarbitone, e.g. 7·5 mg. (⅛ gr.) or potassium bromide, e.g. 75–150 mg. (1¼–2½ gr.) twice daily may have a beneficial action on heart rate. Vitamin E as alpha tocopherol (50 mg. daily) is advantageous. Sugar or glucose in the diet may be beneficial.

Prognosis. Always poor if the stage of failure is reached as compensation is seldom achieved. It is good in those cases seen during middle life if treatment can be tolerated.

Tachycardia

A very rapid heart rate, at times uncountable, is often present in aged cats. Its significance is difficult to assess. If symptoms are attributable to this cause and digitalis is not tolerated procaine amide might be considered as it has been known to be beneficial in the dog; suggested dose 100 mg.

In some cats which have a weak rapid pulse the heart sounds on auscultation are compatible. It is difficult to describe but is probably best called a light tapping sound, giving the impression that the myocardium is atonic and undergoing rather useless contractions. In such cases Vitamin E (50 mg. or more daily as alpha tocopherol) can be beneficial.

From the indefinite nature of these descriptions it becomes obvious that there is little reliable information of a clinical nature available on cardiac abnormalities in the cat.

REFERENCES

Bentley, M. A. W. (1964) Personal communication.
Collett, P. (1930) *Bul. de la Soc. des Sci. Vet. de Lyon.* **33**, 136.
Freak, M. J. (1956) *Vet. Rec.* **68**, 816.
Gilmore, C. E. *et al.* (1964) *Path. Vet.* **1**, 161.
Holzworth, J. *et al.* (1955) *Cornell Vet.* **45**, 468.
Joshua, J. O. (1957) *Vet. Rec.* **69**, 146.

SUGGESTED FURTHER READING

Anonymous. (1958–59) *Iowa State Coll. Vet.* **21**, 95. (Aortic thrombosis in a cat.)
Bardens, J. W. & Walker, J. S. (1962) *Small An. Clin.* **2**, 247. (Removal of a thrombus from the external iliacs in a feline.)
Block, J. & Boeles, J. (1957) *Acta. Physiol. Pharmacol. Neerl.* **6**, 95. (The electrocardiogram of the normal cat.)
Detweiler, D. K. (1961) *Cardiology.* Vol. V. New York. McGraw-Hill. (Cardiovascular disease in animals.)
Hamlin, R. L. (1960) *J. Amer. Vet. Medical Association* **136**, 359. (Radiographic anatomy of the normal cat heart.)

Joshua, J. O. (1959) *Vet. Rec.* **71**, 941. (Some clinical aspects of cardio-vascular disease in cats and dogs.)

Shouse, C. L. & Meier, H. (1956) *J. Amer. Vet. Medical Association* **129**, 278. (Acute vegetative endocarditis in the dog and cat.)

Tashjian, R. J. *et al.* (1963) *Sci. Proc.* **100**, Annual Meeting Amer. Vet. Medical Association, 113 (Feline cardiovascular studies—a preliminary report.)

Gilmore, C. E. *et al.* (1964) *Path. Vet.* **1**, 18. (Bone marrow and peripheral blood of cats; technique and normal values.)

Holzworth, J. (1963) *An. N.Y. Acad. Sci.* **108**, 691. (Neoplasia of blood-forming tissue in the cat.)

Simpson, C. F. & Jackson, R. F. (1963) *J. Amer. Vet. Medical Association* **142**, 282. (Aortic sclerosis in a cat.)

Holzworth, J. (1956) *J. Amer. Vet. Medical Association* **128**, 471. (Anaemia in the cat.)

Bloom, F. (1937) *Vet. Med.* **32**, 1. (Unilateral exophthalmus associated with leukaemia in a cat.)

Eyestone, W. H. (1951) *J. Nat. Cancer Inst.* **12**, 599. (Myelogenous leukaemia in the cat.)

Meier, H. & Patterson, D. F. (1956) *J. Amer. Vet. Medical Association* **128**, 211. (Myelogenous leukaemia in a cat.)

Meier, H. & Gourley, G. (1957) *J. Amer. Vet. Medical Association* **130**, 33. (Basophilic (myelocytic) or mast cell leukaemia in a cat.)

Holzworth, J. & Meier, H. (1957) *Cornell Vet.* **47**, 302. (Reticulum cell myeloma in a cat.)

Holzworth, J. (1960) *J. Amer. Vet. Medical Association* **136**, 47. (Leukaemia in the cat. I. Lymphoid malignancies.)

Ibid. **136**, 107. (Leukaemia in the cat. II. Malignancies other than lymphoid.)

Chapter 13

URINARY TRACT

Kidneys

Congenital abnormalities of the kidneys are occasionally seen, usually unilateral and cystic in nature in which case the lesion may only be detected incidentally at spaying or post-mortem. Obviously life cannot be sustained in the presence of severe bilateral abnormalities.

A case of unilateral hydronephrosis and hydro-uneter in an 8 week old kitten has recently been reported; removal of the affected kidney was successful and the kitten was apparently normal two months after surgery.

Nephritis

Chronic interstitial nephritis histologically similar to that seen in dogs is quite common. Its aetiology is not known. The presence of significant levels of leptospiral agglutinins has not been correlated with evidence of renal disease and in the present state of knowledge nephritis in the cat cannot be attributed to leptospiral infection.

Age Incidence. It occurs mainly in older cats although animals in middle life which have survived the febrile stage of the hepatic/renal syndrome may develop signs of kidney disease.

Symptoms. Are usually somewhat insidious in onset. Increase in water intake, decrease in appetite, playfulness and energy, and loss of body weight are typical. Vomiting occurs occasionally. Constipation is a frequent accompaniment. Salivation, sometimes blood-stained and dysphagia also occur when uraemia supervenes. The dysphagia and salivation are due to the presence of ulcers which occur more commonly in the post-pharyngeal area rather than on the gums and inside the lips as in the dog and hence are not easily visible. Temperature is normal or subnormal. Signs include dehydration, buccal ulcers, uraemic odour (distinctly ammoniacal in the cat) and frequently pallid mucous membranes. On palpation the kidneys are often smaller than average and the irregular pitted surface can occasionally be detected; there may be disparity in size between the two organs.

Although the condition is a chronic one and usually progressive it is not uncommon to meet cats in which remissions and exacerbations of clinical symptoms occur, thus treatment is usually warranted.

A glomerulo-nephritis associated with Fe LV infection has been recorded by Cotter et. al. 1975. All subjects had high F.O.C.M.A.

antibodies indicating recent Fe LV infection with symptoms of proteinuria, hypoproteinaemia, oedema and uraemia.

Diagnosis. Based on the clinical evidence in association with urinalysis. Urine examination: Since the specific gravity of cat urine varies within wide limits of normality with the frequent occurrence of concentrated urines (1·040+) there is not always an obviously dilute urine in nephritis cases. Values of 1·030 and 1·040 are not uncommon in confirmed nephritics.

Protein is usually present, rarely in large quantity, and should be detected by the sulpho-salicylic acid test; experience shows that the chemically impregnated paper strips are markedly unreliable for cat urine giving frequent false positives and exaggerated values. Glucose should be tested for routinely, to eliminate diabetes mellitus (glycosuria associated with renal disease has not been found in the cat). Microscopic examination of sediment for casts is also helpful.

Treatment. Since cats are usually extremely selective feeders even when having a normal appetite it is not easy to persuade sick cats which are partially or completely anorexic to accept a changed diet. Whenever possible the proportion of protein should be temporarily reduced and that which is fed must be of good quality and easily digestible. Hydrolysed proteins are very valuable for nephritic cats, especially those with which glucose is incorporated. The intravenous injection of hydrolysed protein is feasible but cats which are sufficiently ill to require intravenous feeding are unlikely to survive. Similarly when dehydration is present to a degree necessitating fluid therapy the prognosis is very grave.

Vitamin supplements, especially of B complex and C, should be administered. Intramuscular, intravenous or even subcutaneous (diluted 1 in 2 normal saline) injection of suitable vitamin preparations are most useful, e.g. Parenterovite (Vitamins Ltd.).

The empirical use of hexamine by mouth, 300 mg. (5 gr.) b.d. or t.i.d., is justified by results although apparently having no rationale. Many cats show marked clinical response to treatment with hexamine and Vitamin B complex tablets with return of appetite, decrease in water intake and improvement in general condition. In these circumstances it is justifiable to adopt an apparently illogical line of therapy.

Since there is no evidence that bacterial invasion plays a part in chronic interstitial nephritis of the cat antibiotic therapy is not called for and sulphonamide therapy is probably actually contra-indicated.

Prognosis. In mild cases short-term prognosis can be reasonably optimistic but the long-term outlook is seldom good since recurrences with eventual renal failure are to be expected.

Cats with nephritis are liable to rapid deposition of soft dental calculus, parodontal diseases and gingivitis. Any cat presented with a dirty mouth of obviously recent development should be subjected to a thorough clinical examination including urinalysis before dental treatment is attempted.

In some cat sepsis cases bacteraemia with spread of pyogenic organisms to various organs can occur, consequently a bacterial nephritis can be encountered but is more properly regarded as a complication of cat sepsis than true renal disease; other organs are usually involved simultaneously. Vigorous antibiotic therapy, e.g. with chlortetracycline, may be effective.

Renal involvement appears to occur in the hepatic/renal syndrome described elsewhere since the kidneys are often palpably enlarged and painful. Proteinuria, which is usually present, is not necessarily related to the renal damage as it may occur when inflammation of other parenchymatous organs such as liver co-exists.

Neoplasia

The kidneys are a very common site for sarcomata, usually lymphosarcomata but occasionally of other types. Metastasis from other organs is not uncommon and in the series reviewed two such cases occurred, one a metastasis from a ceruminous carcinoma and the other a probable metastatic deposit from a leiomyosarcoma.

Lymphosarcoma occurs in all age groups although commoner in older cats; kidney involvement may be uni or bilateral.

Symptoms. The clinical picture in the early stages is often vague and indefinite. There is usually some loss of energy, appetite and weight. Increased thirst is common but not invariable. Vomiting occurs occasionally.

Signs. Kidney enlargement is common but not invariable. When palpable enlargement occurs there may be disparity in size of the kidneys and sometimes the irregular bulging of the tumour masses can be felt.

Urine examination is not diagnostic; urine is usually dilute to correspond to the polydipsia but proteinuria is only an irregular finding. Haematology is unlikely to be helpful in diagnosis.

Prognosis. Hopeless. Euthanasia to be advised; the rarity of unilateral primary renal neoplasia in this species makes nephrectomy a usually futile proceeding.

Subcapsular Renal Haemorrhage

This occurs not infrequently following street accidents in which a non-fatal crushing force has been applied to the abdomen, e.g. bicycle accidents.

There will be evidence of shock, abdominal discomfort and blood loss which is not rapidly progressive. The lesion is often palpable. If the capsule is ruptured a rapidly fatal internal haemorrhage occurs.

Treatment is symptomatic, to counteract shock and limit further haemorrhage by the injection of suitable coagulants. Absolute rest is essential to obviate the risk of further bleeding. In all accident cases in which the trunk has been involved careful palpation is advisable as detection of a subcapsular kidney haemorrhage will indicate delaying surgical intervention for such things as fractures or ventral herniae.

Prognosis is good, resorption commencing from about the tenth day and being complete in 3 weeks.

Renal Infarction

Areas of infarction are not uncommon in cat kidneys and can often be attributed to a previous arterial thrombosis. For this reason prognosis in such cases should always be guarded with reference to this possibility. There is no treatment. Small infarcts may not cause symptoms but large areas of kidney tissue subjected to cessation of blood supply will cause evidence of renal insufficiency. Cats showing such signs after a thrombosis episode should be destroyed.

Bladder

Cystitis

Inflammatory conditions of the bladder are very common in all age groups, usually due to bacterial infection. According to Smith (1964) *Escherichia coli* and *Proteus* spp. share the bacterial aetiology of cystitis in the cat. Whilst the condition is essentially a sporadic one it has been noted that there is an increased frequency of cases during or immediately following a fall of snow which has lain at any depth. It seems possible that actual chilling of the ventral abdominal wall may be a factor in precipitating active infection in the adjacent urinary bladder.

Cystitis is an important disease from the aspect of differential diagnosis since, failing adequate clinical examination, it may easily be confused symptomatically with urethral obstruction or one of the forms of constipation.

A hyperacute form of cystitis is recognised, almost certainly associated with one type of bacterial invasion; from one such case a heavy pure culture of haemolytic *Escherichia coli* was obtained but far more evidence is required before concluding that this is the organism to be incriminated. (Smith.) It is characterised by massive haemorrhage into the bladder, early necrosis and rupture of the bladder wall with evidence of severe toxaemia. There is a high mortality rate, death occurring within 24–96 hours.

Symptoms include frequent straining, inability to pass urine, restlessness and crying due to acute abdominal pain, inappetence, vomiting and early collapse. According to the stage at which the case is first seen temperature may be raised or sub-normal.

Inability to pass urine is almost certainly due to the admixing of large quantities of blood and desquamated epithelial cells making a relatively thick mixture which cannot pass the narrow feline urethra. Obviously in such cases the bladder is distended, tense and painful; the bladder wall becomes rapidly extremely fragile due to the acute inflammatory change and normal pressure may easily cause rupture. However, in many cases using great care bloody fluid may be expressed via the penis in sufficient quantity to confirm patency of the urethra. In other cases investigation under general anaesthesia is required when passage of a suitable probe (or piece of nylon) will demonstrate that there is no urethral obstruction.

The condition is so rapid in onset that treatment is usually of no avail and the cat either dies or is destroyed in extremis within 72–96 hours. Attempted treatment will be antibacterial (antibiotics, preferably broad-spectrum) together with such emptying of the bladder as is possible. Vesical paracentesis is contra-indicated on two grounds, the undesirability of risking introduction of infected urine into the peritoneal cavity and the absence of contractility of the much changed bladder wall so that the puncture may continue to leak. Ideally drainage of the bladder via a suitable urethral tube followed by irrigation and introduction of antibiotic solutions is indicated but such attempts usually fail as the maximum diameter tube which can be introduced into the feline urethra is not adequate for a free flow of the grossly thickened urine.

The common form of cystitis is much less acute. Symptoms are those of constant straining to urinate, usually with the passage of a few drops of urine which may be bloodstained. Normally house-clean cats often squat in odd corners of rooms attempting to micturate. The penis may be partially extruded. The cat may cry out while straining. As a rule the cat remains well, apart from the distress occasioned by repeated straining; appetite is unaffected and there is rarely increased thirst. Temperature is occasionally slightly elevated.

Such a history received about any feline patient indicates the necessity for an early clinical examination to eliminate urethral obstruction as the cause. Either sex may be affected. Differentiation from faecal retention is necessary.

On examination it is usual to palpate a tightly contracted empty bladder which may be sensitive on pressure, the thickened walls of which can be detected. In mild cases the bladder may remain thin-walled but is seldom more than one third full. *E. coli* and *Proteus* spp.

Treatment. By antibacterial drugs; those found to be particularly valuable include chlortetracycline (50–100 mg. b.d. or t.i.d.) and the low-dose sulphonamide sulphamethoxypyridazine. In cases where pain and distress are evident due to repeated straining symptomatic antispasmodic treatment is of value, e.g. a mixture containing potassium citrate and tincture of hyoscyamus administered three or four times daily.

Response is usually good with recovery within 7 days but recurrences are common. Due to the small calibre of the urethra irrigation and introduction of antibiotics direct into the bladder is not easily practicable as it is in the dog.

Prognosis. Short term good, long term probable recurrence. Frequent recurrence sometimes results in increasing severity eventually necessitating euthanasia.

It is of interest that on post-mortem examination there is macroscopic evidence of inflammation but rarely any sign of the sabulous material which many people consider to be associated with cystitis.

Feline Urolithiasis

By O.F. Jackson, Ph.D. M.R.C.V.S.

Feline urolithiasis/Urological Syndrome (FUS), a terminology current since 1972, tends to group together indiscriminately cystitis, urethritis, vesicular calculi, haematuria, dysuria, polyuria, sabulous plug, matrix plug and any form of calculus causing partial or total urethral obstruction. However, it is clearer if the various conditions are dealt with under separate headings rather than as the umbrella term of 'FUS.'

Urethral Obstruction

Premonitory signs of urethral obstruction in an entire or castrate male include increased frequency of micturition, frequently with lapse of housetraining habits, and increased grooming attention to the preputial area.

Signs of urethral obstruction are repeated and sometimes continuous attempts at micturition with postural adaptation to effect increased intra-abdominal pressure. Thus, the normal relatively upright squatting posture with low placement of hocks and perineum is replaced by an arched-crouch with hocks more elevated, and straining is often accompanied by crying or signs of distress (contrast Figs. 24 and 25). In between straining efforts, the cat may retain a guarded posture and move with obvious reluctance.

Signs Found On Examination. Include a palpably hard and distended bladder, sometimes tumefaction or ulceration of penis and prepuce due to excessive grooming and in some cases the presence of a white, sabulous plug on preputial hairs.

Treatment. Must be aimed at immediate relief of obstruction, with supportive nursing, and the prevention of recurrence in the long term. Attempted relief of obstruction by medical means, including the use of tranquilizers and antispasmodic drugs, such as atropine and pancreatic extract, is rarely successful, but gentle urethral massage or 'milking' for a couple of minutes may successfully relieve obstruction caused by sabulous or matrix material. Manual pressure on the bladder should be avoided because of the danger of rupture.

In the event of failure of more conservative techniques, urethral catheterisation and irrigation of the anaesthetized subject is indicated, avoiding the use of specifically renally excreted anaesthetic agents

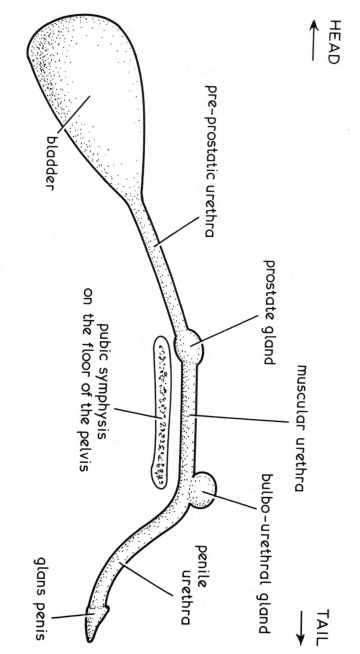

HEAD

TAIL

bladder

pre-prostatic urethra

prostate gland

pubic symphysis
on the floor of the pelvis

muscular urethra

bulbo-urethral gland

penile
urethra

glans penis

FIG. 23   Urinary system (male)

169

such as Ketamine (Vetalar, Parke Davis). Sterile water, normal saline or preferably sodium acetate/acetic acid buffer (Walpoles solution-- Arnold's Vet. Products Ltd.) may be employed to flush out, break up or dissolve plugs. Sterile, blunt lacrimal duct cannulae are convenient for lavage of the penile urethra, but longer nylon tom-cat catheters ('Jackson' Tom-cat catheter, Arnold's Vet. Products Ltd., Reading) are required for deeper penetration.

Commonest points of obstruction are at the tip of the penis and at the level of the bulbo-urethral glands (Fig. 23), but attempted catheterization of the extruded penis almost invariably meets resistance at the point of urethral passage over the pubic brim, though this can be negotiated by release of the penis and application of tension caudally on the prepuce to straighten the urethra.

Advancement of the catheter beyond the obstruction is not uncommon, though an accompanying 'gritty' sensation may indicate mucosal damage likely to become the focus of subsequent scarring and stenosis. For this reason, every effort must be made to unblock the urethra entirely. Sabulous material is readily dissolved by Walpole's solution, while micro-calculi are not [Jackson (1970] and should be flushed back into the bladder by repeated lavage.

Following relief of urethral obstruction, the bladder should be emptied by gentle suction via the catheter rather than by manual expression and may afterwards, in the case of crystalluria, be flushed with Walpole's solution or in the case of bacterial cystitis with a solution of crystalline penicillin. In the event of failure of catheterization to unblock the urethra, a temporary relief of pressure may be achieved by bladder paracentesis after which catheterization is occasionally feasible. With the subject immobilized, to prevent undue damage to the viscus, paracentesis with a 22 gauge needle can be carried out through a suitably prepared site some 2cm cranial to the pelvic brim.

In certain cases, emergency urethrostomy may be necessary to restore urine flow, but ideally this technique should be carried out as an elective procedure when the subject and its urethral tissues have recovered from the acute obstructive episode.

Treatment of the systemic effects of obstruction is aimed at correction of acidosis and high plasma potassium levels resulting from renal obstruction of 12-24 hours or more duration. Symptoms clinically manifest are of hypothermia, depression and elevation of blood urea. As well as the provision of comfort and warmth, rapid treatment essential to combat the life-threatening changes [Burrows and Bovee (1977)] is based on administration of sodium bicarbonate at 0.5-2.Om equivalents per kilogram body weight either by slow intravenous injection over 5-10 minutes or by infusion in a balanced electrolyte solution (Lactated Ringers). The volume of electrolyte to be administered intravenously is estimated on the basis that volume in ml. = percentage dehydration x body weight in pounds x 5. Treatment of hyper-

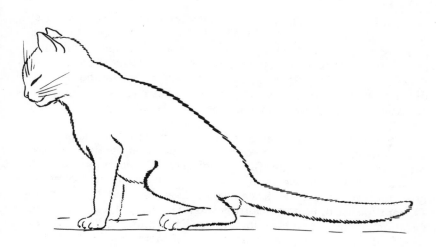

FIG. 24   Normal position assumed during urination

FIG. 25   Straining caused by obstruction

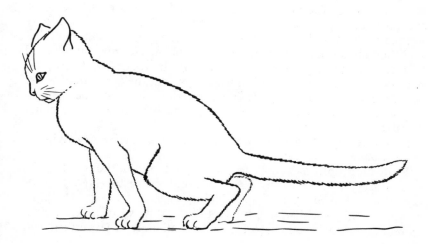

kalaemia by the use of insulin and dextrose has been described [Schaer (1975)].

Attention to fluid balance is especially important in the few cases which undergo diuresis following relief of obstruction, an effect possibly attributable both to clearance of accumulated metabolites and to transient loss of effective powers of urine concentration by proximal renal tubules. Whereas balanced electrolyte solution may initially be administered, the possibility of excessive loss of sodium and potassium in the long term must be considered [Green and Scott (1975)].

Since bacterial cystitis may be both cause and effect of the obstructive episode, all cases should receive routine antibiotic therapy, preferably with drugs specifically indicated by microbiological examination and sensitivity testing of urine, but avoiding such potentially nephrotoxic agents as Kanamycin, Neomycin and Gentamycin. Therapeutic use of urinary acidifiers should be delayed in case of complication of existing acidosis and urinary antiseptics should be chosen with caution, especially avoiding the use of Methylene blue which is known to cause haemolysis in cats.

Prevention of recurrence of urethral obstruction in the short term may be achieved by leaving a urinary catheter in situ for several days. This may be secured by suturing to the prepuce, and is of particular value in long-standing cases in which secondary bladder atony exists. To prevent interference with the catheter an Elizabethan collar should be fitted and to prevent undue urine soaking a secondary polythene drainage tube should be attached to the catheter.

Prophylactic treatment to prevent recurrence of obstructive episodes in the long term is difficult, given lack of understanding of the basic aetiology. The prime candidate for FUS has been shown to be the lazy, obese, neutered male fed dry cat food and having only limited fluid intake [Walker et al. (1977)] and so manipulation of diet and fluid intake should be attempted in control. This may be achieved by feeding a higher proportion of high moisture foods (meat, fish, tinned foods, etc.); dry cat foods must not be fed; the addition of water to food at the rate of 40 ml per 200g, the addition of salt and the provision of gravy, water and milk with which to quench the thirst created.

Prevention of obesity and enforcement of an active life style are regrettably not practicable.

Medical prophylaxis may be attempted and although struvite crystalluria per se is not the cause of urethral obstruction, reduction of crystalline deposits by urinary acidification may be helpful. Chlorethamine (Ethylene diamine, Intervet Laboratories Ltd.) methionine, ammonium chloride and ascorbic acid are all more or less effective in this context.

The use of megoestrol acetate to reduce incidence of cystitis has

172

been described but its prophylactic usefulness in control of obstruction though reported [Evans (1976)], is difficult to evaluate.

In the case of repeated recurrence of obstruction, or of severe urethral damage and stenosis, surgical urethrostomy is indicated. Several techniques have been described, including implantation of a silicone shunt [Skelcher and Steele (1978)], preputial urethrostomy, the suturing of preputial skin to urethral mucosa [Christensen (1964), Biewenga (1975)], and prepubic urethrostomy [Mendham (1970), Snow (1972)], this latter having the disadvantage of some loss of sphincter control due to urethral nerve damage. The commoner operation of perineal urethrostomy, initially described by Carbone (1963) and repeatedly modified [Denny (1972), Long (1977), Gaskell et al. (1978)], is preferred by this author who favours transection and exteriorization of the penis at the level of the bulbourethral glands (Gaskell et al. (1978)].

The Neurogenic-Bladder Syndrome

This presents as atonic distension of the bladder with an urethral dribble of strong smelling urine and a cystitis associated with urinary retention. On examination, the distended viscus is palpable and easily expressed.

This atony commonly occurs in males as a sequel to prolonged overdistension secondary to total urethral obstruction, but may occur in either sex due to lower spinal nerve lesions which are usually of accidental origin, but sometimes of spontaneous occurrence in tail-less (Manx) cats.

Treatment. Aims at initial relief of symptoms to allow time for recovery of tonal control and prognosis varies with aetiology. The introduction of an indwelling catheter successfully prevents overfilling of the viscus, as described in management of urethral obstruction.

In the case of sacro-sciatic nerve damage, regular and prolonged nursing including manual emptying may be indicated, and the use of parenteral neostigmine (0.25mg) on alternate days, or Ubretid (Berk Pharmaceuticals) (1.25mg) given orally may assist.

The use of specific antibiotics in control of the resultant cystitis is indicated and megestrol acetate (Ovarid, Glaxo) has also proved useful in this respect.

Hansen (1977) suggests that some cases are caused by a persistent urachus which can be corrected surgically.

Vesicular Calculi

Vesicular calculus formation in the cat is rare and commoner in the female than the male [Frost (1958)]. The common crystal in a series of 14 cases examined by crystallography was struvite, magnesium ammonium phosphate hexahydrate (Jackson).

Presenting symptoms resemble those of chronic cystitis.

Treatment. Removal by cystotomy of all calculi, followed by a prolonged course of therapy with a specific antibiotic in an attempt to prevent recurrence.

Prophylactic measures such as the replacement of dehydrated foods by foods of high moisture content and attention to fluid intake by provision of milk, gravy and fresh water drinks reduces the risk of recurrence and has proved effective in two queens that had a second vesicular calculus episode before these prophylactic measures were instigated.

REFERENCES

Biewenga W.J. (1975) *J. Am. Vet. Med. Assoc.,* **166(5)**, 460-462. (Preputial urethroplasty for the relief of urethral obstruction in the male cat).

Bloom, F. (1957) *N. Amer. Vet.* **38**, 114.

Burrows C.F. and Bovee K.C. (1977) *J. Am. Vet. Med. Assoc.* In Press.

Carbone M.G. (1963) *J. Am. Vet. Med. Assoc.,* **143**, 34. (Perineal urethrostomy to relieve urethral obstruction in the male cat).

Christensen M.A. (1964) *J. Am. Vet. Med. Assoc.,* **145**, 903. (Preputial urethrostomy in the male cat).

Cotter S.M.; Hardy W.P.; Essex M. (1975) *J. A.V.M.A.* **166**, 449.

Denny, H.R. (1972) *Vet. Annual* 13th Ed., 133-140. (The surgical techniques for urethrostomy in the male cat).

Evans J.M. (1976) Personal Communication.

Frost R.C. (1958) *Vet.Rec.,* **70**, 765-766. (Cystic calculi in the cat).

Gaskell C.J. (1973) *Vet Annual* 14th Ed., 139. (Urolithiasis in cats: treatment).

Gaskel C.J., Denny H.R., Jackson O.F. and Weaver A.D. (1978) *J. Small Anim. Pract.* In Press. (Clinical management of the feline urological syndrome).

Greene R.W. and Scott R.C. (1975) Feline Urolithiasis Syndrome. In: Textbook of Veterinary Internal Medicine (Ed. by S.J. Ettinger), p. 1568. W.B. Saunders Company, Philadelphia.

Hansen J.S., (1972), *Vet. Med. Small Anim. Clin.* **67**, 1090. (Persistent urachal ligament in the cat).

Jackson O.F. (1970) *Vet. Rec.* **87**, 667. (The use of sterile walpole's buffer solution pH 4.5 as a diagnostic agent and a treatment of struvite urolithiasis in the cat).

Jackson O.F. (1971) *J. Small Anim. Pract.* **12**, 555. (The treatment and subsequent prevention of struvite urolithiasis in cats).

Johnston D.E. (1974) *J. Small Anim. Pract.* **15**, 421. (Feline urethrostomy—a critique and new method).

Long P.D. (1977) *J. Small Anim. Pract.* **18**, 407. (A technique for perineal urethrostomy in the cat).

Mendham J.H. (1970) *J. Small Anim. Pract.* **II**, 709-721. (A description and evaluation of antepubic urethrostomy in the male cat).

North, D.C. (1978). *J. Small Anim. Pract.* **19**, 237-240.

Osborne C.A., Hardy R.M. and Finco D.R. (1972) Therapeutic and Prophylactic After Care of Cats with Cystitis, Urethritis, Urethral Obstruction Syndrome. Procs. 39th Ann. Meeting Am. Anim. Hosp. Assoc., 182.

Parks J. (1975) *J. Am. Anim. Hosp. Assoc.,* **11**, 102. (Electrocardiographic abnormalities from serum electrolyte imbalance due to feline urethral obstruction).

Schaer M. (1975) *J. Am. Anim. Hosp. Assoc.,* **11**, 106. (The Use of regular insulin the treatment of hyperkalaemia in cats with urethral obstruction).

Skelcher, P.B., Steele R.B.T. (1978) *Vet. Rec.,* **102**, 98. (Use of a silicone shunt for the surgical relief of feline urethral obstruction).

Smith, J.E. (1964) *J.Small An. Pract.* **5**, 517.

Smith, J.E. (1964) Personal communication.

Walker A.D., Weaver A.D., Anderson R.S., Crighton G.W., Fennell C., Gaskell C.J. and Wilkinson G.T. (1977). *J. Small Anim. Pract.,* **18**, 283. (An epidemiological survey of the feline urological syndrome).

SUGGESTED FURTHER READING

Pierson, D. L. & Grollman, S. S. (1960) *Acta Anat.* **40**, 385. (Absence of one kidney and abnormal development of the uterus in the domestic cat.)

Whitehead, J. E. (1961) *Small An. Clin.* **1**, 307. (Urolithiasis in the feline.)

Bloom, F. (1960) Gamma Publications Inc. New York. (The urine of the dog and cat; analysis and interpretation.)

Chapter 14

REPRODUCTIVE SYSTEM

Before considering diseases of the reproductive organs it is necessary to consider certain facts of the sexual cycle of cats. It is essential to appreciate that the cat is a highly sexed animal with a relatively brief period of sexual quiescence annually, usually between late September and the last week of December. It cannot be too strongly emphasised that the segregation of entire cats of either sex which prevents a regular breeding life is to be condemned; it can be regarded as tantamount to cruelty. For this reason the neutering of the vast majority of cats to be kept as household pets is to be recommended especially in urban and suburban areas where the opportunities for sexual activity are very limited due to unbalanced sex ratios, which can lead to considerable nuisance from noise and spraying.

There seems to be comparatively little written concerning the sexual behaviour and cycles of the cat living a free existence. Nearly all the literature refers to cats kept in captivity either as experimental colonies or in breeding catteries in which there are some significant deviations from the state of affairs prevailing in the free-living cat. From observation of ordinary cats living an uncontrolled existence in an average suburban area and from prolonged practice experience, the following points emerge:

1. *Breeding season.* This starts usually in the week after Christmas as may be deduced from the behaviour of entire toms and the incidence of cat bite sepsis; thus the early litters are likely to arrive during February. Its duration is variable, the main breeding season for many female cats finishing in May or June (litters born July and August) while others show an oestrus cycle as late as July–August with correspondingly late litters; an unusually mild autumn may result in a final cycle during September. From late September to the third week in December most cats of both sexes are relatively quiescent.

2. *Puberty.* There is a marked difference between the sexes and a great deal depends upon the time of year at which an individual kitten is born.

It is not uncommon for kittens to have their first oestrus cycle at $3\frac{1}{2}$ months, concrete evidence of this being the presence of 28 day foetal units in kittens presented for spaying which were known positively to be only $4\frac{1}{2}$ months old at that time.

On the other hand the first cycle in kittens born in March–April may be delayed until the following spring, being then 10–12 months of age. Climatic conditions may have some bearing on this, cold summers tending to delay sexual maturity until the following year.

Although the number of litters born annually to ageing cats may be reduced, queens continue to show oestrus cycles well into old age, 14–15 years being well recognised.

Puberty in the male is seldom reached before 10–12 months of age and in some subjects is not attained until the second spring after their birth, making some toms 18–20 months of age before breeding activity is shown. At this point it may be mentioned that many male cats towards the end of the breeding season (July–August) show a marked deterioration in general condition with loss of bodyweight, poorness of coat and a somewhat hidebound feel of the skin; the abdomen is often somewhat tucked up and the large kidneys characteristic of breeding males are not only very easily palpable but may be visible as 'swellings' in the flank, for which owners may seek advice. Entire males are often presented to veterinary surgeons at this time of year for general unthriftiness, the fear occasionally being expressed by owners that the cat is tubercular.

3. *Signs and periodicity of oestrus*. Visible physical signs such as vulval swelling or discharge are minimal, in fact often impossible to detect. Occasionally slight moistness and oedema of the vulval labiae may be noted but no reliance can be placed on these signs.

Evidence of oestrus is simply the behaviour of the cat herself. Many normal free-living females simply stay out for prolonged periods and may be absent for several days. Others show restlessness and increased vocal activity particularly in the Siamese in which the constant calling during oestrus may be well nigh intolerable. This increased vocal expression has given rise to the usual term applied to oestrus in the cat by laymen, i.e. 'calling'. Some cats, especially kittens during their first oestrus cycle when they may be too nervous or inexperienced to go out to seek males will indulge in constant rolling and crying which often causes emergency calls to veterinary surgeons to attend a cat that is 'writhing in agony'. A very small minority of queens are of such nervous disposition that they will neither go out to seek males nor permit the entry of males to their own territory. These, together with the very few physiologically sterile cats and those kept in enforced segregation form the bulk of pyometra cases met in feline patients.

In view of the absence of obvious physical signs of oestrus and the fact that behavioural changes may pass unnoticed in cats at liberty, the exact normal periodicity of oestrus cycles remains to some extent a matter for conjecture. It is usually described as being a 3 weekly cycle with active oestrus occupying 1 week of this time. It seems probable that during the breeding season queens which do not become pregnant remain in a constant state of 'potential' oestrus with waves of varying intensity from apparent quiescence to obvious 'calling'. These waves occupy some 7–10 days of alternating intensities but if during the period of apparent quiescence contact with a tom is permitted frank oestrus is stimulated very rapidly. Pseudo-pregnancy only occurs following a sterile mating or an artificial stimulus which simulates coition.

The return of oestrus following kittening is variable, some females remaining anoestrus throughout lactation whereas others become pregnant within 7—10 days of parturition or at any subsequent stage during lactation. This again is proved conclusively by the number of cats which are spayed when nursing kittens of some 6 weeks of age and are found to be as much as 28–35 days pregnant. Mating behaviour may be modified in nursing queens which often appear to be in a state of conflict between their maternal duties and sexual instincts; the prolonged stage of courtship is often omitted, the female remaining away from her litter only a sufficient time for very brief courtship and mating to occur. The obvious signs of oestrus such as calling and restlessness are often suppressed.

4. *Mating behaviour.* Prolonged courtship by several males before eventual acceptance of one is usual, the queen remaining out for hours or days at a time, not even necessarily returning for food, during which time she is surrounded by several males making tentative advances which are repulsed until the stage of selection and acceptance is reached. This period may vary from 12–96 hours. This is followed by a period of some 24 hours during which service from one male may be accepted several times. It is highly probable that this period of courtship is required to stimulate follicle development to the stage when rupture (ovulation) will follow the stimulus of coitus—the so-called trigger ovulation. The significance of this lies in the difference between natural and controlled mating, the latter only permitting contact at selected intervals, and may account for the usual high fecundity of street cats as compared with the irregular breeding so often complained of by pedigree cat breeders

The full co-operation of the queen is essential to the act of coition, i.e. the appropriate posture must be adopted. This comprises flexing of the hocks with the feet placed somewhat behind the cat resulting in raising the perineum to an almost horizontal position and correspondingly tilting the vulval orifice from a vertical to horizontal plane to permit introduction of the penis of the male, hence forced matings in the cat are not feasible.

Gestation

Is classically described as being 63 days but the usual variation tends to be in the direction of a longer rather than a shorter period, i.e. 64–66 days. Kittens born before the fifty-sixth day are unlikely to survive. Categorical figures for duration of pregnancy are only available for captive cats in which the date of service is accurately known and for those very rare street cats which, lacking modesty, copulate under their owners' noses!

Diagnosis of pregnancy. Palpation. Abdominal palpation being easy in the cat this is the simplest method and may detect very early foetal units, i.e. 19–22 days. It is usually accepted that ovulation occurs at some 24–30 hours post-coitus and fertilized ova enter the uterus 5 days later, implantation probably taking place at 13–14 days.

At 19–22 days the foetal units are felt as pea-sized enlargements in the uterine cornua; at 28–32 days they are tensely spherical and easily palpable, some 2–2·5 cm. in diameter. By 35 days the constrictions between units are disappearing, the units themselves becoming ovoid and less tense and hence less easily palpable. Abdominal distension becomes evident when the cat is pregnant with multiple foetuses at some 33–40 days. Foetal heads and outlines are palpable from 49 days (at which stage the skeleton is becoming radiographically visible) and remain so throughout the remainder of pregnancy.

Nipples, especially in primigravidae, often become turgid, pink and erectile from some 16 days post-coitus. Mammary development is palpable during the last few days of pregnancy.

Appetite usually remains good or is increased; behaviour may be unchanged or become more tranquil and affectionate.

MANAGEMENT DURING PREGNANCY AND PREPARATIONS FOR KITTENING

Since this book purports to deal mainly with the individual household cat rather than the more specialized problems of catteries it is proper to say that provided the cat is receiving a reasonable diet little need be done during pregnancy. The solely raw meat and water diet which is beloved of some cat breeders is not adequate and is to be strongly deplored. Increased appetite is better catered for by increasing the number of meals and ensuring that constituents are highly nutritious rather than giving a larger single meal. Vitamin supplementation during the latter half of pregnancy is wise if not essential.

Normal exercise, jumping and climbing are continued until term. It is highly desirable that the cat should have some provision made in late pregnancy for a suitable place to have her kittens. A box inside a cupboard is ideal, e.g. the lower part of a dresser, as all cats seek cover and at least semi-darkness for parturition.

Normal parturition

Since cats have been less subjected to mutation by man, problems of parturition are less common than in many other domestic species. Furthermore the independent relationship of cat to man eliminates the emotional dependence so often seen in dogs and thus obviates the problems associated with conflicts between natural instincts and, acquired emotional ties. It is interesting to note that in the Siamese cat which approximates most closely the canine temperament in certain respects, first stage labour is occasionally accompanied by undue apprehension and even hysterical behaviour.

First stage labour is less obvious in objective signs than in the dog and is usually only manifest by a desire for solitude and repeated sorties to the place selected for kittening; some bed-making usually takes place. Occasionally the latter part of first stage is accompanied by panting.

Second stage is marked by the commencement of visible voluntary straining initiated by engagement of the presenting part, usually the head, of the foetus in the pelvic inlet. With the exception of the more flattened face of the Long-haired (Persian) types foetal head shape is uniform, thus engagement rarely presents problems. Posterior presentation is fairly common and may be regarded as normal but if it occurs in the first foetus to be delivered may cause some delay in full initiation of voluntary straining and thus result in slower delivery. 5–30 minutes straining usually effects delivery; time intervals between foetuses are variable but usually comparatively short, 10–60 minutes. It is important to recognise that in the cat a variant of normal occurs in the form of interrupted labour; part of the litter is delivered normally and easily and there is an interval of 12–24 hours during which time the queen behaves as though parturition is completed yet there are obviously further foetuses still in utero. Examination in such patients fails to show any abnormality: the queen is well, restful and eating, the kittens already born are progressing normally, there is no evidence of obstructive dystokia and none of the foetuses still in utero is yet approaching the pelvic inlet. No interference is called for in such cases; second stage labour is resumed within 12–24 hours and delivery of the remainder of the litter completed without any difficulty. The reason for this interrupted type labour is not known.

Third stage labour, expulsion of foetal membranes, is normally repeated with or after each delivery but sets of membranes may be held up and delivered after a further one or two births. It is rarely that assistance is needed in separating the umbilical cord, most queens being perfectly well able to sever the cord and subsequently eating the membranes.

Abnormal Parturition. Dystokia

Prolonged first stage

Very occasionally considerable apprehension with inhibition of the normal progress of labour is seen, usually in the Siamese. The cat may refuse to be left alone, following the owner and crying constantly; such behaviour may verge on hysteria and in these cases ataractics such as chlorpromazine (10 mg. intramuscularly) are most valuable in allaying apprehension and allowing parturition to proceed.

180

Uterine inertia

Very rare in the cat. The intermittence described above does not appear to be in any way related to a secondary inertia. Inertia is occasionally associated with low litter numbers, especially the single foetus pregnancy.

Cases have been seen in which second stage labour apparently proceeds normally with reasonably strong, regular contractions until the head is delivered; the cat then rests on its laurels making no attempt to expel the trunk of the kitten, resting with the foetal head fully delivered through the vulva; in such cases it is necessary to complete delivery with manual assistance if asphyxia of the kitten is to be avoided. This condition has been seen mainly in highly temperamental Siamese.

Abnormalities of the maternal pelvis

Almost invariably the result of fracture of the pelvis in a street accident with displacement and distortion on healing. It is highly desirable that all female cats having a fractured pelvis should be spayed as soon as possible thereafter to terminate any existing pregnancy and prevent future breeding. Vaginal neoplasms are rare and have not been recorded as causes of dystokia.

Foetal causes of Dystokia

Oversize is comparatively rare in the cat and is usually relative only. Foetal monstrosities (hydrocephalus, anasarca) have been seen.

Malpresentations do occur and cause obstructive dystokia, mainly lateral deviation of the head. The fact that the birth canal of the cat is so small renders manipulation and correction of abnormal postures difficult or impossible.

Treatment of Dystokia. Medical treatment is extremely limited being confined to appropriate tranquillisation or sedation during abnormal first stage and the very occasional use of ecbolics.

Ecbolics are not indicated in the interrupted labour mentioned under normal parturition. They may be used with discretion in cases of relative oversize to augment the force of normal contractions but care must be taken to see that obstructive dystokia does not exist.

Manipulative treatment is confined to assisted delivery in cases of partial delivery previously described and additional traction, preferably by fingers, but if essential, by Rampley's sponge forceps applied to a presented part, in cases of relative oversize. Digital correction of abnormal posture can occasionally be achieved.

Surgical treatment is the method of choice in many cases, both Caesarean section and Caesarean hysterectomy being well tolerated in the cat.

Caesarean section is the method to be performed in all early cases where putrefaction is not already occurring. Anaesthesia is preferably by volatile agent by open mask, e.g. halothane, ether, trilene, preceded by medication with atropine and pethidine or promazine.

The flank approach is ideal and the surgical technique is routine.

Caesarean hysterectomy is indicated in cases where future pregnancies are undesirable, e.g. obstructive dystokia due to fractured pelvis or when neutering is requested by the owner at the time of parturition necessitating surgical treatment. It is well tolerated in this species and is not contra-indicated.

Whilst the quick recovery from volatile anaesthetics is desirable the choice of agent may be widened to include intravenous (never intraperitoneal) barbiturates if live kittens are not required.

The flank approach is again the method of choice, ovarohysterectomy being performed by the routine technique taking care to ligate the ovarian and middle uterine arteries adequately with catgut. Total ovarohysterectomy at term does not interfere with the institution and maintenance of lactation.

Complications of the Puerperium

Retention of foetal membranes

Not a common occurrence but it should be suspected in any cat which shows evidence of malaise or abdominal discomfort in the 24–72 hours following parturition. Temperature may be slightly raised, appetite poor and the presence of a brownish vaginal discharge noted; abdominal palpation discloses the thickened section of uterus from which the membranes have not been expelled.

Treatment is by administration of stilboestrol (0·5 mg. orally or subcutaneously) and/or small doses of posterior pituitary extract or oxytocin (2–3 units intramuscularly). Routine antibiotic cover is advisable.

Metritis

Occasionally occurs within 3 days of parturition being completed. The cat is obviously ill, may ignore her kittens, is off food, dull and has an increased desire for water; vomiting may occur. A purulent brownish vaginal discharge is present in variable quantity; on palpation the uterus is slightly thickened and may be sensitive to pressure. Temperature is usually moderately raised 39·2–40° C. (102·5–104° F.).

Treatment is by antibacterial drugs, sulphonamides or antibiotics, e.g. penicillin. In view of the desirability of attaining a rapidly effective blood level the use of crystalline penicillin for the first dose is advisable. Failure of quick response to penicillin indicates recourse to a broad spectrum antibiotic, e.g. chlortetracycline or oxytetracycline.

Mastitis

Acute suppurative mastitis occasionally occurs during the period 2–14 days post-parturient.

Usually only one gland—commonly posterior or penultimate—is involved. The lesion is hot and painful causing the cat to be distressed by the conflict between her desire to suckle her kittens and the pain occasioned by doing so. On examination a mammary gland is found to be enlarged, indurated, hot and painful; localisation of pus may result in pointing and rupture. Anorexia, dulness and fever are present.

Antibacterial therapy together with local application of heat and expression of pus (incision if necessary) are usually quickly effective. It may be necessary to devise some form of bandaging to prevent kittens attempting to suckle the infected gland. The usual course is for secretion of milk to cease in that gland for the remainder of that lactation.

Lactation Tetany

Although not a common occurrence in the cat the condition has recently been well documented by Lawler (1963) and others. Age incidence is not significant, recorded cases having occurred in cats between 14 months and 5 years of age. Usually the cat is nursing a biggish litter (5 or 6 kittens) and the time of onset of tetany varies from 17 days to 8 weeks post-kittening.

Symptoms comprise inco-ordination especially of forelimbs, tetanic spasm of muscles and the onset within a few hours of collapse or even coma. A variety of other signs have been noted by various observers, e.g. dry sclera, dry mouth, dilation of pupils and rapid or panting respiration.

Treatment is by intravenous and/or subcutaneous injection of a suitable calcium preparation, usually 20 per cent calcium borogluconate. The intravenous dose should not exceed 2 ml. augmented by 2–5 ml. subcutaneously. Response is usually spectacular. Dosage may be repeated in 24 hours if deemed advisable, by the subcutaneous route only. Kittens should be removed, reduced in number and/or augmented feeding instituted. Any queen which has had an attack of lactation tetany should subsequently be allowed to rear only a relatively small number of kittens, not exceeding four.

Abnormalities of pregnancy and parturition such as uterine rupture, torsion and prolapse are not uncommon and have likewise been well documented recently (see references).

The signs may be those of an abdominal catastrophe and exact diagnosis may only be made at laparotomy.

Any evidence of severe illness in late pregnancy, during or immediately following parturition, is an indication for early emergency laparotomy when the exact cause will be ascertained. It is usually necessary to perform ovaro-hysterectomy which again is surprisingly well tolerated. Dramatic recoveries following extremely serious uterine lesions are the rule rather than the exception, thus attempted operation is always to be advised.

All grades of severity are seen from the 'acute abdomen' to mild local symptoms such as vaginal discharge. Uterine prolapse is obvious, abdominal palpation may reveal abnormality but its exact nature can often not be ascertained, e.g. whether foetuses are intra- or extra-uterine.

Preparation must be made for whatever surgical technique is called for when the nature of the abnormality becomes clear at laparotomy.

This group of conditions admirably illustrates the great resistance and recuperative powers of the cat in face of extreme abdominal disaster, thus prognosis is always reasonably optimistic unless the patient is shocked or collapsed when presented.

Castration and Spaying

The neutering of cats of both sexes is the commonest surgical procedure carried out in practice. While the term castration may be properly applied to the removal of gonads in either sex it is proposed to adhere to the terms castration for the male and spaying for the female.

Castration

As previously indicated is a highly desirable operation in the vast majority of male cats. The effects of castration if performed before puberty are to prevent the development of secondary sex characters such as the hypertrophy of the skin of the cheeks and the characteristic but unpleasant odour of tom cat urine; increased amounts of fat are often laid down both in generalised subcutaneous distribution and in specific localities such as the inguinal folds. Sexual instincts are abolished thus straying is minimised and fighting usually markedly decreased; the latter statement is deliberately modified as some neutered cats retain a strong sense of territory and may attack intruders. It is generally believed that neutering decreases hunting instincts; observation suggests that this is more a matter of inherited behaviour rather than sexual status, cats coming from known hunting strains usually continuing to be excellent vermin killers even after castration. It may well be that in cats which have only a moderately developed hunting instinct this can be decreased by neutering. The point is of some importance in relation to advice regarding castration of cats kept on business premises to deal with vermin and it seems that it is more important to ensure that the cats concerned come from known hunting strains rather than to maintain them entire; the latter has the disadvantage that spraying, the stench of cat urine and absence on breeding expeditions often militates against their usefulness and is undesirable in such places as food shops.

AGE

Although it is customary to castrate kittens before puberty it cannot be too strongly emphasised that cats of any age can be safely and advantageously castrated.

It is physically possible to castrate kittens as young as 6 weeks of age since testes are often present in the scrotum within 3 days of birth.

Owing to a legal requirement (now no longer in force) that general anaesthesia be induced for castration of kittens over 6 months of age it has become customary to recommend that it be performed prior to 6 months. Anaesthesia is now required for castration of cats of all ages so that the choice of age can depend on other criteria.

The age of 4–5 months is ideal for most kittens by which time the testicles are adequately developed but not yet functional so that the blood supply is minimal. Some of the pure breeds such as Siamese, Burmese and Abyssinian are less well developed than corresponding 'alley' cats of the same age and castration may be deferred a further 2–3 weeks. The advantage of leaving castration as long as is easily practicable is that it permits the development of some masculine character in the head; the contention regarding urethral development is not proven but could be a further reason for not castrating too young.

Adult cats, as previously stated, can be castrated at any age but it is highly desirable to select the period of sexual quiescence, viz. late September to Christmas, whenever possible. The reason for this suggestion is to minimise shock, both physical (highly active vascular gonads) and psychological (sudden abolition of sexual instinct in mid-breeding season). Adult cats settle well after castration with decrease in incidence of cat bite sepsis, less wandering and improved bodily condition. Many owners who have been reluctant to consent to castration in an adult cat have volunteered the opinion that the cats seem 'happier' as a result.

ANAESTHESIA

This is a difficult question particularly in the light of changed legislation and there must be many shades of opinion regarding it. Since the predominantly painful stimulus is the traction on the spermatic cord during separation and not the incision of the scrotum which, if done precisely with a sharp knife, is of minimal duration and pain it becomes obvious that analgesia of skin and distal cord is not enough. The only logical conclusion is that general anaesthesia must be induced which in young kitten castration somewhat resembles taking a sledge-hammer to kill a gnat.

The choice of anaesthetic agent, anaesthesia now being obligatory, must rest with the clinician, sensible criteria being that it shall be easily and rapidly induced with minimum voluntary resistance, that recovery shall be smooth and rapid and that peripheral vasodilation shall not be a feature. At the present time halothane by open mask, despite its cost, is probably the best choice.

All adult cats must be anaesthetised both on humane grounds and for proper restraint, quite apart from legal considerations. The quick recovery from volatile agents is to be preferred but occasionally intravenous thiopentone sodium will be the agent of choice, the tendency for peripheral vasodilation being of no importance as proper steps for adequate haemostasis are essential in older cats.

Surgical technique

Kittens. In short-haired cats the use of copious surgical spirit on the scrotum is adequate but in long-hairs some removal of hair is desirable and this is better accomplished by plucking than clipping. The scrotum is incised precisely, the primary incision usually severing tunica vaginalis reflexa at the same time; the testicle is grasped and the cord separated by traction. This method usually means that some 3–6 cm. of spermatic cord come away with the testicle thus separation is occurring at approximately inguinal canal level. Any fat and/or tunica vaginalis protruding through the scrotal incision should be trimmed away so that there is no possibility of tissue remaining. The scrotal wound is not sutured. The procedure is repeated on the other side the whole occupying only a matter of seconds. In young kittens with poorly developed testes great care must be taken in grasping the testicle prior to incision that the penis is not damaged. The statement is self evident but it is not unknown for amputation of the penis to occur during castration.

Adult cats. Basically the technique is similar but greater care must be taken over hair removal and cleansing of the scrotal skin. The main problem is that of satisfactory haemostasis and a wide variety of methods is adopted.

Simple forci pressure with two pairs of Spencer Well's artery forceps applied closely adjacent to one another and subsequent twisting off of the cord between the two by rotation of the more distal forceps is adequate in young adult cats with large but relatively inactive testes.

Once breeding has commenced the testes become more vascular and even in the quiescent season the calibre of blood-vessels is quite considerable. Methods of haemostasis used in such cats are severing the cord by actual cautery, ligating with cat gut, knotting the cord itself or by the application of specially designed clamps.

No cat, young or old, should be castrated unless it is in good health and free from any lesion of cat bite sepsis. Failure to observe this simple precaution can lead to serious infection in the scrotum.

If, as occasionally happens, an owner insists on castration before an infected lesion is completely healed the prognosis must be suitably guarded and the operation performed under pre- and post-operative antibiotic cover.

Complications. Rare in average cases. One case has been seen in a young kitten (the usual 4–4½ months) in which haemorrhage occurred and continued despite treatment and terminated fatally in 3 days when the abdomen was found to be filled with virtually unclotted blood; the case was presumably one of haemophilia. In adults haemorrhage can follow inadequate haemostasis. Infection of the scrotum in adult cats if proper surgical cleanliness is not observed or if a septic lesion exists, is another hazard.

The development of sexual alopecia due to sudden withdrawal of androgen has been seen in one cat castrated just after Christmas when testicular activity was probably rapidly increasing.

Cryptorchid Castration

Feline testes are often palpable in the scrotum at birth; thus it seems

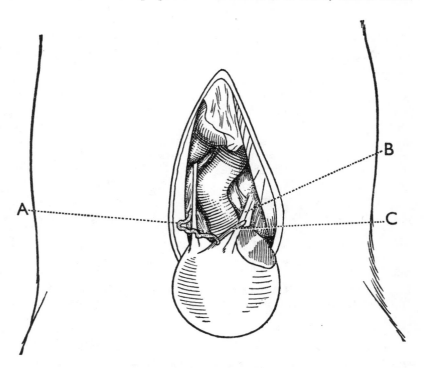

FIG. 26 Technique of cryptorchid castration; urinary bladder is reflected posteriorly through incision showing:
    A. Slack convoluted vas deferens attached to the undescended testis.
    B. Fold of peritoneum associated with ureter.
    C. Tense vas deferens attached to descended testis.

clear that early descent is normal. Unilateral retention of a testicle either in the inguinal region or abdomen is occasionally met.

Kittens presented with one descended testicle (no case of bilateral cryptorchidism can be recalled) may be left entire until 8–10 months of age by which time it may be taken as pretty certain that further descent will not occur.

It is very unwise to remove one descended testicle. If for any exceptional reason this is done a careful record *must* be kept of the side from which the testicle was removed.

Operation for removal of both normal and ectopic testes should be strongly recommended as nothing is more disconcerting than an apparently neutered cat with all the habits and disadvantages of an entire.

If the retained testicle is inguinal operation is by obvious and simple methods.

There is equally a simple and pleasing technique for the removal of abdominal testes.

Under general anaesthesia the cat is restrained on its back and the incision made in the mid-line with the posterior commissure 0·5–1·25 cm. anterior to the pelvic brim, as for cystotomy. The bladder is brought out of the incision and reflected backwards; a tense fold of peritoneum with much fat is associated with the ureters and between these can be readily recognised two white tubular structures with no fat, the vasa deferentia. The vas to the descended testicle will be tense and obviously entering the inguinal ring; that attached to the abdominal testicle is slack, often a little corrugated, and traction on it brings into view the spermatic artery and usually the testicle. The vessel is ligated, the vas sectioned and the testicle removed. The normal testicle is then dealt with routinely.

In the rare cases when traction on the cord does not bring the ectopic testes into view it may be assumed that the gonad is actually incarcerated in the inguinal canal. Ligation and section of spermatic artery and vas will result in functional castration and eventual atrophy of the testicle.

Spaying

Cats can be spayed at any age; it is physically possible at 7–8 weeks and well tolerated in aged subjects. It can also be performed during pregnancy with ease to 28 or 30 days and without apparent adverse effect as late as 49 days.

The spaying of female cats is a highly desirable operation in all cats which cannot be permitted to lead a regular breeding life. It is inhumane to keep entire female cats in enforced segregation which may, apart from humanitarian considerations, result in disease in later life, i.e. pyometra.

AGE

Owners often ask if a cat should be allowed to breed one litter before being spayed. There seems to be little advantage in this, the disadvantages of spaying kittens before puberty not being comparable to the similar situation in the bitch, e.g. infantile vulva leading to intractable perivulval dermatitis; the conformation of the feline vulva does not predispose to this condition. Surgically the ideal age is $3\frac{1}{2}$–$4\frac{1}{2}$ months, the majority of kittens of this age not being sexually mature thus the blood supply to uterus and ovaries is minimal and ligation of vessels not required. It must be emphasised, however, that some kittens may have an oestrus cycle at 3½ months, and be found as much as 28 days pregnant when spayed at 4½ months. The signs of this first heat are often not noticed by the owner hence even careful enquiry may fail to elicit the fact that the animal is already sexually mature.

In the case of kittens and cats over 5 months careful enquiry should always be made in an attempt to ascertain the cat's sexual status since many owners delay arranging for operation until the nuisance of the first oestrus occurs when they will keep the cat in and seek an immediate appointment. All possible steps should be taken to avoid spaying cats in oestrus. Not only are blood-vessels greatly engorged necessitating careful ligation but the uterus itself is vascular, foreshortened, thickened and extremely friable making the approach to the vaginal end both difficult and hazardous. Operation should be refused for cats on heat and advice given to allow the cat freedom to get mated, to telephone for a further appointment when the cat has settled (usually quite obvious to the owner) and arrange to operate at 7–10 days of pregnancy. It is *not* sufficient to await the more quiescent part of the oestrus cycle since, in the absence of impregnation, the uterus will retain its erectile, vascular character rendering surgery difficult.

Anaesthesia

A volatile agent should preferably be selected, e.g. ether, halothane, trichloroethylene, since the duration of the operation is so short and the prolonged recovery time associated with barbiturates is unnecessary. Pre-anaesthetic medication with atropine and/or promazine is a matter of personal choice and decision. It is not essential but will obviate the copious salivation occasionally seen and mitigate the period of voluntary struggling during induction.

Many practitioners, however, prefer barbiturate anaesthesia despite prolonged recovery times and the possible consequence of peripheral vasodilation; if barbiturates are selected the choice will be between intravenous thiopentone or pentobarbitone sodium or the latter intraperitoneally or even orally, the latter routes having the disadvantage of irregular response to an arbitrarily assessed dose.

PREPARATION

Sex must be checked; failure to carry out this routine precaution will result in totally unnecessary laparotomies on male cats. Should this unfortunately occur it cannot be too strongly emphasised that the owner should be told the truth. Allowing the owner tacitly to accept the fact that the cat is a female can result in untoward sequelae such as the subsequent presentation of the cat in later life with urethral obstruction when the veterinary surgeon unthinkingly remarks that this is quite a common condition in neutered males, only to be told by the owner 'but it is a female, you spayed her 6 years ago'. Difficulties arise in the case of stray females taken in at over 5 months of age and it is impossible to decide whether they have already been spayed; the owner must be advised either to wait and see if oestrus or kittens ensue or to allow exploratory laparotomy—most prefer to take the latter course.

Clipping of the appropriate area of the flank may be undertaken in the conscious, medicated or anaesthetised patient as conditions indicate. Shaving is unnecessary if a fine clipper head is used. An adequate area to permit surgical cleanliness *must* be clipped; pandering to owners by preparing a 'key-hole' site is surgically improper; it must be clearly understood that despite its apparent triviality spaying comprises total ovarohysterectomy and as such is a major operation demanding a proper surgical approach.

When anaesthetised the bladder should be emptied by pressure, a suitable bowl being held to catch the urine expressed from the vulva; failure to make this a regular feature of spaying routine results in punctured bladders as an occasional but totally unwarranted complication.

It is desirable that food should have been withheld for 12–18 hours prior to operation.

Technique

A. KITTENS

Approach via the left flank (the right flank may be selected by left-handed surgeons) is the method of choice.

The kitten is hobbled and tied down in lateral recumbency with fore and hind limbs fully extended; this is essential for correct location of the landmark for incision. Football bootlaces make excellent hobbles for cats and kittens.

The clipped area is cleaned with spirit or other agent of the veterinary surgeon's choice and drapes are applied.

The exact siting of the incision is vital to speedy operation. The site is best located by recognising firstly the external angle of the ilium, secondly the great trochanter of the femur and then completing an isosceles triangle when the remaining angle of that triangle will be the site for incision. This method allows for varying sizes of cat, the vertical distance below the external angle of the ilium being necessarily greater to form an isosceles triangle in larger cats.

A small skin incision, which should never need to exceed half an inch in kittens, is made obliquely downwards and backwards through the predetermined point; subcutaneous connective tissue is divided and it is permissible to excise a small amount of subcutaneous fat to expose the fibres of the external oblique muscle. Frequently a blood-vessel which bleeds freely for a few seconds but which does not require ligating is incised with the fat. The external oblique is incised in the direction of its fibres which exposes internal oblique; this, together with the usually closely adherent transversalis, is picked up tent-wise in forceps and

190

incised. The uterine horn is located by recognising and picking up the pad of retroperitoneal fat which is characterised by its homogeneous appearance and relatively fixed nature as compared with the mobile lobular omentum. The broad ligament of the uterus is attached to the under surface of this fat, withdrawal of which through the incision will bring into view the membranous broad ligament on its ventro-medial aspect. The uterine cornua and/or ovary is thus drawn into the incision. The horn is picked up and the left ovary drawn through the incision and upwards, exposing the fairly long ovarian ligament. A pair of Spencer Well's artery forceps is applied as low down as possible on this ligament, and a second pair applied immediately above; both can be easily placed well below the ovary. The second pair is used to separate the ligament by torsion, the under pair being left clamped *in situ* for a few seconds longer. The left ovary and horn is then drawn backwards horizontally, parallel with and close to the draped hind limb. This will bring into view the bifurcation of the uterine cornua and the right horn is picked up in dressing forceps and drawn through the incision. The right ovary is brought through the incision and dealt with similarly to the left. Both uterine horns are then picked up and artery forceps applied as far posteriorly as possible by pressure of the forceps down into the flank rather than traction upwards on the uterus; in most cases it is possible to place the forceps well below the bifurcation and often posterior to the cervix thus achieving panhysterectomy which is desirable. Separation at the vaginal end is performed identically with that used for the ovaries, crushing and torsion being adequate for haemostasis. The abdominal incision is repaired in one, two or three layers. Experience shows that linen thread is an ideal suture material for all layers, no untoward sequelae ever having been noted to follow its use in many thousands of cases. The use of antibacterial topical application or antibiotic cover should be unnecessary.

B. OLDER CATS

The technique used is identical except that haemostasis by ligation of ovarian and middle uterine arteries is necessary. No tissue reaction has ever been noted using linen thread for ligatures but in pregnant cats with very large blood-vessels catgut is a better choice. According to the size and character of the uterine body the ligature may be an encircling one, including both arteries, or by individual ligation of each middle uterine vessel on the lateral aspect of the uterine body including a small portion of uterine tissue in each ligature.

The initial incision must be gauged to suit the circumstances e.g. 28 day pregnancy and will usually be some 1·25–3·5 cm. in length. For repair of incisions over 1·25 cm. in length fine catgut, (00 or 0) is to be preferred for internal sutures. Light bowel clamps (Doyens) should be used at the vaginal end rather than artery forceps.

The necessity for careful ligation of vessels increases the time taken for operation very considerably. Whereas a practised surgeon will complete a kitten spay within 3 minutes it is seldom that an adult cat can be dealt with in less than 10–12 minutes.

COMPLICATIONS AT OR AFTER OPERATION

1. A cystic condition associated with either or both ovaries. This is occasionally met in cats of all age groups including young kittens. Inability to draw an ovary through the usual abdominal incision arouses suspicion; it is often necessary to enlarge the incision considerably before the ovary can be exteriorized.

2. Congenital anomalies of the uterus.

(a) Absence of uterine body, both cornua continuing posteriorly into the pelvis ununited and entering the vagina as separate structures; this condition is occasionally met and may cause some dismay when the bifurcation cannot be located.

It may be possible to locate the right cornu via the initial incision but it may be necessary to perform a double-flank operation and deal with this cornu and ovary by a right flank approach.

(b) Absence of one cornu.

On rare occasions one uterine cornu is vestigial in development and represented by a ligamentous structure only. Care must be taken in such cases to remove both ovaries.

3. Breaking of a horn during operation.

Most likely to occur in cats found to be in or near oestrus, the fragile tissue being easily torn or cut by artery forceps no matter how carefully applied. Haemorrhage is seldom serious but steps must be taken to remove the separated cornu and related ovary then or later.

POST-OPERATIVE

Haemorrhage is rarely serious and only likely to occur in haemophiliac kittens or older cats in which haemostasis has been inadequate.

Wound infection is likewise rare if proper surgical cleanliness is observed. The occurrence of infection in a number of spay wounds during a relatively short period is a signal for a critical assessment of technique, operating premises and equipment. The handling of a case of cat sepsis during the 24 hours prior to spaying, no matter how carefully the surgeon scrubs up, often results in infected wounds. When it is impossible to avoid doing spays after a 'dirty' cat case has been handled gloves should be worn and/or antibiotic cover supplied.

Spay appointments should not be made during any serious epidemic of feline enteritis in the practice area.

Persistence or recurrence of oestrus behaviour is occasionally reported following spaying. In most cases this can be traced to faulty surgical technique but sometimes there can be no doubt as to the correctness and completeness of operation and such cases remain unexplained.

One case has been seen in which cervicitis occurred in an adult cat spayed after breeding in which panhysterectomy had not been achieved, the cervical secretion was apparently sufficient to attract males whose constant attentions to the non-receptive female caused her to become neurotic and as the owners would not permit further surgery euthanasia was performed.

Granulomata of the ovarian or vaginal stumps have not been seen.

If for any reason an ovary with or without uterine horn is not completely extirpated at initial operation the advice should be to re-operate on the appropriate side about a month later, the owner being clearly informed that oestrus on pregnancy in the remaining organ can occur.

Although in cases due to congenital anomalies no possible blame can attach to the surgeon it is none the less a pleasant gesture to modify or even remit the fee for re-operation depending on circumstances.

Sexual alopecia in spayed females is uncommon and urinary incontinence has not been seen.

Pyometra

The incidence of pyometra varies considerably in different localities being highest in those areas where unspayed queens are prevented from breeding by enforced segregation. In most places female cats are either neutered or allowed to breed freely and in such the incidence of pyometra is very low. It is essentially a disease of the older non-breeding female hence queens which are either physiologically sterile or those failing to get mated due to abnormally timid temperament are particularly prone. The condition, as distinct from endometritis, is usually acute.

Symptoms. General depression and malaise, failure of appetite, abdominal distension, vomiting and thirst are all features of the disease. Abdominal distension occurs with remarkable rapidity and reaches an advanced degree within 24–48 hours. Temperature is usually raised.

The combination of severe illness and abdominal distension in a non-breeding queen are often enough to justify a firm diagnosis. The distended uterus can frequently be clearly palpated. Most cases are closed but vaginal discharge of pus occasionally occurs, the flow being usually less copious than in open pyometra of the bitch.

Differential diagnosis will relate mainly to cardiac, hepatic and chylous ascites.

Treatment. Surgical only, by early ovarohysterectomy. The technique is as for spaying, via a left flank incision of 5–6·5 cm. in length, ligation of ovarian and middle uterine vessels being essential and preferably by catgut.

The uterus is tensely distended with pus and usually very thin-walled hence great care must be exercised in opening the abdomen and handling the organ.

Prognosis. Good if early operation is performed.

Endometritis

Whilst it is appreciated that pathologically there may be a close relationship with pyometra the two syndromes are clinically fairly distinct, endometritis being much less acute and may even be chronic.

Clinical sub-divisions of endometritis are possible.

A. In the younger non-breeding queen a low grade endometritis is often seen. It is most likely to occur in pedigree show cats in which breeding is deliberately deferred. Age incidence can be from 2 years onwards.

Vaginal discharge is common varying from a viscid mucus to frank pus hence a common symptom is frequent licking of the vulva. In long-haired breeds soiling of the 'trousers' may be noted. General ill-health is variable: during remissions it may be normal but during more acute phases (which often follow an oestrus cycle) appetite is lost or decreased, the cat is dull and disinclined to move about, temperature may be raised to 39·2–39·4° C. (102·5–103° F.), vomiting and thirst are occasional.

The uterus is frequently palpable being enlarged and thick-walled.

The disease may persist weeks or months during which oestrus periods of variable frequency and intensity occur.

The condition is slowly progressive and eventually causes a marked deterioration in condition and even death.

Treatment. Surgical, by ovarohysterectomy. Medical treatment is not effective. Advice to spay is often resisted by owners who still hope to breed from the cat at their own convenience. Such cats will not breed.

Prognosis is good unless owner resistance causes too much delay.

B. In older breeding queens of all types a syndrome is clearly recognised comprising the following stages:

1. Decreased litter numbers.
2. Neo-natal deaths and stillbirths.
3. Abortions, increasingly early.
4. Fairly acute endometritis.

Several complete breeding cycles are usually completed before the clinical picture clarifies. It is almost certainly due to a low-grade bacterial infection of the uterus progressive endometrial changes causing the changing stages described. In both endometritis and pyometra the role of *E. coli* is important (Smith, 1964), haemolytic staphylococci are occasionally involved.

Once recognised, treatment is by ovarohysterectomy which is well tolerated even in really aged cats (13 years +) hence prognosis is good.

C. Tuberculous endometritis; this is not common but the uterus is an organ not infrequently involved in feline tuberculosis which is itself becoming steadily less common.

A case has been seen in a young Siamese queen (ca. 9 months) which

194

showed abnormal discharge at and after her first oestrus cycle. Advice to spay was resisted as the owner wished to breed from the cat but persisting discharge, loss of condition and some fever necessitated surgery. The uterus was thrown into spiral rugae and was tensely thickened, partly due to oestrus. A rapid improvement in general health followed operation but within a few weeks fatal tuberculous peritonitis supervened. Regrettably vaginal discharge was not examined for tubercle bacilli pre-operatively as specific infection was not suspected.

Male Genitalia

TESTES

Are frequently absent and thus comparatively rarely the seat of disease. Neoplasia is rare but in one 13-year-old cat an embryonal carcinoma was found in the left testis and interstitial cell nodular hyperplasia in the right.

PROSTATE

Atrophic in neuters hence is not a source of trouble. Freak (personal communication) records the case of a 10-year-old cat with an enlarged prostate which showed the classical picture of interference with defaecation as seen in the dog.

PENIS

Involved indirectly in urinary obstruction when the penile urethra is involved. The penis becomes bruised and haemorrhagic after attempts at digital relief but spontaneous return to normal quickly occurs.

Female Genitalia

Neoplasia

Neoplasia of uterus and vagina is not common. Obviously the former can occur only in entire females. Vaginal tumours have been recorded in entire queens.

In the neoplasm series surveyed one fibromyoma of the uterus of a 12-year-old cat occurred and one vaginal fibroma in a 9-year-old. Wolke has recorded vaginal leiomyomata in cats of 8 and 14 years causing mechanical interference with defaecation.

MAMMARY GLAND

Mastitis has already been described and is usually the acute condition seen during lactation. Chronic inflammatory lesions such as are seen in the bitch are extremely rare.

Neoplasia

Neoplasms of the mammary glands occur reasonably frequently, mainly in entire females with a regular breeding history but some occur in spayed females and cases have been recorded in castrated males.

The commonest site is the anterior (pectoral) glands and the majority are malignant, (carcinomata or adenocarcinomata); metastasis is common. Peak age incidence is about 12 years.

The lesion is often not noticed until ulceration, necrosis and surface infection have occurred when the owners attention is drawn to it by frequent washing by the cat or the foul smell. The tumours are usually flattened and plaque-like and often cratered, particularly after skin ulceration has occurred.

Treatment is by early surgery, mastectomy being the technique of choice.

Prognosis is always guarded in view of the high incidence of malignancy and early metastasis. Spread is via the axillary lymphatic node and vessels or haematogenous direct to lungs.

Any cat with a mammary tumour should be carefully examined for evidence of local lymphatic or pulmonary secondaries before treatment is discussed and advised.

The following are details of the six cases of mammary neoplasia occurring in the quoted series:

Age	Sex	Site	Histology
1. 16 years	♀	Penultimate mamma.	Adenocarcinoma.
2. 12 years	♂	Right penultimate nipple and mamma.	Cystadenoma resembling mammary neoplasm.
3. Aged	♀	Not noted.	Adenocarcinoma and lung metastasis.
4. 12 years	♀	Right axillary mamma.	Carcinoma metastasis in lymphnodes, lungs and pleura.
5. —	♀	Abdominal mamma.	Adenocarcinoma.
6. 12 years	♀	Left axillary mamma.	Adenocarcinoma.

It will be noted that of the above six cases two are atypical as regards sex and two as to site, case 2 being unusual in both respects but despite this the usual picture is as previously described.

REFERENCES

Lawler, D. C. (1963) Vet. Rec. **75**, 811.
Smith, J. E. (1964) J. Small An. Pract. **5**, 517.
Wolke, R. E. (1963) J. Amer. Vet. Medical Association **143**, 1103.
Freak, M. J. (1963) Personal communication.

SUGGESTED FURTHER READING

Lactation tetany
Dildine, S. C. (1929) Vet. Bull. U.S. Army **23**, 220.
Gardner, D. E. (1957) New Zealand Vet. J. **5**, 110.
James-Ashburner, P. W. (1961) Vet. Rec. **73**, 884.
Milnes, D. M. (1963) Vet. Rec. **75**, 1341.
Vigue, R. F. (1953) Vet. Med. **48**, 70.

Uterine torsion, rupture, prolapse etc.
Allen, G. S. (1964) *Vet. Rec.* **76**, 355.
Arnall, L. (1961) *Vet. Rec.* **73**, 750.
Boswood, B. (1963) *Vet. Rec.* **75**, 1044.
Lewis, M. R. W. (1954) *Vet. Rec.* **66**, 243.
Luckhurst, J. (1961) *Vet. Rec.* **73**, 728.
Newman, M. A. H. (1961) *Vet. Rec.* **73**, 680.
Newman, M. A. H. (1961) *Vet. Rec.* **73**, 1269.
Philcox, R. A. & Pepper, R. T. (1964) *Vet. Rec.* **76**, 386.
Thompson, F. G. A. (1961) *Vet. Rec.* **73**, 892.
Wilkinson, G. T. (1951) *Vet. Rec.* **63**, 470.
Young, R. C. & Hiscock, R. H. (1963) *Vet. Rec.* **75**, 872.

Dow, C. (1963) *Vet. Rec.* **75**, 141. (The cystic hyperplasia-pyometra complex in the cat.)
Bignozzi, L. (1955) *Veterinaria Milano* **4**, 9. (Cystic mastitis in a cat.)

197

Chapter 15

HERNIAE

Hernia

Diaphragmatic rupture and hernia has already been dealt with (see Diaphragm); inguinal hernia is rare and no case of scrotal hernia has been seen in 24 years of practice experience. Of the congenital herniae umbilical is quite common as is acquired ventral hernia.

Umbilical hernia

Both small and large ringed umbilical herniae are seen, the latter being fairly common with the ring some 1–13 cm. in length. The contents are fat, omentum and frequently small intestine. The defect is frequently first noticed when the cat is presented for spaying although occasionally advice is sought for this alone. Figures of sex incidence are not available but experience suggests that it is commoner in females.

The small ringed herniae (ring less than 0·5 cm.) are of no consequence and seldom demand treatment.

Large ringed cases neither incarcerate nor strangulate but in view of the jumping propensities of the species with the possibility of tearing of the ventral abdominal skin on objects such as projecting nails or wire surgical correction is advisable. It is both feasible and practical to undertake hernia repair at the same time as ovarohysterectomy is performed, but it must be emphasised that spaying via the hernia opening is not possible without considerable extension of the mid-line incision posteriorly; it is far better to spay via the usual small flank incision and repair the hernia at the appropriate site.

Anaesthesia is as for spaying and the technique is the usual one for umbilical herniorrhaphy, taking care to enlarge the ring sufficiently to prepare an elliptical opening for suturing and to freshen the muscle edges by removal of the peritoneal sealing of the lips of the ring. Results are excellent.

Ventral Hernia

Rupture of the musculature of the abdominal wall is quite common in the cat as a result of external violence and results in the development of ventral herniae.

Any part of the abdominal wall may be involved, common sites being the anterior and more superior part of the flank and the insertion of the rectus abdominis into the pubic brim.

The signs are those of a suddenly developed swelling, usually asymmetrical in character; there may be a history of accident. Palpation of the swelling sometimes results in the easy recognition of coils of small intestine in a subcutaneous position and frequently the torn edges of the muscles can be accurately detected.

Differential diagnosis must exclude haematoma and abscess formation, also localised or diffuse lipomatosis since these are sometimes described by owners as having been 'sudden' in onset. Careful examination should be made to eliminate other injuries or lesions which may have resulted from the trauma, e.g. sub-capsular kidney haemorrhage, as this will have a bearing on the timing of surgical treatment.

Treatment is surgical and is usually eminently satisfactory even in extensive defects. Operation should be undertaken as soon as possible having regard to shock and other lesions so that muscle retraction and scarring is minimal.

Under general anaesthesia a generous incision is made over the defect and the rents in the muscle or muscles clearly recognised. Herniated viscera are returned to the abdomen and the torn muscle edges freshened if necessary and sutured with catgut or linen thread. All muscle layers must be carefully examined as the defects are not necessarily superimposed on one another. Extensive 'darning' is often necessary.

When the rectus abdominis is torn from the pubis, omentum and small intestine may track down the loose subcutaneous tissues on the medial aspect of the thigh creating what could reasonably be described as a femoral hernia. Even at this difficult site with little anchorage for sutures repair is usually successful. Prognosis is therefore good.

Chapter 16

THE SKIN

Skin diseases in animals present the veterinary surgeon with many problems in daily practice and the cat is no exception in this respect. As is customary these will be considered under the conventional divisions of parasitic and non-parasitic diseases.

Parasitic Skin Diseases

1. Fleas

Many cats are parasitised by fleas, mainly *Ctenocephalides* spp. but also occasionally the human flea *Pulex irritans* and the species infesting birds and hedgehogs, *Ceratophylus* spp., is occasionally involved. The striking fact clinically is that the severity of infestation bears little relationship to the severity of symptoms in that cats carrying a really heavy burden may show minimal signs whereas a single flea may produce almost maniacal response in others.

Symptoms include scratching and biting and in some cases extreme hyperaesthesia of the posterior dorsum resulting in most exaggerated response if this area is stroked or scratched. Sudden jumping and constant twitching of the skin of the trunk by panniculus activity are also seen. The cat often 'growls' for no apparent reason.

Symptoms may be so bizarre and severe that owners flatly refuse to believe they can be due to something so mundane as flea infestation! Whilst the dorsum, especially the more posterior part, is the region most commonly involved all areas of the body may harbour fleas, frequent sites being the soft fluffy hair of the inside and back of thighs and the head and under the chin.

Diagnosis is based on finding the parasites themselves or their excreta; the deep 0·5-1 cm. of coat harbouring variable quantities of these hard, shiny, blackish spherical bodies sometimes so copious that it is difficult to reach the skin. The finding of even one speck of typical excrement is sufficient to warrant a firm diagnosis. In many cases the fleas remain in the cat's bedding only visiting the host tissues to feed hence detection of the fleas themselves is not always easy. Cats of any age and under any management can be infested, including quite young kittens still in the nest.

In many cases the coat and skin remain apparently unaffected but in some individuals alopecia and broken hairs are common. Whilst the exaggerated response to a light infestation shown by some individuals may be a form of hypersensitivity reaction, the so-called 'flea allergy' as seen in the dog very seldom occurs.

Treatment. Is by the use of appropriate parasiticides, carefully selected and used in the light of the cat's habit of grooming by licking with consequent risk of ingestion of toxic dressings. D.D.T. (Dicophane) should *never* be used on cats which are very susceptible to its toxic effects; neither should dieldrin ever be used. Derris remains a very valuable agent for eliminating fleas but should be used only as a dry dusting powder. Gamma benzene hexachloride is also useful and as well as being used as a dusting powder, it may be used occasionally as a medicated shampoo (0·05 per cent suspension) but in such form is preferably used on a limited part of the body only although combined with equal parts of sulphur it has been used safely as a shampoo for the whole body. Gamma BHC has the disadvantage of causing some increase in the activity of fleas before killing them hence reports of intense skin irritation of short duration following application of gamma benzene hexachloride preparations have been received.

Pybuthrin (pyrethrum synergised with piperonyl butoxide) is also valuable as a dry dusting powder for use on cats for which it is regarded as particularly safe.

All dressings should be repeated at 7–10 day intervals and attention should be paid to cleaning and disinfestation of sleeping places. In dealing with flea infestations it is essential that the whole body shall be effectively dressed otherwise fleas will simply migrate to 'safe' areas. Dusting powders should be applied by careful sprinkling all over the body, subsequent working in of the dressing by massage with the spread fingers against the lie of the coat and finally rubbing over the hair, with the lie of the coat, with a clean duster or chamois leather to remove excess powder from the hair surface and so avoid undue ingestion of the powder.

It must be remembered that elimination of fleas and lice is an essential part of treatment for infestation with *Dipylidium caninum*.

2. Lice

A relatively rare infestation in the cat and then usually by the biting louse *Felicolla substrata*.

Symptoms of skin irritation and, in very heavy infestations, anaemia, may be seen.

Treatment is as recommended for fleas.

3. Ticks

In some localities infestation with ticks, *Ixodes* spp., is common in cats probably with hedgehogs as the natural host, and can thus occur in urban as well as rural areas.

Whilst any part of the body may be involved the head, ears and neck are the common sites. Occasionally a single engorged tick is seen but not infrequently examination reveals 30–40 parasites in various stages of engorgement. The ears, forehead, top of skull and parotid region are all frequently found infested.

A common history is that the cat has suddenly developed a 'growth' or 'cyst' on its head; examination discloses the extremely characteristic parasite.

Treatment varies according to the number of parasites found. A single tick is often dealt with by applying a swab of ether or chloroform to cause the tick to release its hold so that withdrawal of the embedded head is facilitated. Even so the head is often detached during removal. The result of the deep attachment of the tick is formation of a smallish granuloma which is slow to resolve; when necessary resolution may be assisted by application of non-staining Iodine Ointment. Owners should always be warned that a small persistent swelling will result. An alternative and equally effective treatment is to apply a paste of gamma BHC in water to the tick and leave it to fall off. Suitably diluted gamma BHC suspensions may be applied to the whole head and neck in severe cases and in patients in whom infestations are recurrent regular (10–14 day) dressing with this agent will prevent attachment of ticks during the relevant period.

4. Harvest Mites. (*Trombicula autumnalis*)

Infestation with this parasite is even more localised than in the case of ticks hence in some practice areas it is never seen while in others it is a well recognised problem. Attacks occur mainly in warm damp conditions. The parasite causes intense pruritus and tends to attach itself to areas of thin relatively hairless skin, e.g. the interdigital fossae, where they may be seen as clusters of orange red dots. Treatment with gamma benzene hetrachloride and/or sulphur is efficacious.

5. Mange Mites

Otodectes, Notoedres and Cheyletiella are the mites of importance in cats.

Otodectes cynotis has already been dealt with under the heading of ears.

Notoedric Mange

This is a moderately common and usually relatively mild disease nearly always confined to the head and neck. In the mildest cases lesions are confined to the thinly furred area of skin between the ears and eyes.

Symptoms noted are frequent washing of this area and scratching. On examination the area is found to be virtually hairless and a scratch reflex can usually be evoked.

In more severe cases the convex surface of the pinna, the top of the head and the back of the neck may be involved; rarely the condition spreads over the withers and down the dorsum. In chronic neglected cases the skin becomes bald, thickened and corrugated and self-inflicted lesions may become secondarily infected with pyogenic organisms with resultant ill-health.

Treatment by gamma benzene hexachloride (0·05 per cent) and/or sulphur as a wash to affected areas twice weekly is usually readily effective. In the very localised cases first described application of ordinary sulphur ointment may be sufficient. Only in severe cases is dressing of the whole body necessary.

Diagnosis is based largely on the distribution of lesions with pruritus and may be confirmed by routine skin scrapings.

Prognosis is usually good.

Cheyletiella parasitivorax

Infestation with this parasite causes no signs or lesions in the cat but is of importance since it may cause a severe and obscure pruritus in humans.

The mite is not a burrower hence it may be demonstrated in combings from infested cats.

In any case where in-contact humans develop a highly irritable rash on the forearms and chest (parts which will come into contact with a cat which is sitting on its owner's lap) which is said to resemble scabies, the cat should be examined for presence of Cheyletiella. Whilst not common it is sufficiently frequent to warrant emphasis as a possible cause of skin disease in man.

The parasite is readily eliminated by use of gamma BHC and sulphur preparations.

Blow Fly Strike

Although not common, cats are occasionally subject to blow fly strike by *Lucilia sericata*; this is more likely to occur in aged cats which are sluggish in mental and/or physical reaction.

The perinaeum is the usual site when it has become soiled by urine or faeces but slow-healing infected wounds or abscess cavities may likewise be attacked.

The cat shows great discomfort and even pain, is extremely restless and often apparently cannot locate the source of irritation. There is a characteristic odour in these cases associated with the activities of larvae which are initially surface feeders but later burrow into the tissues causing severe inflammation, serous exudation and eventually cavitation. The struck cat may rapidly become severely ill and even after removal of the maggots the necrotic areas are extremely slow to heal.

Treatment. Usually necessitates anaesthesia in order to clip the affected area thoroughly and remove all larvae. A very large area usually requires clipping as maggots may be found in the hair some distance from the main focus. Creams containing gamma BHC are most helpful in dealing with this peculiarly revolting lesion. Subsequently, supportive

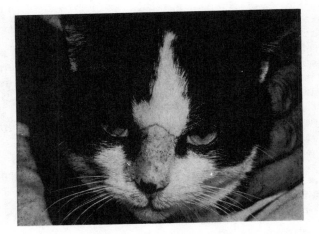

FIG. 27 *M. Canis*. Natural Infection. Lesion before start of treatment. (Reproduced by courtesy of the editor, Journal of Animal Technicians)

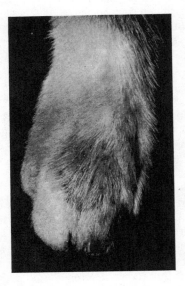

FIG. 28 *M. Canis*. Spontaneous infection

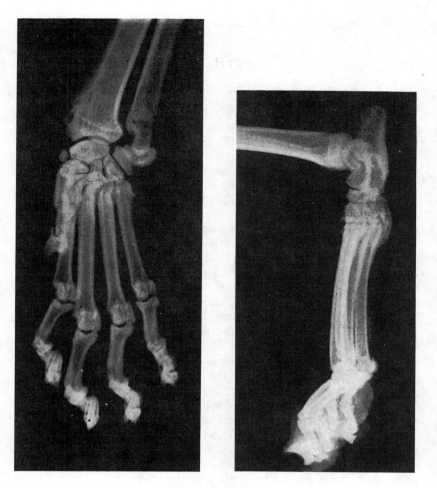

RHEUMATOID ARTHRITIS

FIG. 29 Rheumatoid Arthritis. (*left*) Carpus of 8-year-old castrated male Siamese showing peripheral changes of medial aspect lower end radius and increased joint spaces in carpus

FIG. 30 Rheumatoid Arthritis. (*right*) Tarsus of same cat showing periarticular changes ankylosing hock

treatment and routine attention to the damaged tissues is all that is required

Ringworm in cats

(C. J. La Touche, L.A.H.(Dublin), M.C.Path., M.Sc., M.I.Biol.)

Ringworm in cats, more especially in kittens, is a superficial fungal infection which involves the skin as well as its appendages: the hair, whiskers, and occasionally even the claws. Only the horny layer of the skin, the stratum corneum, is affected, but this includes also the intrafollicular stratum corneum, moreover, while the deeper layers of the skin are not invaded, a deep-seated inflammatory reaction may sometimes result from infection. The dermatophyte fungus, *Microsporum canis* Bodin is the most frequent etiologic agent in ringworm occurring in cats. The infection due to this species presents in either of two clinical forms: acute which is more frequently encountered in kittens, or chronic, found more frequently in adult cats. In the acute form, in adults and kittens, the local reaction appears to vary according to the individual or the strain of *M. canis*, some infected animals exhibiting a severe inflammatory response, with erythema, scaling and serous exudation as well as the breaking off of hair and depilation; others exhibit merely some matting of the scales due to exudation of serum in addition to the breaking off of hair and depilation. Even in the same individual, lesions vary in appearance because they are in different stages of their evolution. In the chronic form, scaling and thinning of the hair may be the only indications of infection on superficial examination. Indeed some infected cats exhibit even less naked eye signs of infection, the hair being only dull in patches. Finally, there may be no naked eye signs at all. These cats are 'carriers' and may carry their infections for many months or even years. The most frequent sites in which lesions may be found are: the head, the back, the tail, the inner aspect of the thighs and the paws. A frequent finding is mottling of the bridge of the nose due to punctate lesions, or thinning of the hair of the eyebrows or ears, and all these sites may be involved in the same animal. During an examination of a suspected animal no part should be neglected, and it is therefore advisable to examine in the particular order which is the same each time. A good site to start with is the head. Diagnosis by the unaided eye is unreliable, as thinning of the hair and scaling may be due to other causes. Other aids, such as the use of the Wood's lamp and microscopical examination make for certain diagnosis. The Wood's lamp is a source of ultraviolet light filtered by glass impregnated with nickel oxide. This enables the examiner of a suspected animal to detect infection by *M. canis* in hair, whiskers or claws, because when these structures are invaded by the dermatophyte a substance is produced in them which emits a pale but bright green fluorescence. The lamp should be held over the cat in such a way that light emitted from the side of the bulb shines on the part being examined. This is made possible by having one side of the lamp-shade cut away. Such an examination enables the observer to detect even traces of infection represented by only a few hairs, whiskers or claws. Very occasionally false fluorescence manifested by a green colour also, may be seen. For this reason, when possible, fluorescent hairs should be checked microscopically for evidence of infection. This can be done without difficulty by mounting such hair in a drop of 10 per cent caustic potash solution on a glass slide which is then placed on the stage of the microscope and examined successively with low and high magnification lenses. Air bubbles can be dispersed from the hair by slightly warming the slide over the flame of a spirit lamp. Infected hair shafts will be seen to be surrounded by a sheath made up of innumerable, minute, closely-packed, refractile (shining) granules (spores) associated with underlying threads, in and on the hair. At times oil drops on the hair may be misleading, but these may dissolve away by washing the hair in a little ether before mounting it in the caustic potash solution.

Ringworm in cats may be caused by another dermatophyte, the granular variety of *Trichophyton mentagrophytes* (Robin) Blanchard, which is commonly found on mice. It also causes scaliness and depilation with more or less exudation of serum, but hair infected with this dermatophyte does not emit a green fluorescence. Microscopical examination of suspected hairs and scales should therefore of necessity be carried out. The microscopical appearance of hairs infected by this dermatophyte is somewhat similar to that provided by hairs infected by *Microsporum canis*, although the spores making up the sheath around the hair tend to be somewhat larger than those produced by *M. canis*; moreover, on careful examination, chains of these spores may be seen on the surface of the hair or forming part of the sheath. Much depends on the stage of development of the fungus on the hair; at an early stage, chains are seen quite easily; at a late stage, with difficulty.

Lastly, cats, on rare occasions, present with a skin disease known as mouse favus. This is so called because the mouse is the natural host and the lesions it develops as a result of infection include the characteristic fungal crusts, known as scutula which are also seen in the lesions of human favus. These scutula are also found in the lesions developed by cats which have been in contact with mice infected by the etiologic organism *Trichophyton quinckeanum* McLeod and Muends, also thought to be merely a variety of *T. mentagrophytes*.

Treatment of these diseases is, as a rule difficult and often impractical. First of all it is time-consuming, and for this reason is expensive, both for the owner and for the veterinary surgeon. Until it is completely cured, a cat so infected remains a potential source of infection for humans. Indeed most ringworm in cats is detected usually only after one or more humans have developed ringworm. Furthermore, a veterinary surgeon would be reluctant to take over a cat with ringworm because of the risk of its spreading to other animals—cats and dogs—in his care. It is obvious therefore, that, unless special conditions are provided, treatment of a cat with ringworm should not be considered. However, despite these considerations, circumstances might arise when treatment might be thought desirable. The treatment of choice is griseofulvin administered orally in the dosage of about 60 mg./kg. daily. As this drug is usually dispensed in the form of tablets, these should be subdivided as required and may be crushed before being administered. Most kinds of topical applications are unsatisfactory as the vehicle in which they are contained fails to penetrate into the hair follicles adequately enough to bring the fungicide in contact with all the fungal parasite. In cases where lesions are minimal it helps sometimes to epilate fluorescent hair or non-fluorescent hair in lesions, because this diminishes the amount of infective agent present. Dry shampooing is also a useful supplementary measure. Treatment with griseofulvin may have to be continued for 2 months or more, but the doses may be reduced to 2 or 3 weekly after the first 2 weeks. The response is very variable. The treatment is the same for the various types of ringworm which occur in cats. Destruction of cats only suspected of having ringworm is all too common and is to be deplored, not only because of the emotional factor involved, but because this action may destroy valuable evidence as to the source of the infection, or may be misleading in so far as some other cat might have been the source of infection for the human patient.

In the past in Britain, human ringworm due to *Microsporum canis* was wide-spread, although more so in some districts than in others. In cities such as Bristol, Birmingham and Leeds, the incidence of infection due to this species amongst children was so high as to be a matter for concern for public health and educational authorities. In fact, in Leeds, a campaign for the elimination of the animal reservoir was started in 1950, with after several years, the gratifying result that ringworm of this type had very significantly diminished, and has now virtually disappeared from the community of that city. Doubtless, also, the provision of better housing conditions has been a contributory factor in diminishing the incidence of ringworm of all types among humans and animals, as also has the increasing awareness of its epidemiology among school medical officers and others concerned with child welfare and education. However, despite these favourable trends, constant vigilance, not only in schools, amongst those responsible but also in catteries and pet shops by owners of these establishments, is the only safeguard against the spread of this disfiguring and socially distasteful disease.

SUGGESTED FURTHER READING

La Touche, C. J. (1957) Ringworm in cats due to *Microsporum canis* Bodin. In Worden, A. N. & Lane-Petter, W. *U.F.A.W. Handbook on 'The Care & Management of Laboratory Animals'*, 2nd ed. 526–32. U.F.A.W.

La Touche, C. J. (1955) *Vet. Rec.* **67**, 578–9. Onychomycosis in cats due to *Microsporum canis* Bodin.

La Touche, C. J. & Forster, R. A. (1963) Sabouraudia, **3**, Pt. 1, 11–13. Chronic infection in a cat due to *Trichophyton mentagrophytes* (Robin) Blanchard.

La Touche, C. J. (1960) *Trans. of St. John's Hospital Dermatol. Soc.* Griseofulvin in natural and experimental infections in cats and chinchillas.

La Touche, C. J. (1961) *Advances in Small Animal Practice*, **2**, 90–3. London, Pergamon Press. Fungi as skin parasites of domestic pets.

La Touche, C. J. (1955) *Vet. Rec.* **67**, 666–9. The importance of the animal reservoir of infection in the epidemiology of animal-type ringworm in man.

Rebell, G., Timmons, M. S., Lamb, J. H., Hicks, P. K., Groves, B. S. & Coalson, R. E. (1956) *Amer. J. of Vet. Res.* **17**, No. 62, 74–8. Experimental *Microsporum canis* infections in kittens.

Uvarov, Olga (1961) *Vet. Rec.* **73**, No. 11, 258–62. Recent advances in the treatment of skin diseases with special reference to griseofulvin.

Georg, Lucille K., Roberts, C. S., Menges, R. W. & Kaplan, W. (1957) *J. Amer. Vet. Medical Association*, **130**, No. 10, 427–32. *Trichophyton mentagrophytes* infection in dogs and cats.

Kaplan, W. & Ajello, L. (1959) *J. Amer. Vet. Medical Association*, **135**, 253–61. Oral treatment of spontaneous ringworm in cats.

Non-parasitic Diseases

1. Miliary Eczema

This is probably the commonest problem of the cat, other than sepsis, with which the veterinary surgeon has to deal; it is not an easy one.

The name is probably a misnomer since the lesions are scarcely eczematous but miliary is comparatively accurate in view of their size and type. The essential condition is so often complicated by other factors such as hypersensitivity, parasitic infestations and secondary bacterial invasion that it is not easy to get a clear picture of an uncomplicated case. To use a very brief generalisation, histologically the lesions are of a non-specific inflammatory nature often associated with the presence of mast cells in some number.

Clinically the lesions are papular in nature sometimes with pin-point serous or pustular oozing but more commonly capped by a small scab. The number present is very variable, from less than ten to uncountable lesions; pruritus is virtually invariable and the degree bears no relation to the number or type of lesions present.

The commonest site is the skin of the dorsum, particularly posteriorly just above the base of the tail; occasionally the only area affected is under the chin and down the under surface of the neck. In severe cases the whole body surface may be covered with lesions whereas in mild cases very careful and thorough finger-tip palpation is necessary to locate any eruptions. Hair loss is usual in the worst affected areas.

Licking and nibbling is more common than scratching but naturally either may occur according to the location of the irritation.

In advanced cases generalised hair loss occurs, the undercoat being completely lost and only scanty numbers of harsh and often broken guard hairs remain. At this stage the papular eruptions are clearly visible.

In some cases the whole body surface feels warm and moist as though generalised sweating were occurring; in others, areas of erythema, plaques of skin characterised by serous oozing and less commonly pustule formation are seen. In chronic cases skin thickening is usual.

Whilst general health cannot usually be said to be affected some cats are greatly distressed by the constant irritation and in really advanced long-standing cases a degree of emaciation may be seen.

Aetiology. This is a highly controversial matter and no cast-iron case can be made for any one theory. Hypotheses put forward include:

1. *Hormonal origin.* Protagonists of this theory maintain that the disease occurs almost entirely in neutered cats and that response to administration of androgens is good.

The fact remains however, that cases are regularly seen in entire males and females and since these comprise a relatively small proportion of the cat population seen by veterinary surgeons it is dangerous to generalise without carefully worked out percentages of both sexes and neuters thereof. The condition is not typical of other hormonal dermatoses and response to androgen therapy is so varied that it seems improbable that it is of solely endocrine origin.

2. *Parasites.* Protagonists of ectoparasites as the cause of a high proportion of skin disease in animals believe parasitism to be the essential factor despite failure to demonstrate such infestation.

It is true that the use of gamma BHC/sulphur washes is usually a very valuable therapeutic measure but it needs to be used in conjunction with other treatment to be fully effective hence it seems unlikely that miliary eczema is purely of parasitic origin.

3. *Diet.* Miliary eczema has been referred to as 'fish eaters skin' due to the fact that many affected cats are fed solely on fish. But so are many completely unaffected cats! Additionally, severe cases are regularly seen in cats on a most adequate mixed diet in which fish is a very minor constituent.

The response to administration of biotin is sufficiently good in many cases to justify thoughts as to the role of this vitamin in aetiology. It is probably not true to assume a frank deficiency in such cases since many diets would seem adequate in every respect but rather to question whether certain individuals are suffering a deficiency due to inadequate utilisation as an idiosyncratic factor rather than low intake.

Other dietary supplements are less effective than biotin in producing adequate response.

4. *Hypersensitivity.* It is tempting to blame an allergic response for miliary eczema and the claims for the value of antihistamine and anti-inflammatory drugs (especially corticosteroids) are based on this assumption; this response is almost certainly non-specific and there is

little evidence to support this view although hypersensitivity is a frequent complicating feature.

Metabolic factors may be implicated and it is of some interest to record that one very severe and extremely chronic case of miliary eczema in a castrated male short-haired cat which had been in existence over 8 years resolved spontaneously a few months before the animal developed diabetes mellitus.

Psychological reasons have been put forward as possibilities, e.g. boredom, since some patients improve markedly in a changed environment.

The truth is probably that the fundamental aetiology of the syndrome is still not identified and that all the factors mentioned may be involved, with dietary considerations predominating.

Treatment. None is specific despite many and varied claims. The administration of Megoestrol Acetate ('Ovarid', Glaxo.) is now probably the most effective treatment, but response is alleviative rather than curative and is apparently related to the immuno-suppressant effect of progestational agents. Another somewhat empirical line of approach is parenteral administration of biotin, together with regular washing of affected areas or even complete bathing with a gamma BHC and sulphur suspension of appropriate dilution (0·05 per cent) at 3–14 day intervals according to the need. Parenteral rather than oral administration of biotin is strongly advised on the assumption that faulty utilisation rather than frank deficiency is involved.

Diet should always be considered carefully and a suitable mixed protein intake advised including a fair proportion of raw or lightly cooked liver. White fish should be reduced, raw white fish prohibited, and oily fish such as herring and mackeral substituted. Vitamin supplementation, especially of A, B complex and C is advisable.

Antibacterial drugs to deal with pyogenic infection and antihistamines or corticosteroids to alleviate pruritus can be helpful, remembering the possible idiosyncratic response of the cat to the former group.

Hormonal treatment by testosterone implants is disappointing in miliary eczema cases which are not complicated by co-existence of an endocrine type alopecia.

Occasional dramatic response to griseofulvin has been met despite failure to demonstrate a fungal cause. Dosage is within the range 50–200 mg. daily in divided doses and is usually well tolerated. Response is prompt, within 7–10 days, and failure to respond within this period is an indication for withdrawal of the drug. Relapse in responded cases often follows withdrawal and administration may need to be continued over long periods or repeated at frequent intervals.

The percentage of cats responding to griseofulvin is small but the treatment is so spectacularly successful in these few that its exhibition is justified in any intractable case.

Topical applications other than gamma BHC/sulphur shampoos are seldom indicated since effective dressing in the cat is not easy unless self-interference is eliminated by application of an Elizabethan collar. The use of such restraining devices as collars and protective jackets may be helpful in obviating the complications and exacerbations caused by licking, biting and scratching but can scarcely be said to be a very constructive approach to this exceedingly difficult problem.

Prognosis. Always most guarded as to cure but reasonably good for temporary improvement. Much depends on the perseverance of the owner and the degree of co-operation which can be obtained from the cat to adjustment of diet, wet dressings and drug administration.

Endocrine Deficiencies.

1. *Sexual Alopecia.* This may be seen in neuters of both sexes in adult and ageing cats.

The signs are a non-pruritic hair loss commencing inside the thighs and groins and extending over the ventral surface of the abdomen and up the back of the thighs progressively. In severe chronic cases the baldness may extend up the flanks. Lesions are bilaterally symmetrical.

The skin is free of lesions and any hair remaining is of a soft fluffy character.

Androgen therapy by implantation of 25 mg. testosterone pellets is usually effective in both sexes; oestrogens should *not* be used as treated cats may be attractive to males and pestered by them for weeks or months. Oral administration and injection of androgens are not usually satisfactory.

Implants may need to be made at intervals of 3–12 months according to the duration of response.

2. *Hypothyroidism.* This is not a very clear cut entity in the cat but needs to be considered. Obesity is little guide but excessive sluggishness and decrease in quantity and quality of coat over the trunk are suggestive. Lesions are less localised and less frank alopecia occurs than in sexual alopecia.

Thyroid extract sicc. in a dose rate of 60–120 mg. ($\frac{1}{2}$–1 gr.) daily is often effective in restoring vitality and improving quality of hair coat; pulse or heart rate should be regularly checked during periods of thyroid administration, tachycardia being an indication for prompt withdrawal.

Allergic Dermatoses

Although apparently not so common as in the dog, skin lesions due to hypersensitivity in cats quite definitely occur. The difficulty of diagnosis lies in the fact that allergic dermatosis may be a primary condition or a secondary complicating factor of other underlying skin abnormalities such as miliary eczema. Lesions are not diagnostic in character but pruritus is usually severe and causes constant licking and biting; this results in areas of hair loss on various parts of the body, particularly the limbs, with evidence of inflammation in mild cases and with the development of plaques of serous, oozing lesions which may become scabbed over temporarily and occasionally invaded by pyogenic bacteria.

Unlike the dog allergens seem to be more commonly alimentary rather than contact and foodstuffs which have been incriminated include milk and all products of avian origin; the latter naturally creates considerable problems in cats which are natural bird hunters! Very occasionally a violent allergic response to penicillin therapy is seen. At present diagnosis is mainly based on trial and error by adjusting diet to exclude serially particular items; skin tests are of little value but serological methods being developed show promise.

Treatment comprises identification and elimination of any dietary factor incriminated and the use of suitable antihistamine drugs—always remembering the feline idiosyncracy to this group; corticosteroids will suppress inflammation and irritation, e.g. betamethasone 0·075–0·125 mg. b.d.

It is important that the possibility of hypersensitivity be borne in mind in any intractable skin condition characterised by pruritus and the development of plaque-like lesions and also as a possible complicating feature of other entities. Curiously enough although severe symptoms may be shown by cats infested by fleas the aptly termed acute 'flea allergy' so often seen in dogs appears to be infrequent.

'Lickers Skin'

The syndrome to which the above decidedly colloquial term has sometimes been applied is a quite clear cut clinical entity from the point of view of recognition but the lesions are non-specific and the aetiology probably multiple and equally non-specific. At the same time recognition is essential if adequate treatment is to be applied. The lesions are highly characteristic although quite variable according to the stage at which the patient is first presented. Typically, lesions occur mainly on the inner aspect of the thighs, also on the posterior aspect of the hind limbs above the hock but in advanced cases may be found elsewhere.

The owner's attention is usually attracted by the excessive licking of affected parts; at first this is assumed to be normal washing but the continuous and vigorous licking is soon recognised as being indicative of skin irritation. The lesions are essentially ulcerative in nature and a well-developed one will have thickened, reddened raised edges surrounding a roughly spherical area of skin from which the epithelium is denuded; it may even be cratered. Lesions vary from a few millimetres to 2 cm. in diameter and adjacent ulcers may become confluent with resultant very large areas of ulceration. The central surface may be scabbed, raw or oozing serous or purulent discharge.

Whilst bacteriologically and histologically lesions are non-specific, it seems proper to regard the condition as a low grade bacterial invasion of the dermis with the development of non-healing ulcers.

Treatment. It cannot be too strongly emphasised that purely topical treatment is useless except in a very early single lesion which is rarely seen. Neither is prevention of licking by suitable restraint the answer, although it may be a necessary adjunct.

Treatment must be local and general. Systemic treatment comprises antibacterial therapy, e.g. chlortetracycline 200–300 mg. daily in divided doses,with corticosteroids in low dosage introduced after several days on antibiotic. Vitamin supplementation is helpful.

Local treatment comprises attention to the lesions under general anaesthesia on one or more occasions as required. This consists of curetting each lesion very vigorously; it will be found that a coating of very soft granulation tissue lies quite thickly over the ulcer and this must be removed. A suitable solution of antibiotic and corticosteroid (usually penicillin and/or streptomycin with betamethasone) is injected under each lesion, the needle being introduced via normal skin adjacent to the ulcer, and subsequently the area is cauterised with 10 per cent solution of or even solid silver nitrate. Treatment must be continued until all lesions are completely healed and the cat is totally ignoring the areas involved; this usually means a course occupying 2–5 weeks. Response to this vigorous combined therapy is usually good.

A good response has also been achieved following application of cryosurgical techniques.

Prognosis is good for the immediate result but guarded as to recurrence. Some patients are cleared permanently.

Dietetic Factors

Clear cut dietary deficiencies are not readily recognisable in household cats unless one is prepared to accept a solely nutritional factor as being responsible for miliary eczema (see page 209). A general poorness of coat condition characterised by scurfiness, dryness and sparseness of guard hairs and deficiency of undercoat will often respond favourably to vitamin supplementation; if possible A, B, C and E should be provided in such supplements. Despite the fact that cats synthesise Vitamin C the desire of town cats to seek fresh vegetable matter is interesting and it seems wise to ensure that some natural source of this vitamin is available to all house or cattery-bound cats.

Skin Tumours

True neoplasms of skin are quite common in the cat (twenty-one in this series) as also are other tumour-like lesions, many of which show a tendency to spontaneous regression. The appended list illustrates the diversity of lesions found in the twenty-one cases quoted: together with the difficulty of making a clear-cut histological diagnosis in many.

Clearly a histo-pathological prognosis is highly desirable in all cases of tumour-like lesions surgically excised. It is improbable that ordinary clinical examination will be much guide to the nature of the lesion.

Recently Wilkinson has drawn attention to the occurrence of granulomatous lesions associated with an acid-fast bacillus morphologically resembling *Mycobacterium tuberculosis* in the cat; in all his cases euthanasia was performed. White records an apparently similar but

	Age	Sex	Site	Histology
1.	11 year	♂	Skin behind shoulder.	Epidermal inclusion cyst.
2.	10 year	♂		Basal-cell carcinoma, probably of hair follicle epithelium origin.
3.	7 year	♂		? Sarcoma.
4.	13 year	♂		? Sarcoma.
5.	10 year	♀	Skin behind right ear.	Myxoma.
6.	Adult cat.		Skin of hock.	Reticulosarcoma or granuloma.
7.	11½ year	♂	Left Carpus.	? Sarcoma.
8.	11 year	♀	Right inguinal fold.	Basal-cell carcinoma.
9.	10 year	♂	Skin behind shoulder.	Melanotic basal-cell carcinoma.
10.	8–9 year	♀	Skin of back.	Undifferentiated: malignant.
11.	10 year	♂	Inner aspect hock.	Haemangioma.
12.	17		Skin over mamma.	Adenocarcinoma.
13.	11 year	♂	Skin, multiple.	Undifferentiated epithelial tumour.
14.	17 year	♂	Scrotal skin.	Fibroma.
15.	9 year		Skin of breast.	Basal-cell carcinoma.
16.	14 year	♀	Skin back of neck.	Baso-squamous epidermal tumour.
17.	15 year	♀	Edge of ear flap.	Spindle cell tumour. ? Neurofibroma.
18.	8 year	♂	Skin under chin.	Pigmented basal-cell tumour, benign.
19.	11 year		Skin, forelimb.	Spindle-cell sarcoma.
20.	13 year	♂	Skin of back.	Baso-squamous carcinoma.
21.	8 year	♀	Skin, upper cervical area.	Melanotic epidermal tumour.

bacteriologically and histologically unconfirmed case in which there was regression following treatment.

The author has on record a similar case in which, unfortunately, after biopsy it was lost sight of, hence no follow-up or bacteriological investigation could be undertaken but it is believed spontaneous resolution occurred. Biopsy material from two skin lesions was examined which proved to be granulomatous in nature consisting of endothelioid cells with microscopic areas of caseation. Smears showed numbers of acid fast organisms morphologically resembling *M. tuberculosis*.

The tremendous range of proliferative lesions of the feline skin makes any definitive statements as to aetiology, nature and prognosis inadvisable. Each case needs full investigation and it is clear that this is a field for considerable research.

REFERENCES

White, K. (1964) *Vet. Rec.* **76**, 900.
Wilkinson, G. T. (1964) *Vet. Rec.* **76**, 777.
Wilkinson, G. T. (1964) *Vet. Rec.* **76**, 833.

SUGGESTED FURTHER READING

Head, K. W. (1958) *Brit. J. Derm.* **70**, 399–408. (Cutaneous mast-cell tumours in dog, cat and ox.)
Joshua, J. O. (1958) *Vet. Rec.* **70**, 193. (Non-parasitic skin diseases of the dog and cat.)
English, P. B. (1960) *Aust. Vet. J.* **36**, 85. (Notoedric mange in cats, with observations on its treatment with malathion.)
Clark, M. L. (1958) *Vet. Rec.* **70**, 502. (Cheyletiella parasitivorax infestation in the cat.)
Thornton, G. W. (1963) *Cornell Vet.* **53**, 144. (Diagnosis and treatment of common skin disorders of the cat.)
Cotchin, E. (1957) *Vet. Rec.* **69**, 425. (Neoplasia in the cat.)
Cotchin, E. (1956) *Brit. Vet. J.* **112**, 263. (Further examples of spontaneous neoplasms in the domestic cat.)

Chapter 17

THE SKELETAL SYSTEM

Damage to the skeletal system of cats is far commoner than the un-initiated believe, fractures and tendon damage both being reasonably frequent. Fractures associated with the head have been dealt with earlier. Disease of bone may occur as a complication of cat bite sepsis but this latter is so important a topic that both it and its sequelae are dealt with in a separate section.

It has previously been noted that cats are good surgical subjects and of no system is this more true than the skeleton. The repair of bones and tendons provides great scope for a surgeon's ingenuity and enterprise and all operations are well within the capability of any small animal surgeon of average ability; such surgical enterprise is usually more than justified and quite remarkable recoveries occur in the most unlikely cases, such is the cat's ability to adapt and compensate apparently gross mechanical defects. It is to be strongly urged that an attempt should be made to repair bones and tendons whenever it is within the bounds of humane considerations to do so.

General Considerations in Fracture Treatment

Despite the above optimistic generalisations there are certain limiting factors which must be clearly recognised and accepted. Cats are unable to tolerate heavy external splintage such as substantial plaster casts particularly on the hind limbs; the interference with the strongly developed balancing mechanisms causes considerable disorientation. Even comparatively light appliances create some disturbance causing the patient to adopt postures which appear to be distressing; for this reason it is wise to retain as in-patients cats to which casts have been applied for the few days required to enable the animal to adapt, otherwise owners may become unduly perturbed and even request euthanasia. It may well be that the Zimmer Finger Splint ($\frac{1}{2}$ inch width), to the use of which Sumner-Smith (1964) has drawn attention, will prove to have a place in the external fixation of feline fractures. On the credit side is the fact that cats, unlike dogs, seldom interfere with dressings such as plaster casts.

Methods of internal fixation are also subject to some limitations but intramedullary pinning of suitable bones (femur, tibia, humerus) is extremely easy; a straightforward femur pinning can be completed in approximately the time needed to spay an adult cat! On the other hand plating is seldom feasible due not only to the small calibre of the bones but to the convexity of most diaphyses of long bones, the surfaces of which will rarely accept a plate; even so the use of human finger plates is worth exploring in exceptional circumstances. In several bones the epiphyseal lines are much convoluted and in kittens with epiphyseal separations the epiphysis and diaphysis can be fitted together like pieces of a jig-saw puzzle during open reduction; it is often sufficient to wire these cases with temporary external fixation as a support for a short time at suitable sites, e.g. lower end tibia.

In the author's experience fractures of the hind limbs and pelvic girdle are far more frequent in cats than fore-limb fractures, but according to various workers in the field of small animal orthopaedics relative incidence between limbs and bones differs widely. An interesting table showing this occurs in a paper by Carter, 1964.

Various fairly common fractures and methods of treatment applicable are outlined below with only brief details of technique included.

Pelvis

Fractures of the pelvis are common usually as the result of crushing in street accidents. Ordinary clinical examination is often sufficient for diagnosis, disparity in length of limbs, crepitation and movement frequently being elicited during routine examination. Radiography will confirm diagnosis. It is necessary to suggest that radiographs should be viewed optimistically; even severe pelvic fractures heal so well that quite horrifying radiographic appearances may be disregarded so long as complications, such as that described by Freak (1962) of laceration of rectum by a bone fragment, are excluded by careful examination if damage to pelvic organs is suspected.

Treatment simply comprises rest for 14–28 days, preferably in a confined space such as a cage in a cattery.

If owners insist on nursing pelvis fractures at home advice should be given to make a suitable cage out of a tea chest. Confinement to a room is *not* sufficient. Adequate dietary intake should be ensured.

It is essential that in all cases the sex of the patient be checked by the veterinary surgeon in order that advice to spay may be given in the case of entire females. It is appreciated that in the case of strays, entirety of the female is not easy to confirm and exploratory laparotomy may well be justified to avoid the risk of future dystokia.

Femur

A common bone fractured, the usual sites and types occurring, viz. neck, shaft, supracondylar and epiphyseal.

Femoral neck. The most difficult femur fracture to treat. It occurs mainly in young cats and kittens (usually under 1 year) since violence of the type causing injury at this site usually results in hip luxation in adult animals. Radiography is necessary for precise diagnosis.

There is no generally agreed method of treatment which is entirely satisfactory, the disparity in size between proximal and distal fragments and the muscle stresses applied to the latter making effective immobilisation virtually impossible. The bone is of insufficient calibre to permit satisfactory internal fixation such as transfixion screwing. Simple immobilisation by confinement or the strapping of the limb in full flexion are probably the best methods at present available and many cats adapt remarkably well to apparently severely distorted femoral neck repair.

Shaft. Fractures of upper third, mid-shaft and lower third are all easily, effectively and speedily repaired by intramedullary pinning. Under general anaesthesia the fracture site is exposed and the pin introduced at this point; the technique must include care to embed the pin firmly in the dense bone of the distal epiphysis; a pin of $\frac{3}{32}$ inch diameter is suitable for most cases. In simple cases the cat is often using the limb well within a few days of operation and even in those in which a severely comminuted fracture results in virtual absence of a significant part of the shaft function is regained remarkably rapidly. Contracture of the posterior thigh muscles occurs in some patients but usually resolves to some extent with adequate exercise. The pin may be removed in 4–6 weeks in most cases.

Supracondylar and lower epiphyseal fractures. Owing to the relatively small size of the distal fragment and the muscular pull exerted on it considerable displacement is invariable and methods of external splinting useless. Ordinary intramedullary pinning is only very occasionally satisfactory since the small fragment tends to be pulled or even torn off the pin. Oblique transfixion screwing can be applied in a few cases, particularly late inadequately treated ones in which displacement has not been properly reduced and soft tissue repair is already taking place.

In recent cases, however, retrograde pinning with over-reduction of the fracture is extremely satisfactory and the technique comparatively simple. Under conditions of extreme surgical cleanliness a suitable skin incision is made to expose the stifle joint which is opened and the patella displaced laterally or medially to permit access to the anterior aspect of the trochlea. A suitable pin, pointed at both ends, is inserted in the notch between the insertions of the cruciate ligaments, through the epiphyseal fragment which is then levered into a position of slight over-reduction. The pin is driven upwards through the proximal fragment and out through the skin in the usual manner and is then withdrawn until the point of the pin in the distal fragment is virtually flush with the articular cartilage but is not out of sight. The pin is cut off in the region of the hip in the usual manner. An appropriate antibiotic (an intra-mammary cerate is eminently satisfactory) is introduced into the opened stifle joint, the patella replaced, the joint capsule sutured and other tissues closed routinely. A light plaster cast designed to maintain the stifle in moderate extension for some 10–12 days post-operatively is useful. The pin is removed from the upper end of the femur routinely in 4–6 weeks. Results are usually good once any ankylosis of the joint resulting from the interference and muscle contracture due to disuse are compensated or overcome.

Tibia
Fractures of the fibula are not discussed separately since a stable tibia is sufficient to immobilise it. The usual sites of tibia fracture are the shaft and lower epiphysis. Whilst external fixation by plaster cast would be perfectly satisfactory in many cases, the feline intolerance of hind limb appliances already referred to makes this method seldom practicable.

Intramedullary pinning is again simple and satisfactory and is rather easier than in the dog since the medullary cavity is less curved. The pin is introduced from the proximal extremity of the tibia rather than at the fracture site; if the latter method is used the pin often emerges at a point which causes considerable interference with stifle movement. The pin can be inserted lateral to the inferior patella ligament without opening the joint capsule, the fracture is aligned by open reduction and the pin guided on into the distal fragment. The pin is cut off as flush as possible with the upper end of the tibia to preserve maximum joint function and hence may not always be accessible for removal; this does not appear to be a great inconvenience and the implant may be left *in situ*.

In one 14½-year-old cat whose tibia was pinned (in the belief that the animal was several years younger!) excellent healing resulted with little if any diminution in function due to the pin which was left *in situ* until the patient's death some 2½ years later.

Separation of the lower epiphysis. This is a relatively uncommon fracture which may be caused when the kitten becomes suspended by a hind limb while climbing. Owing to the extreme convolution of the epiphyseal line proper reduction can only be achieved by the open method when the two fragments can be fitted together in an interlocking manner. Fixation by drilling and wiring and subsequent temporary immobilisation by a light plaster cast extending only one inch above and below the joint can be most successful. (Joshua 1957).

Fractures of the tarsus would only be seen in severe crushing accidents when coincidental lesions are likely to dominate the clinical picture. Metatarsals and phalanges may likewise be fractured by crushing type accidents but associated injuries can be less severe in which case immobilisation in a light plaster or strapping may be adequate.

Forelimb
The common fractures are those of humerus and radius and ulna.

Humerus

Almost invariably shaft fractures and then not common.

These are amenable to intramedullary pinning, the fracture site being exposed via a lateral approach and the pin introduced at this site. Nerve damage caused by the violence to which the fracture was due, giving rise to signs of radial paralysis may be in existence at the time of operation, but it can also arise during operation from stretching of the musculo-spiral nerve during reduction.

Post-operative paralysis is one of the hazards of humerus pinning but many cases resolve within 3–6 weeks.

Radius and Ulna

A much less common fracture than in the dog although some clinicians regard it as being of fairly high incidence. Non-union does not appear to be a serious problem and most cases are satisfactorily treated by closed reduction and application of a plaster cast, tolerated quite well on the forelimb.

The carpus, metacarpals and phalanges. Similar remarks apply as to the equivalent regions of the hind limb.

The Spine

The spine may be fractured at any level in severe accidents involving crushing or sudden propulsive violence fore or aft. Such fractures are usually comminuted (from heavy crushing) or compressed. Clinical signs will vary with the level of the lesion and the degree of damage to the cord and include coma, spasticity, paresis and paralysis or any combination of these states. Sometimes crepitation is detected during routine clinical examination but more often fracture is deduced from the severe spinal signs. Radiography is a definitive diagnostic aid but frequently the evidence of cord damage is so obvious and great that euthanasia is decided upon regardless of precise diagnosis of fracture. Heroic surgery to decompress the cord and restore some integrity to a fractured spine is probably never justified in this species since the protracted period of recumbency is not well tolerated.

Sacrococcygeal Fracture

This is a relatively common fracture due to falls or blows from behind; often the type of accident is not known, the cat merely coming in showing the typical signs.

Pain may or may not be a feature of these cases but there is often inability or difficulty in sitting. The tail hangs flaccid and cannot be raised in response to stroking. Pain is elicited by manipulation of the tail, crepitus may be detected and the lesion can be demonstrated radiographically.

Treatment. In a proportion of cases spontaneous recovery occurs, the main difficulty being hygiene. Since the cat cannot raise the tail when urinating and defaecating the ventral surface becomes badly soiled and regular attention is necessary to prevent complications arising from this cause. In some cases in which the degree of separation is considerable something more is needed than simple rest. It has been found possible to apply a plaster cast over the posterior dorsum and encircling the base of the tail for about 1½ inches, taking care to leave the anus free, which both immobilises the fracture and supports the proximal part of the tail in a horizontal position, minimising or eliminating soiling. Such a cast is surprisingly well tolerated.

Prognosis in most cases is reasonably good.

The Tail

Fractures of the coccygeal vertebrae accompany many traumatic lesions of the tail especially crushing through being shut in doors. In most cases the soft tissue injuries are more significant than the fracture, loss of skin and blood supply being particularly serious. It is rarely necessary to treat the fracture as such.

Luxations

Dislocations of the hip, patella, hock and jaw have been seen, the first being by far the most common. Shoulder and elbow luxations have not been seen but this is not to say that they do not occur.

Hip Luxation

Occurs more commonly in cats over 9 months of age when the epiphyses are fused. The lesion may co-exist with fractures of the femur or pelvis and is always due to external violence. Dysplastic conditions of the hip do not appear to exist.

The signs are typical. Severe unilateral hind limb lameness, often complete carrying of the leg, undue prominence in the region of the hip due to the displaced great trochanter, disparity of distance between tuber ischii and great trochanter of the two sides, shortening of the limb (¼–1 inch) with reduced mobility and pain on attempted flexion and extension. The luxated femoral head can often be detected per rectum through the obturator foramen. The luxation is most commonly upwards and forwards.

Radiography confirms diagnosis.

Treatment. Manual reduction under general anaesthesia is usually easily accomplished, the well moulded spherical femoral head in the cat and the deep acetabulum forming a functionally good ball and socket joint on which to work. The capsular and round ligaments are usually ruptured hence reduction may be difficult to maintain. If the dislocation recurs repeatedly on manipulation or after recovery from anaesthesia reduction should be maintained by strapping the limb in full flexion for 7–14 days. Whether strapped or not the cat should be confined to a cage for several days; strapping is remarkably well tolerated once the cat has adjusted to it.

Prognosis is quite good. It is relatively seldom that irreducible luxations persist resulting in the formation of a false joint.

Patella

Congenital patella luxation is now apparently common in the 'Rex' varieties. Patella luxation does occur but is infrequent and experience suggests is usually traumatic. Often the unusual stress causing the luxation has not been observed and can only be assumed. The cat is found to be suddenly and severely lame on one hind limb; the lesion is readily detected on routine examination, the patella luxating easily but painfully, usually to the medial aspect. The acuteness of the condition usually results in early attention being sought thus the stretching of superior and inferior patella ligaments, so often a feature of recurrent patella luxation in the dog, is rarely present and prompt treatment is usually effective. This comprises early immobilisation of the stifle after careful reduction of the dislocation, preferably by a light plaster cast despite the disadvantages referred to earlier; occasionally strapping with an adhesive bandage such as Elastoplast is sufficient. Care must be taken that the patella is securely in the proper place during application of the cast and the best position of the joint is usually found to be moderate flexion at which angle the ligaments are sufficiently tensed to maintain the reduction. Analgesic drugs are seldom necessary but may be prescribed if pain is persistent. 10—18 days immobilisation is usually adequate. A good result may be expected.

Hock

Dislocation of the tarsus must be a very unusual condition but has been seen (Joshua 1957). The deflection of the limb below the tarsus is obvious but there is far less mobility than in separation of the lower tibial epiphysis; it is more likely to occur in adult than young cats.

Reduction may be easy but maintenance is difficult. A method of transfixion pinning which was successful in one case has been described (*vide supra*) in which a $\frac{3}{32}$ inch stainless steel intramedullary pin was introduced from the posterior aspect of the os calcis, driven across the tibio-tarsal articulation and upwards into the medullary cavity of the tibia. Reinforcement by a light and small plaster cast was necessary in the case described, the patient being exceptionally fat (about 11 kg. (24 lbs.)) but is probably not required in average subjects.

Dislocation of the temporomandibular joint has been described in another section. Whilst dislocation of any joint can theoretically occur, those described appear to be the most likely.

Luxation of an interphalangeal joint is not uncommon; the distortion of the digit is obvious but the lesion needs to be confirmed radiographically in some cases to eliminate the possibility of fracture.

Reduction is simple and light strapping for a few days usually enough to maintain it.

Vertebral luxations may co-exist with fractures of the spine and from the practical point of view differ little from spine fracture in severity, effects and outcome.

Osteogenesis Imperfecta

Whilst ordinary bone abnormalities analogous to rickets seem uncommon in cats a more distinct entity does occur as a result of a diet deficient in calcium causing rarefaction of bone and spontaneous fractures. Experience supported by reported evidence makes it clear that the Siamese cat is particularly prone to osteogenesis imperfecta. This may be due to the curious propensity of many Siamese cat breeders to rely solely or largely on a raw meat and water diet; not only are their own cats and kittens maintained on this type of diet but the continuation of this unbalanced method of feeding is ensured by the advice given to purchasers of kittens, often reinforced by the statement that Siamese cats will not take milk. Scott has reported in several communications (see suggested further reading) the effects of feeding a diet in which the calcium and iodine intake is deficient resulting in an abnormal calcium phosphorus ratio.

Signs. These are rather characteristic in naturally occurring cases but even so they are not always recognised immediately for what they are. As a rule no abnormality is noticed until really active movement starts, i.e. between 6 and 16 weeks, but occasionally owners do remark that, in retrospect, affected kittens have been less active than average. It is the occurrence of spontaneous fractures which causes the typical signs of sudden lameness or paresis associated with considerable pain. The feature of these fractures is the presence of intense pain but there is often absence of certain cardinal signs of fractures such as mobility at the fracture site, distortion of the limb and crepitation. This lack of characteristic signs is due in part to the types of fracture which tend to be folding or impacted and to the grossly abnormal bone which has no rigidity.

It may be impossible to diagnose fractures by ordinary clinical examination. Affected kittens are otherwise usually in good bodily condition and eat well.

Diagnosis. It cannot be too strongly emphasised that any kitten between 6 weeks and 6 months which shows evidence of skeletal pain and/or weakness of sudden onset, particularly Siamese, Siamese crosses and similar types, should be subjected to thorough radiographic

224

examination. Radiography should preferably extend to the whole skeleton and not be confined to the part suspected; frequently numerous fractures are demonstrated in one kitten, many of which would have been unrecognised clinically.

The X-ray appearance is characteristic, the whole skeleton showing evidence of calcium lack with marked rarefaction. The cortices of long bones are very thin and ill-defined.

Fractures may be found at all stages of healing from very recent to completely healed lesions.

On post-mortem examination severely affected bones can be folded between the fingers like thick paper and are easily cut with scissors.

Treatment. Some cases are so advanced by the time a firm diagnosis is made and fractures so numerous that euthanasia is considered to be the best course but in early cases or those in which rarefaction is comparatively slight, response to treatment may be good. Diet must be suitably adjusted and calcium administered orally to redress the calcium phosphorus imbalance; adequate Vitamin D intake should be ensured to make certain that available calcium will be fully utilised.

More important than treatment of the individual is a form of prophylaxis by spreading the doctrine of adequate balanced feeding to all cat owners, especially those with breeding catteries or long-term boarders such as quarantine kennels. It is essential to combat the idiotic vogue for meat and water feeding whenever it is encountered.

Prognosis. Good in mild cases, e.g. kittens of 5 months of age with a single fracture or if early recognition is possible; poor in advanced cases with numerous fractures.

Neoplasms of Bone

According to Cotchin (1956, 1957) tumours of bone comprised about 8 per cent of the cat neoplasms surveyed and included osteogenic sarcomas, chondrosarcomas and the occasional sarcoma of giant and spindle cells. The bones affected in order of frequency appear to be humerus, femur, head bones (chiefly jaw), pelvis, scapula, radius and vertebral body, the latter four sites being rather rare. Age incidence showed no particular trend cases occurring in all age groups from 2–20 years.

In the series of cat neoplasms mentioned elsewhere in this book five cases of tumour associated with bone appear; age and sex was known in only two cases. They were as follows:

1. 8 year ♀ Osteosarcoma of zygomatic ridge; lung metastases.
2. 8 year ♂ Sarcoma arising from periosteum of humerus.
3. Osteolytic sarcomas respectively of femoral cortex and adjacent to the thoracic spine.
4. Osteogenic tumour of low malignancy in the hard palate.
5. Spindle cell sarcoma of lower end femur.

Number 3 is of particular interest as this appeared to be a case of multiple primary sites.

The signs are usually those of a slowly increasing firm swelling often accompanied by lameness when limb bones are involved. The tumour has often attained a quite considerable size by the time attention is sought, probably due to the absence of obvious pain or systemic signs, the owner being lulled into a sense of false security. A firm swelling of some duration (4 weeks plus) which is in any way connected with the skeletal system, especially in the region of the head, humerus or femur, should be regarded as highly suspicious of bone tumour and steps taken to make a firm diagnosis. Radiography and biopsy are the obvious means available. Feline bone tumours are not always so radiologically distinctive as are many canine cases but radiography may well incriminate bone as the tissue of origin. Surgical removal of a representative slice of tumour tissue in certain cases and a histopathological examination will be diagnostic.

Metastasis tends to occur rather late in the course which accounts for the relatively low percentage of metastases reported in the series quoted, viz. 6 of 26 in Cotchin's cases and 1 of 5 above.

Treatment is seldom feasible, limb amputation not being, in the author's view, either ethically or aesthetically acceptable in the cat. X-ray therapy and limb perfusion have yet to be evaluated. Euthanasia is usually required.

Tendons

Tendons are often involved in soft tissue damage such as extensive sepsis, accidental wounds and trapping in wire snares, the results of which will be dealt with routinely in each circumstance. The most characteristic tendon lesion seen in cats is rupture of the Achilles tendon, i.e. tendinous portion of the gastrocnemius.

The cause is usually traumatic and includes such accidents as dog bites and suspension by the hind limb in trees etc.

Symptoms are characteristic and comprise dropping of the hock, the cat being severely lame and taking weight on the whole posterior surface of the metatarsal area; the normally tense tendon (hamstring) is slack and the rupture may be palpable; sometimes it is clearly detached from the tuber calcis, detachment of the epiphyseal top of this bone has been seen on one occasion (Joshua 1953).

The only treatment is by surgical repair which is well worth undertaking. Subject to considerations of shock, operation should be performed as soon as possible since contraction of the tendon occurs rapidly making repair more difficult.

A routine surgical approach is made under conditions of extreme cleanliness and the ruptured tendon exposed. In late cases it may be necessary to freshen the tissue. The severed ends are united preferably using non-absorbable material such as monofilament nylon; anchor sutures of silk-worm gut are sometimes helpful; these may be reinforced with numerous catgut sutures. In cases of detachment of the epiphysis of the tuber calcis with the superficial flexor tendon this latter structure may be inserted into the deep flexor as near to the tuber calcis as possible and firmly sutured. Reinforcement by a light, small plaster cast to obviate hock movement is necessary in some cases, e.g. heavy or aged cats. Results are often surprisingly good.

Rupture of the Cruciate Ligament of the Stifle

This lesion is less common than in the dog but does occur. The cause is usually external violence rather than the type of exaggerated spontaneous stifle movement as in dogs. Lameness is severe; very little weight can be taken on the affected limb which appears extremely weak. Whilst pain may be elicited on palpation the characteristic 'feel' of an affected stifle is one of disruption and looseness. On radiography the femur is seen to be riding far back on the tibia. Conservative treatment by immobilisation in a plaster cast results in improvement but soundness is seldom restored.

Vaughan (personal communication) reports the successful treatment of these cases by the insertion of a prosthetic cruciate ligament utilising a strip of skin; the technique is as described for the dog.

A Congenital Skeletal Deformity

A curious congenital abnormality has been recognised. It is often not noticed until the kitten is presented for castration or spaying and is often strikingly obvious when the animal is hobbled out on the operating table for the latter purpose. It comprises a considerable foreshortening of the long bones of the fore-limb, especially humerus, radius and ulna. Affected cats often show a marked degree of kyphosis (roach back) in addition.

It may occur in any type of cat but of the pure breeds has been mainly seen in Long Hairs. The functional significance seems to be minimal but it is a deformity which should be watched and ruthlessly eradicated if it shows up in pedigree cats; one or two cases of osteo-arthritis have been seen in older cats which appeared at that stage to have unusually short forelimbs hence the abnormality may have some significance in being a predisposing factor in some joint pathology.

Intervertebral Discs

Protrusions of intervertebral discs is known to be quite common in the cat but their clinical significance is not so easy to establish. King (1958) found dorsal protrusions in twenty-six of 100 cats examined at random, ninety-one discs being involved.

Both Type I and Type II protrusions occur. The distribution of protrusions is discussed by the same author who found the cervical region most commonly affected; the lumbar region is also frequently involved, especially discs L4–5 and L5–6; the thoraco-lumbar region shows a somewhat low incidence.

The existence of disc protrusions was easily confirmed in practice by post-mortem examination but it is more difficult convincingly to correlate clinical signs and disc lesions. This, in view of the moderately frequent occurrence of posterior paresis, locomotor ataxias and inco-ordination in ageing cats, is surprising. Most clinicians agree that paraplegia of sudden onset comparable to that seen so commonly in disc protrusions in the dog is rare in the cat. King suggests that the neural canal of the cat may be more roomy than that of the dog hence comparable lesions will not necessarily produce similar clinical signs. Be that as it may it is singularly difficult to recognise clinically intervertebral disc syndromes in the cat.

On the other hand Milnes (1959) has recorded three cases in which signs and the presence of disc lesions may reasonably be said to be correlated; the clinical signs included forelimb lameness, hind limb inco-ordination, thoraco-lumbar pain and posterior paresis.

In the present state of knowledge the most that can be said is that in ageing cats showing evidence of obscure lameness, muscle pain and spasm, posterior paresis or inco-ordination which cannot be attributed to other causes, intervertebral disc protrusions should be considered as a possible aetiology.

There is scant reference to treatment of these cases thus both therapy and prognosis must be based on what is known in other species, e.g. analgesics (remembering the idiosyncracy of the feline to aspirin and nynalgin), rest, administration of Vitamin B complex and possibly infra-red irradiation.

Arthritis

Arthritis is considerably less common than in the dog and has received correspondingly little attention in the literature but does occur.

Osteo-arthritis

This is comparatively uncommon. Probably the most frequently affected site is the spine spondylitis having been seen on a number of occasions. Again correlation of clinical signs and lesions is difficult, exostoses and even ankylosis having been detected radiographically in cats showing no clinical abnormality. Painful arthritis of the cervical region has been met as has a degree of ankylosing spondylitis resulting in the cat being rigidly fixed with the spine from skull to tail in extreme flexion.

In grossly overweight cats (usually neuters) or those showing the foreshortening of limbs described above, degenerative arthritic changes occasionally occur in the limbs in later life. Hips, shoulders and elbows are amongst the joints affected.

Clinical signs include lameness and unwillingness to jump or walk.

In extreme cases the cat will reluctantly totter a few steps and then lie down. Pain is elicited on flexion and extension of affected joints; crepitation is occasionally detected; the joint and associated periarticular tissues are not usually noticeably enlarged.

Treatment is aimed at weight reduction, elimination of joint concussion by avoiding jumping and the use of suitable anti-inflammatory and analgesic drugs (with the usual limitations). Phenylbutazone (25–50 mg. once or twice daily) is often well tolerated; corticosteroids may be given in the usual dosage bearing in mind the disadvantages of prolonged administration, or gold salts by injection, viz. sodium aurothiomalate (Myocrisin, May and Baker) may be tried. Gold is moderately well tolerated by cats; blood dyscrasias have not been encountered but should always be looked for during a course of gold therapy. Suggested dosage is half that used for dogs, i.e. 5 mg. test dose, 10 mg. weekly for 6 weeks followed by 25 mg. weekly for a further 4–6 weeks; it is administered by deep intramuscular injection preferably using alternate hind limbs. Response is variable from none to good; if there is no response at all after the fifth injection it is unlikely to occur and gold should be discontinued.

Septic Arthritis

This is fairly common sequel to cat bite sepsis in the region of a joint and is dealt with fully in another section.

Tuberculous Arthritis

Whilst not common this specific joint infection does occur and on public health grounds requires recognition since the discharge may be literally teeming with organisms. The condition is fully dealt with under Tuberculosis in another chapter.

'Rheumatoid Arthritis'

This heading is given in inverted commas to indicate that the name may not be acceptable universally. A small but significant number of cats has been seen showing a syndrome having many features in common with rheumatoid arthritis in man and from this point of view the term seems justified. These features include multiplicity of joints involved, early and more severe lesions in the smaller joints such as carpus, tarsus and carpo-metacarpal articulations, increased joint spaces, increase in synovial fluid and primarily peri-articular rather than articular changes including associated soft tissues.

The author has diagnosed the condition in some half dozen cats and emphasises that the most critical assessment of any suspect case is essential before even a tentative diagnosis of rheumatoid arthritis is made; the label should not be lightly applied to every case showing multiple joint changes.

The age incidence has been late middle age, i.e. 8 years plus.

The condition has been seen in a somewhat chronic and insidious form and in no case could be related to a previous infection. Oral sepsis has been present in some of these patients but in no case has treatment of the infected foci resulted in alleviation of the joint condition.

The clinical signs are predominantly, reluctance to walk and jump progressing to almost complete refusal to move. Lameness in a limb or limbs has occasionally been noted. Mild malaise with partial or complete anorexia is common; in the later stages severe loss of weight occurs and patients become quite emaciated. Temperature is often slightly elevated →39·2° C. (102·6° F.).

Clinical findings include some or all of the following:

Marked pain on flexion and extension of affected joints.

Multiplicity of joints involved, never only one. The small joints show earliest and most severe changes although all may eventually be affected. The forelimbs have been frequently the more severely involved.

In the early stages there may be no visible or palpable change in the joints but later peri-articular swelling occurs (comprising both exostoses and soft tissue enlargement); joint spaces are increased, this is particularly noticeable in carpus and tarsus; there is an increase in synovial fluid which is often turbid in appearance (as much as 1 ml. has been withdrawn from the carpus in one patient). Heat and pain on pressure often exist.

Considerable hypertrophy of the claws has been seen, probably due to active inflammation in various associated structures.

Laboratory tests have disclosed mild non-specific anaemia in some patients and leukocytosis although the latter has not been invariable.

The following are the findings in a recent case in an 8-year-old castrated male Siamese.

Blood	Urine
R.B.C's 5·92 mill.	Blood −ve
W.B.C's 58,600	Protein −ve
Hb 9·5	Sugar −ve
P.C.V. 32 per cent	Ketones −ve
M.C.V. 53 Cu/u	Bile salts −ve
Differential:	Bilirubin −ve
Polymorphs—93 per cent	Specific gravity 1042
Lymphocytes—5 per cent	pH 6·5
Eosinophils—2 per cent	*Deposit*: fat droplets + +ve

A number of R.B.C's containing Howell Jolly bodies were present. The synovial fluid contains a large amount of protein, a few R.B.C's and polymorphs were present.

No growth obtained on culture of synovial fluid.

Radiography shows changes to be peri-articular rather than articular.

Diagnosis. Is based on a critical assessment of clinical, laboratory and radiographic findings. Whilst it should never be lightly made it is warranted in cats which over a period of several months show a progressive polyarthritis having a number of the features previously described.

Treatment. Despite apparent absence of success any infected focus such as teeth should be vigorously dealt with by routine methods.

Otherwise treatment has been mainly by corticosteroids. Gold, which is spectacular in a similar condition in the dog, gives disappointing results.

Trial and error methods may be necessary to determine both which corticosteroid and what dose is optimal for any individual. Prednisolone, triamcinolone and betamethasone have each proved most suitable for different individuals.

Once response is obtained dosage should be reduced as rapidly as practicable to a minimum maintenance level. Although it was found possible to withdraw the drug after several months treatment in one cat, in most cases it has proved necessary to continue therapy for life, symptoms returning as soon as the drug is withdrawn. Several cats have been maintained symptom free for some years including one on as little as 0·5 mg. prednisolone daily but which relapsed immediately on complete withdrawal.

Prolonged corticosteroid therapy is clearly undesirable in many respects but there is no doubt that a few patients have been given an increased expectation of life by its use; euthanasia becomes essential otherwise.

Prognosis. This may be moderately optimistic in cases presented and recognised early but even then only as regards suppression of symptoms. Cure has not been obtained with the possible exception of the one case in which symptoms did not recur on cessation of a prolonged course of treatment. Advanced cases already showing some evidence of emaciation and general ill-health merit a very guarded to poor prognosis. A sufficient number has been controlled by corticosteroid therapy to warrant an attempt being made to treat all cases.

Hypervitaminosis A

Cats appear to be particularly susceptible to a high level of Vitamin A in the diet; this arises when cats are fed a diet containing large amounts of liver.

Exostoses are formed which can produce anrylosis. The main site is the vertebral column, especially the cervical area. Cases are seen in which the new bone formation is so extensive that the vertebral column becomes fused in a flexed position. Affected cats show an increasing loss of mobility with consequent muscle atrophy. In extreme cases, the cat can be picked up in the thoraeo-lumbar region and remain absolutely rigid in a curved sitting position. Exostoses have also been seen affecting the limbs but this is less common.

In advanced cases, treatment is of no avail. One case has been seen showing a fluctuation in signs. The cat was solely liver fed and would become progressively less mobile; she would then refuse all food for periods of up to 6 weeks—this history seemed to be entirely reliable—in the later stages of this self-imposed starvation mobility gradually returns, the whole sequence being repeated at about six monthly intervals. Radiography during a period of immobility showed widespread early exostoses, the limbs being mainly affected. It seems doubtful if advice regarding diet was followed and the case was lost sight of due to the owner's removal.

Muscle

Various muscles are involved in cat bite sepsis lesions which will not be considered here; equally, muscle is damaged in many forms of trauma. Sprains and tears attributable to spontaneous activity are strikingly rare although ligaments and tendons associated with joints are subject to the usual injuries of these regions. Ischaemia of a given muscle or muscle mass may follow arterial thrombosis and result in replacement by fibrous tissue. Obscure and indefinite muscle lesions and apparent myasthenias have also been seen.

In one case a 9-year-old spayed female cat showed a syndrome comprising malaise and lameness which persisted over several weeks; during the latter part of the course progressive emaciation occurred. The only significant clinical finding was an obvious change in certain muscles, viz. the triceps of both forelimbs and the biceps femoris in the right hind leg. The change comprised a hardening and contraction of the affected muscle mass. Histologically the lesions showed an extensive myonecrosis, replacement fibrosis with some attempt at muscle regeneration. The cause is unknown. Cowie-Whitney (personal communication) suggests that the condition appears somewhat analogous to traumatic myositis fibrosa or ossificans. It is difficult to visualise how individual muscle masses in different limbs could become affected if the cause was trauma unless from cat bites sustained at these various sites.

In aged cats inco-ordination and posterior paresis are common and in some cases the paresis appears to be due purely to poor muscle tonus sometimes with a degree of atrophy and could reasonably be described as a myasthenia. The hind limbs are mainly concerned, particularly the semi-membranosus and semi-tendinosis muscles. Treatment is rarely of avail although there is occasionally temporary response to vitamin therapy preferably by combined parenteral and oral administration; in the few cases which respond, Vitamin B deficiency may be a factor.

Pansteatitis-"Yellow Fat Disease"
This is a regularly occurring but uncommon disease of cats. Cases had been recorded in the American literature from the mid-1950's and

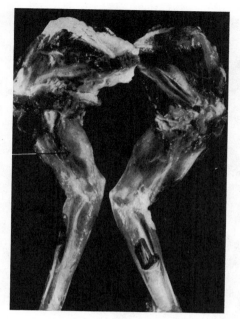

FIG. 31 Forelimbs of 9-year-old spayed female cat showing lesions of myonecrosis and replacement fibrosis in both triceps, the larger lesion in the right

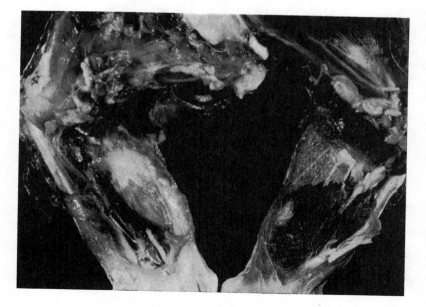

FIG. 32 Close up view of lesions as in FIG. 31

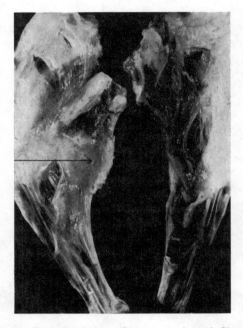

FIG. 33 Extensive lesion of myonecrosis and fibrosis in biceps femoris of right hind limb

from Australia in 1973 but the first case report in the United Kingdom was in 1975 (Gaskell, Leedale and Douglas, 1975) and more recently by Flecknell and Grufydd-Jones, 1978.

The symptomatology described is very uniform, viz. discomfort on handling, temperature rise, lethargy and inappetence.

Initially, the condition was ascribed to a diet mainly of oily red fish such as tuna and pilchards but has now been recognised in cats receiving a white fish diet.

Most cats showed pain on abdominal palpation; the painful areas of fat may have a nodular feel. Haematology shows a neutrophilia with a shift to the left. Reports regarding the value of radiography for diagnosis vary. A firm diagnosis is based on biopsy of a suitable specimen of fat; the changes include fat cell necrosis and infiltration with neutrophil leucocytes; foreign body giant cells may be seen.

Treatment comprises elimination of fish from the diet, administration of Vitamin E, corticosteroids and antibiotics.

Prognosis is good, although progress may be somewhat slow; some improvement may be seen within 7 days, but at least 4 weeks should be allowed for full recovery. Relapse should not occur provided the diet is kept free or very low in fish. Owner co-operation and patience is vital since difficulty may be met in persuading patients to accept the changed feeding regime.

REFERENCES

Carter, H.E. (1964) *Vet. Rec.,* **76,** 1412.

Cowie-Whitney, J. (1963) Personal communication.

Flecknell, P.A., and Grufydd-Jones, T.J., (1978), *Vet. Rec.,* **102,** 149.

Freak, M.J. (1962), *Vet. Rec.* **74,** 985.

Gaskell, C.J., Leedale, Alison, H., and Douglas, S.W. (1975), *J. Small An. Pract.,* **16,** 117.

Joshua, J.O. (1957), *Vet. Rec.,* **69,** 929.

Joshua, J.O. (1953), *Vet. Rec.,* **65,** 174.

King, A.S. *et. al.* (1958), *Vet. Rec.* **70,** 509.

Milnes, D.M. (1959), *Vet. Rec.* **71,** 932.

Sumner-Smith, G. (1964), *Vet. Rec.,* **76,** 973.

Vaughan, L.C. (1964) Personal communication.

Hickman, J. (1964) Edinburgh, Oliver and Boyd. (Veterinary Orthopaedics.)

Jonas & Jonas (1964) *J. Amer. Vet. Medical Association* **144**, 1277. (Double-sleeved Jonas splint for lengthening the femur of a cat.)

Beadman, R. *et al.* (1964) *Vet. Rec.* **76**, 1005. (Vertebral osteophytes in the cat.)

Glenny, W. C. (1956) *J. Amer. Vet. Medical Association* **129**, 61. (Canine and feline spinal osteoarthritis (spondylitis deformans).)

King, A. S. & Smith, R. N. (1958) *Nature Lond.* **181**, 568. (Diseases of the intervertebral disc of the cat.)

King, A. S. (1959) *Proc. XVIth. Int. Vet. Congr. Madrid* **2**, 331. (Dorsal protrusions of the intervertebral disc in the cat.)

King, A. S. & Smith, R. N. (1960) *Vet. Rec.* **72**. (Disc protrusions in the cat (in two parts).)

Leonard, E. P. (1961) *Orthopaedic Surgery of the dog & cat* (Philadelphia & London, Saunders & Co.)

Osteogenesis imperfecta.

Coop, M. C. (1958) *J. Amer. Vet. Medical Association* **132**, 299. (A treatment for osteogenesis imperfecta in kittens.)

Henderson, G. L. B. & Keywood, E. K. (1959) *Vet. Rec.* **71**, 317. (An osteodystrophy in Siamese kittens.)

Fagg, R. H. (1959) *Vet. Rec.* **71**, 707. (Osteodystrophy in Siamese kittens.)

Jowsey, J. & Gershon-Cohen, J. (1964) *Proc. Soc. exp. Biol. Med.* **116**, 437. (Effect of dietary calcium on production and reversal of experimental osteoporosis in cats.)

Scott, P. P. (1960) *Brit. Small An. Vet. Ass.* Proceedings **84**. (Calcium and iodine deficiency in meat-fed cats with reference to osteogenesis imperfecta.)

Greaves, J. P. *et al.* (1958) *Proc. Nutr. Soc.* **17**, No 2. (Raw meat and carnivores: the effects of feeding ox heart to kittens.)

Greaves, J. P. *et al.* (1959) *J. Physiol.* **148**, No. 2. (Thyroid changes in cats on a high protein diet, raw heart.)

Chapter 18

NERVOUS SYSTEM

Due to the relative absence of neurotropic virus diseases in the cat conditions such as encephalitis are comparatively rare, a persisting locomotor ataxia and inco-ordination having been seen in one group of cats recovered from infection with one of the feline respiratory viruses and very much resembling post-distemper inco-ordination in the dog. Quite recently a cat showing bizarre neurological signs was shown to have a meningo-encephalo-myelitis involving the entire brain and cord. The lesions were similar to those seen in canine distemper but no relevant history of disease existed. Pyogenic infections of brain and neural canal are not infrequent, usually as a sequel to otitis media or cat bite sepsis.

Damage to nervous tissue of brain or cord can obviously result from accidental injuries; intervertebral disc protrusions have been dealt with elsewhere. Fits are less common than in the dog. Innes has made the point that a great deal is known about the nervous system of the cat owing to experimental work, yet neurologic disease is uncommon in the species. In an article covering many aspects of nervous system disease in all species, Innes states that no form of demyelinating disease has been reported but mentions the possibility that virus diseases during pregnancy may cause effects on the cerebellum of the foetus.

Fits

Although not common, fits are by no means a clinical rarity in cats and do not always take a classical form; they may take the form of un-controlled and violent galloping round a room, often literally 'going up the wall' in so doing and knocking ornaments, etc., off furniture; they may also appear to be a purely temporary loss of consciousness, i.e. a black-out or faint.

Differential diagnosis is thus not easy, particularly as any or all age groups may be affected and great care must be taken in history taking and clinical examination to ensure that no underlying cardiac dysfunction is present. Probably the most reliable evidence that a fit has occurred is the occurrence of an automatic phase after the convulsive or un-conscious phase has passed off, i.e. the cat seems unaware of its sur-roundings, may be apprehensive, has a vacant expression and is totally unresponsive to normal stimuli.

Epilepsy

A number of cats have been seen in which fits commence and continue to occur in an irregular manner and which are ascribable to no obvious cause. The periodicity of seizures and total absence of abnormality in the inter-ictal intervals is similar to the syndrome in dogs which is considered to be epilepsy and which has shown the typical picture on electroencephalography. In the few cases seen, epileptic episodes have commenced during middle life and have persisted. Episodes vary from a very mild almost inapparent momentary vacancy to true convulsive seizures. Periodicity is variable from a single fit every few months to several seizures daily for several days at a time. They usually occur when the cat is resting or even asleep.

Treatment. There is no cure although occasional spontaneous remission may occur. Treatment is aimed at suppressing episodes. Of the drugs used primidone and potassium bromide have proved most successful; the former is apt to cause mild ataxia for 1–2 hours after dosing but is seldom serious; dosage must be estimated for each individual and the minimum maintenance level to obviate episodes established by trial and error, e.g. 60–125 mg. daily in divided doses. As in all conditions of the nervous system adequate Vitamin B intake must be ensured (by regular administration of Vitamin B Complex as yeast or appropriate tablets); this is particularly necessary in this species which is prone to convulsive seizures due to thiamine deficiency or food containing thiaminase (see below).

Fits due to Nutritional Factors. 'Chastek Paralysis'

Cats are highly prone to symptoms related to thiamine deficiency which may arise from one of two sets of circumstances, viz. a diet deficient in thiamine or a diet comprising fish containing thiaminase. A most informative paper describing the whole picture of thiamine deficiency in cats is that of Jubb *et al.* (1956); this article includes a long list of fish in which thiaminase has been detected. In view of the increasing popularity of feeding canned food to cats and the assumption that a high proportion of fish is beneficial these findings are of considerable clinical significance. Summarised, the clinical signs comprise initial anorexia (spontaneous clinical cases are seldom presented in this early stage) with occasional vomiting and salivation; the next phase includes convulsions as the transient feature during the first 24 hours together with ataxia, a high-stepping gait and weaving, with the head held in ventral flexion; placing and righting reflexes are affected. Signs, with the exception of occasional persisting mild ataxia, could be quickly reversed by parenteral administration of Vitamin B complex. This is of particular interest in view of the occasional marked response to Vitamin B therapy in chronic locomotor ataxias of aged cats and suggests that this line of treatment is always worth a trial. In selecting the Vitamin B preparation to be injected it is essential to check that the thiamine content is satisfactory.

Croft records the case of a young cat presented in status epilepticus for electro-encephalography which was subsequently found to be Vitamin B deficient.

From the foregoing it is clear that any cat showing nervous signs whether convulsive, ataxic or abnormal reflexes which cannot be convincingly ascribed to other causes should be carefully investigated for possible nutritional deficiencies. It is essential that all cats should receive a quota of fresh food and that fish containing thiaminase should be rigorously eliminated from the diet.

A form of cerebellar atrophy in kittens now recognized to be a manifestation of FePL virus infection is discussed in more detail in chapter 19 on Infectious Diseases, under the heading, Cerebellar Ataxia.

Stroke

The syndrome known as stroke in man is a not uncommon occurrence in cats in late middle or old age. Whether the signs are due to cerebral haemorrhage or thrombosis is an open question but in view of the comparative frequency of arterial thrombosis it is tempting to hazard a guess that the latter is more likely.

Onset is always sudden, usually in circumstances which preclude accidental injury. Signs are variable from a marked hemiplegia to minor local paralysis confined to the head. In a case of moderate severity the cat is found to be inco-ordinate and often distressed and apparently confused; it may cry out repeatedly. Nystagmus is common. The inco-ordination is found to be unilateral the cat falling or turning always to the same side. Circling does occur but is not a regular feature. Posture tends to be crouching with limbs partially flexed; attempts to move often result in sideways falling. There may be head tilt.

Examination is directed at finding unilateral discrepancies, e.g. absence or decrease in muscle tone, alteration in sensory and motor reflexes in the limbs of one side, uneven pupils and pupillary reflexes, slackness of the posterior commissure of the lips on one side, a drooping ear, ptosis, lack of rigidity of whiskers and decreased whisker twitch reflex. If any degree of facial paralysis is present unilateral dribbling of saliva may occur. Any one or combination of the above signs may be present.

Differential diagnosis must take into consideration otitis media and cerebral abscess; the sudden onset of a stroke is helpful but careful history-taking is essential to make certain that there has been no previous malaise such as would be associated with a cerebral pyogenic focus.

Prognosis depends upon the severity of the neurological signs and may need to be delayed some 7–14 days before a definite opinion can be expressed.

Treatment is aimed initially at assisting the cat to accept and adapt to its disability. Ataractic drugs are contra-indicated because the disorientation already present may be markedly worsened in this species with this group of drugs. Potassium bromide is once again the drug of choice, 150–300 mg. ($2\frac{1}{2}$–5 gr.) twice or even three times daily for the first few days. As in any nervous disease Vitamin B complex should be prescribed.

Nursing instructions must include advice about assisted feeding in cats having any paralysis of tongue or lips since lapping and prehension are affected and cats become quickly discouraged and will then not attempt to eat. Advice must also be given to remove any sleeping-place from which the patient can fall while hemiplegia persists.

Treatment is always worth a trial as many cats make good recoveries and suffer no recurrence over a long period of time.

Incoordination, Locomotor ataxia, Myasthenia

Many old cats show a degree of posterior paresis which is not easily classified as one of the above nor ascribable to a definite cause. As mentioned previously persisting inco-ordination has been seen as a post-virus complication in one group of cats. The term locomotor ataxia is used in a descriptive and not special sense as in tabes dorsalis. Cats are also particularly susceptible to impairment of vestibular function caused by streptomycin but this is a separate issue.

It may be difficult or impossible to decide if the cause of the inco-ordination and/or paresis is of cerebral or spinal origin and if the latter, if it is due to extraneous factors such as disc protrusions. In some cases deficient muscle volume and tone appear to be the only finding. Such cases can but be treated on their merits and all reasonable steps taken to reach a definitive diagnosis. Treatment is quite non-specific comprising multi-vitamin therapy (the B complex and E are important) and attention to nutrition in general.

Prognosis is poor, most cases (despite the occasional inexplicable remission) progressing until euthanasia is necessary. At the same time many aged cats seem to be unworried by their tottering, weaving gait and decreased ability to exercise and adapt readily to an inactive senescence and euthanasia need not always be an immediate or even early recommendation.

What can best be described as 'neighbour euthanasia' is often a problem, i.e. pressure from friends and neighbours by 'talking at' an owner urging that it is unkind to keep an animal alive, and here the attending veterinary surgeon must be prepared, having carefully considered the case, to give a firm decision and the necessary moral support.

Neoplasia

There appears to be little reference in the literature to neoplasia of the central nervous system of cats with any clinical connotation. Cotchin does not mention this system in either his 1956 or 1957 series. Cooper and Howarth describe four lesions in a series of sixty cat brains examined but no clinical details are available. These were all space-occupying lesions such as might have been expected to cause neurological signs and were respectively a diffuse fibrillary astrocytoma and an oligodendroglioma both in the frontal lobe; an early leptomeningioma and a discrete microscopic granuloma.

Whilst the possibility of tumours must not be discarded pyogenic lesions would seem to be both commoner and of more clinical significance.

Peripheral Nerve Damage

Damage to various peripheral nerves can arise in connection with injury and even associated with surgical interventions such as bone pinning, e.g. musculospiral and sciatic nerves.

There is one characteristic and reasonably frequently occurring peripheral nerve syndrome, viz.

Radial Paralysis

This term embraces a set of clinical signs which are easily recognisable although variable in extent according to the level at which damage to the nerve has occurred and is not entirely appropriate in all circumstances.

The cause is always traumatic but the incident may be a street accident, mauling by a dog, being suspended from a fence or tree by a forelimb, incorrect hobbling during operation or as a complication of orthopaedic surgery of the arm or elbow region, i.e. anything which causes severance, contusion or stretching of the nerves of the axillary area. It is perhaps wise to draw special attention to incorrect hobbling during operations. The forelimbs should never be hobbled to the operating table in abduction but always drawn forward in a straight line with the animal's body; forced maintenance in abduction can easily result in radial paralysis.

Signs are typical. There is dropping of the elbow due to paralysis of the triceps muscle and the lower part of the limb is in passive extension with knuckling of the carpus and foot resulting in the dorsal surface of the pes being dragged along the ground. Sensory and motor power may be completely or partially lost.

Prognosis depends upon the extent of nerve damage, e.g. if severed the case is hopeless, contusion merits a guarded prognosis but simple stretching may warrant moderate optimism. Unfortunately there is no immediate criterion by which the extent or type of damage can be gauged, therefore no firm opinion can be expressed at the outset. If improvement occurs within 10 days prognosis is good, if slight or absent at 21 days guarded and if absent at 28–35 days very poor.

Treatment. This is usually of a conservative nature since results of nerve anastomosis are so far not particularly encouraging.

Rest is essential by confining the cat to a small cage or, rest of the affected limb by bandaging or strapping the shoulder and arm to the body wall. The foot must be protected suitably if the dragging is causing excoriation. Vitamin B complex should be prescribed on general principles.

Euthanasia may be necessary in cases failing to recover. Amputation of part or all of the forelimb of a cat is not, in the author's view, morally justifiable.

Special Sensory Organs

Congenital Deafness

This is a well recognised condition occurring in white cats and is due to congenital absence of the organ of Corti and associated cochlear anomalies.

While not all white cats are affected a significant proportion are deaf. Opinions vary as to whether this is more likely to occur in blue-eyed whites or odd-eyed whites!

The evidence of deafness is usually noticed by owners at the age when normal responsiveness should be developing and is clearly absent. Obviously there is no treatment and advice regarding management is the only help the veterinary surgeon can give; curiously enough these deaf cats do not seem to be more accident-prone than others with good hearing and may reach a good age; with increasing traffic hazards, however, this may not continue to be true.

REFERENCES

Cooper, E. R. A. & Howarth, J. (1956) *J. Comp. Path.* **66**, 35.
Croft, P. G. (1962) *J. Small An. Pract.* **3**, 205.
Innes, J. R. M. & Saunders, L. Z. (1957) *Adv. Vet. Sci.* **3**, 33–196.
Jubb, K. V. *et al.* (1956) *J. Comp. Path.* **66**, 217.

SUGGESTED FURTHER READING

Milnes, D. M. (1959) *Vet. Rec.* **71**, 932. (Post-mortem findings in some diseases of the central nervous system in cats.)
Campbell, A. M. G. (1957) *Brit. Med. J.* 1183. (Polyneuritis and illness in cats.)

Chapter 19
DISEASES DUE TO INFECTIVE AGENTS

Written in collaboration with D.E. Jones, B.Sc.; B.V.Sc;
Ph.D.; M.R.C.V.S.

This chapter describes the principal infectious diseases of cats, but septic infections are dealt with separately in Chapter 20 while dermatomycoses are discussed in Chapter 16. Although some feline infectious diseases have been recognised clinically for many years knowledge of their aetiology is far from complete. This is particularly true of feline influenza and feline enteritis, for it is only recently that viruses associated with these conditions have been isolated *in vitro*. On the other hand, it seems probable that more cases of feline infectious anaemia occur in Great Britain than are actually diagnosed, and toxoplasmosis has not yet been recorded in British cats. It is apparent that much remains to be done by both clinicians and research workers before the diagnosis, treatment and prophylaxis of feline infections can be considered to be satisfactory.

Feline Respiratory Virus Infections

These are diseases of cat holding premises, where numbers of animals are brought together. Local epidemics tend to associate with individual animals recently released from such premises and are particularly common during the main holiday and 'cat boarding' seasons. These upper respiratory diseases, generalized under the title of 'cat flu' have recently been intensively studied and are known to be primarily of viral origin. Among causative viruses are the herpes, Feline Viral Rhinotracheitis (FVR) virus and several calici (formerly picorna) viruses (FCV) of which the major serotypes have been isolated. Although non-viral agents are usually involved only in secondary infection, there is evidence that a Chlamydial organism (C. psittaci) is the causative agent of the syndrome 'feline pneumonitis' described in the United States by Baker (1944).

Differentiation of the disease states induced by these agents is not always clinically easy, although, the classic symptoms described for pure experimental infections are distinctive. Mixed infections also occur but it is unclear whether they are more severe than either infection alone.

FVR Infection.

Caused by the virus isolated by Crandell and Maurer (1958) and since demonstrated [Crandell (1973)] to exist as a single serotype. The integrity of the lipo-protein envelope of this virus is essential for intectivity so that risks of viral contamination are low, especially when lipid-solvent detergents are used. A life of the host of approximately 24 hours is postulated and subjects must be maintained in relatively close contact for transmission between them to occur. Viral destruction of target cells commences after an incubation of 2-10 days, causing mucosal necrosis and symptoms of acute inflammation of upper respiratory tract and conjunctivae, with clear ocular and nasal discharges and occasional sneezing.

Lassitude and inappetence with pyrexia up to 104.5°F (40.3°C) are not infrequent as discharges become more copious and mucopurulent, with episodes of paroxysmal sneezing. Excessive salivation may also be a feature, but buccal ulceration is not usual, though, pharyngeal ulceration may develop. Kittens, old cats and Siamese varieties are most susceptible to severe illness. Dehydration and general wastage may be severe, and though natural resolution commences within 7-10 days, recovery may be protracted. A wider range of symptoms sometimes assocated with FVR infection includes bronchopneumonia, abortion, ulcerative keratitis and disorders of the CNS [Povey (1976)] and in some subjects gross necrosis of turbinate structures with sinusitis. In young kittens a fatal disseminated disease may also occur with multi-focal hepatic necrosis.

Following apparent recovery, many animals remain viral carriers and experience occasional episodes of shedding, usually in response to stresses like illness, change of environment or treatment with corticosteroids, and thus commonly in situations in which the animal is in close contact with susceptible subjects, as at cat shows, boarding and veterinary establishment.

Curiously, FVR carriers may themselves occasionally suffer relatively severe symptoms of self-induced illness.

Calici Virus Disease.

This presents variable symptoms of illness, possibly relating to varying pathogenicity of the several viruses and to quantity of exposure. Clinical symptoms relate to necrosis of specific target cells, sometimes causing ulceration of tongue, median nasal septum and nares, or pneumonia which may involve as much as 90% of lung parenchyma [Hoover and Kahn (1975)]. In hyperacute cases, massive influx of oedema fluid and neutrophils to the chest may result in sudden death. More usually, the acute case presents with pyrexia up to about 104.5°F (40.3°C), anorexia, buccal ulceration, salivary drooling and sometimes pneumonic symptoms; the course of illness lasting up to 10 days. In milder cases, there may be little discomfort and only slight buccal ulceration. Calici virus persists for a long time off the host and considerable environmental contamination occurs so that transmission is largely by fomites [Wardley and Povey (1977)] rather than aerosol spread, except under conditions of very close confinement as at cat shows or boarding kennels. Many cats also remain carriers after recovery from clinical illness [Wardley, Gaskell and Povey (1974)] and may be persistent shedders, though, there is evidence that some subjects unpredictably may eventually recover and totally reject the virus.

Signs Found On Clinical Examination. Signs found on examining 'cat 'flu' patients obviously vary with the stage of illness and the aetiological agent. Thus in early cases, the predominant symptom may be sneezing, but in later cases ocular and nasal discharge. In more advanced disease pyrexia is a feature of both FVR and FCV infections whilst the former associates with mucopurulent ocular and nasal discharges that may be so severe as to gum up the eyelids and occlude external nares resulting in noisy respiration and spasms of mouth breathing.

Dyspnoea of advanced calici virus pneumonia is not, however, associated with visible external signs, except possibly salivary drooling secondary to buccal ulceration, though the subject may adopt a charateristic crouching posture with extended head and neck and abducted elbows.

Differential Diagnosis. Of mild forms of 'cat 'flu' from allergic rhinitis and conjunctivitis or contact with irritants is not easy. The full course of the disease aids its diagnosis. Chronic sinusitis and rhinitis, usually originating from previous respiratory virus infection, may also present symptoms confusingly similar to early cat 'flu.

Prognosis. Always guarded, as recovery may be protracted and fatalities may result from inanition as well as generalized systemic disease in some cases [Shields (1977)].

Treatment. Non-specific, though, use of antibiotics for control of secondary bacterial infection is logical. Nursing care is the key to success. The patient must be kept at an even environmental temperature, exudates must be carefully removed and appetite must be tempted by the offering of highly aromatic foods, like kipper and mackerel, to overcome the inevitable loss of the sense of smell associated with the disease. In many cases this course of action is adequate, but in cases of severe respiratory embarrassment due to accumulation of exudates, the use of inhalants may be useful. Vapourizing agents like Compound Tincture of Benzoin (Friar's Balsam) or oil of eucalyptus on hot water are relatively easy to use, or proprietary vapour rubs diluted with 1-2 parts of white soft paraffin ('Vaseline') may be carefully applied around external nares. Occular inflammation may be treated by topical application of antibiotic ointments, but cases of severe conjunctival oedema respond rapidly to instillation of Collosal Argentum, together with adrenalin 1:500,000. Vitamins A and C are usefully employed to hasten mucosal repair, at dose rates of 10,000 I.U. and 1 g. daily respectively. The C vitamin is also thought to assist loosening of tenacious mucous, though proprietary mucolytics may be more effective.

B complex vitamins and particularly B12 seems to aid recovery of debilitated subjects though in many cases the primary requirement is for fluid replacement therapy. This may be supplied in the form of lactated Ringer's solution or 5% dextrose saline, given subcutaneously or intraperitoneally twice daily [Povey (1976)]. In some cases it may also be worthwhile to consider force feeding of emulsified foods via a stomach tube implanted surgically [Lane (1977)].

Prophylaxis. The duration of naturally developed immunity to FVR virus is poor, being at a maximum of approximately 6 months, while to calici viruses it is probably as long as a year in response to some antigenic varieties. Vaccines have been prepared, based on the antigenic capacities of FVR virus and selected, broadly antigenic strains of FCV, there being much common ground antigenically between C-virus strains. Attenuated virus vaccines are available for intranasal instillation or intramuscular injection. The former route is claimed useful for production of zones of local, intranasal immunity, while intramuscular administration is claimed to obviate the risks of viral establishment, passage, re-virulence and dissemination from nasal mucosa. Neither vaccine is proof against the possibility of subsequent subclinical infection and establishment of carrier status.

Interference to vaccine by passively acquired, maternally derived antibodies is thought unlikely beyond 8-9 weeks of age, but 12 weeks is nominated as the age for the final (second) injection of vaccine. An annual booster vaccination is recommended although 6 monthly boosting is advisable for isolated animals in non-endemic areas since acquired immunity is of relatively short duration.

Although it is not absolutely necessary to do so, a feline enteritis (panleucopaenia) vaccine is frequently used as the sterile diluent for suspension of the 'cat 'flu' virus vaccine prepared for intra-muscular injection.

The use of vaccines is probably best confined to rather specific circumstances, for example, the healthy single cat which is about to be exposed to infection of kennelling or admission to veterinary hospital premises, the stud male which is repeatedly exposed to potential carriers, or the establishment of a virus free cattery, when the use of vaccine may be combined with a quarantine policy and the virological and serological screening of inmates.

REFERENCES

Baker, J.A. (1944), J. Exp. Med., 79, 159
Crandell, R.A. (1973), Adv. Vet. Sci. Comp. Med., 17, 201.

Crandell, R.A. and Maurer, F.D. (1958), *Proc. Soc. Exp. Biol. &
& Med. N.Y.,* **97**, 487.
Lane, J.G. (1977), *The Vet. Annual,* 17th issue. 164.
Povey, R.C. (1976) *Vet. Rec.,* **98**, 293.
Shields, R.P. (1977) *JAVMA,* **170**, 439.
Wardley, R.C., Povey, R.C. (1977) *Br. Vet. J.,* **133**, 504.
Wardley, R.C., Gaskell, R.M., Povey, R.C. (1974), *JSAP,*
15, 579.
Hoover, E.A., Kahn, D.E. (1975) *JAVMA,* **166**, 463.

Feline Pneumonitis

This is a disease of doubtful significance considered to exist on a
regional basis rather than world-wide. The causative organism,
Chlamydia psittaci, broadly speaking, bacterial rather than viral, was
initially isolated by Baker (1944) and has subsequently been isolated
only in the United States. The disease produced is protracted and rarely fatal, and though described by Baker to involve.both upper and
lower respiratory tract, has more recently [Ott (1971)] been limited on
the basis of experimental investigation to the naso-lachrymal tract.
The usual pattern of prolonged periods of subclinical or latent infection with occasional flare-ups may represent development of partial
immunity or simply recurrent infection [Cello (1971)] since Chlamydia
are, in general, only weakly antigenic.

Clinical symptoms, described by Baker, include an incubation
period of 6-10 days, followed by a transient pyrexia, the disease being
notably afebrile. Most notable symptoms are increased lachrymation
with conjunctivitis, sometimes becoming mucopurulent. Rhinitis with
increased nasal discharge also occurs.

Paroxysmal sneezing, especially after handling, and development of
a cough, with lower tract involvement including pneumonia, may be
associated with secondary infection since under experimental conditions, these have never been reproduced as part of the primary disease.
In all, symptoms persist for at least two weeks.

Pathology in experimental cases is limited to inflammatory changes
in the upper respiratory tract and conjunctivae.

Differential Diagnosis. May be difficult because of the overlap with
symptoms of the other respiratory diseases. The protraeted and
afebrile nature of this illness, together with its favourable response to
antibiotic, especially tetracycline, therapy is a significant diagnostic
aid.

Prognosis. Good.

Treatment. Most antibiotics, but especially chloramphenicol, tetracyclines and penicillin effects clinical improvement within 4 days.

Prophylaxis. Although the use of attentuated and killed virus vaccines has been widespread in the United States, their prophylactic value is now questioned [Ott (1971)].

REFERENCES

Baker, J.A. (1944) *J. Exptl. Med.,* **79**, 159.
Cello, R.M. (1971) *JA VMA.* **158**, 932.
Ott, R.L. (1971), *JA VMA,* **158**, 939.

Feline Enteritis

Feline enteritis or panleucopaenia, a highly infectious disease of domestic and wild Felidae and certain other species [Povey (1973)], presents clinically in the peracute and acute form, with a high mortality in developed cases and a clinical course of 1 day to 1 week. The viral aetiology of the disease was first clearly demonstrated by Hindle and Finlay (1932) who named it Feline Distemper; but this unsuitable name has been largely discarded. More recently the virus has been classified a parvovirus [Johnson (1969)] and its heat stability and resistance to many disinfectants reported [Johnson (1966)]. The result of experimental infection of germ-free cats suggests the diversity and severity of clinical signs and lesions to be the result of interaction of many factors, rather than of viral damage of host tissues alone [Rohovsky and Fowler (1971)], although this damage itself causes an appreciable degree of illness.

Incidence. The disease has been described in Europe and North America, and the incidence is probably world wide. Feline enteritis is apparently becoming less common in many areas of Great Britain, but remains epidemic in some urban areas. Pet shops dealing in kittens and boarding catteries which do not require prophylactic vaccination as a prerequisite to admission are frequently sources of infection. Despite the extremely thorough veterinary inspection demanded at cat shows, these are also possible sources.

The disease is highly infectious and morbidity is thought to be high; however, many cats become immune to the disease without showing symptoms and it is believed that mild or subclinical infections occur. The mortality rate in cats developing symptoms is high, up to 100 per cent has been quoted by Weipers (1957).

Clinical Symptoms. The incubation period has not been well defined but usually ranges from 4–10 days. Many cats are presented *in extremis*, lying on their sides with the back slightly arched, and giving low moans of pain from time to time. During a local outbreak it is not unusual for an owner to present his cat saying it has been 'poisoned' and that several other cats in the area have also been 'poisoned'.

Appetite is lost early and completely. Depression is profound. Dehydration and loss of body tissues develop with extreme rapidity and a kitten which has been ill only 24 hours may present a picture of extreme emaciation. Washing is in complete abeyance. The cat adopts a sternal posture with the forelegs tucked under the chest, and the head drooping. Normal mobility is lost, but there is sometimes a restless wandering to seek cold surfaces or seclusion. A desire for water is evident but the cat is often unable to take it, remaining poised in the sternal position with the head hanging over a saucer, and making occasional feeble attempts to lap.

The most regular symptom is vomiting, which is usually distressed and apparently painful. The vomitus usually consists only of bile-stained (greenish) fluid; vomiting may occur 2 or 3 times only or be repeated frequently during the first 24–72 hours of illness. Diarrhoea, despite the name of the disease, is not a feature of acute cases, although one changed stool may be passed during the first few hours. Death may occur rather suddenly, from about the fifth day of the infection. In less acute cases secondary infections may occur: pneumonia is not an infrequent complication.

Signs found on Clinical Examination. The temperature is raised (except in dying patients) to 40–41° C. (104–106° F.). The mouth and throat show little evidence of inflammation, but there is a foetid odour or that of vomit. The lips and chin may be soiled with bile-stained material. The eyes tend to become sunken and the cat has an anxious withdrawn expression. The cat is more or less hide-bound due to dehydration from a very early stage. The pulse is rapid and weak. Abdominal palpation almost invariably elicits a cry of pain when the epigastrium is examined.

Pathology. Characteristically there are few gross lesions in the bodies of cats which die of feline enteritis, and in hyperacute cases none may be found. Frequently a localised congestion of a portion of the small intestine (usually in the middle region) is found. In early cases the mucosa is congested: haemorrhage and sloughing have been described in later cases. The mesenteric lymph glands are swollen and moist and may be haemorrhagic. A fluid or semi-fluid bone marrow is suggestive of feline enteritis. Inconstant changes have been described in the spleen, lungs and thymus, and lesions attributable to secondary infections may be present.

On histological examination, striking changes may be detected in the blood from about the fourth day of the infection. Typically a profound leucopenia occurs, but cases in which a relative lymphocytosis and even a leucocytosis occurred have been described. The bone marrow is aplastic. In the presence of signs or lesions suggestive of feline enteritis, the occurrence of eosinophilic intranuclear inclusion bodies (Cowdray Type A) in the intestinal epithelial cells or germinal cells of the lymph nodes may be regarded as diagnostic. These inclusions may be absent if autopsy is carried out some hours after death (Hammon & Enders 1939).

Diagnosis. Diagnosis is based on the clinical picture, typical features being the rapid development of dehydration and extreme illness, vomiting, fever and anterior abdominal pain. An examination of blood films will usually show the presence of leucopenia, but as pointed out above, this is not invariably present. When making blood films it should be remembered that the blood may contain high concentrations of virus. Where positive diagnosis is essential (e.g. in catteries) confirmatory evidence should be sought by post-mortem examination and demonstration of inclusion bodies.

Differential Diagnosis. Bacterial and allergic gastroenteritis and intestinal penetration by foreign bodies are uncommon in cats, but may produce confusingly similar symptoms. The enlarged and palpably turgid small intestine may in some cases be mis-diagnosed as intussusception or soft foreign body. Acute septicaemia must also be considered in differential diagnosis of all severely depressed subjects.

Carpenter (1971) has listed a large number of differentials which may require consideration in the event of atypical symptomatology. Some symptoms, such as otacariasis and bite wound abscesses may be exacerbated by a general lowering of resistance secondary to viral infection. In some cases, gingivitis and palatine ulceration have been encountered and in others respiratory lesions, including pneumonia, and giving cause for problems of differentiation from both feline respiratory virus infections and toxoplasmosis.

In some cases of relatively mild illness various blood dyscrasias may occur, especially anaemia and thrombocytopaenia with resultant haemorrhagic lesions. That absolute reliance cannot be placed on demonstrability or otherwise of a leucopaenia is re-iterated by many who have studied the virus experimentally in-vivo. It is suggested that in many cases a relative leucopaenia may exist for an individual animal without this being apparent on the basis of a single blood count [O'Reilly (1971)].

Cerebellar Ataxia. This ataxic condition of kittens is associated with cerebellar deficiency which has been variously described as aplasia, agenesis, hypoplasia, hypotrophy and dysplasia. It is clinically recognizable between the ages of 8 and 16 weeks, when the persistent unsteadiness and lack of motor control can be distinguished from infant unsteadiness.

Clinical signs include lack of co-ordination, some limb spasticity, a high stepping gait and tendency to topple over. Nystagmus may be present and though appetite is normal, prehension of food and especially the lapping of fluids may occasion some difficulty. Generally all litter-mates are affected though the range of disability within a group is wide and the mildest cases can, within limits, pass as normal.

The aetiology of the condition was long assumed genetic since its congenital transmission was well established, but the chance discovery of the effects of parvovirus infection upon the cerebellar tissues of neonatal hamsters led to re-evaluation of these very similar lesions in ataxic kittens [Kilham, Margolis and Colby (1967)]. The isolation of a transmissible agent capable of reproducing cerebellar damage, when administered in utero or to neonates, quickly followed, and this was eventually established to be feline panleucopaenia virus which, being a parvovirus with selective affinity for mitotic cells, was seen to attack the external germinal layer of the granular cortex giving rise to a 'granuloprival' hypoplasia.

More detailed experimental work has revealed severest clinical cases to correspond to in-utero infection and milder cases to neo-natal infection, with correspondingly less cerebellar damage. Viral isolation studies further reveal that many ataxic kittens, in spite of acquiring passive maternal antibodies, continue to disseminate panleucopaenia virus for weeks or months [Kilham, Margolis and Colby (1971)]. Treatment is impossible and because of the risk of prolonged dissemination of virus, it is advisable to euthanase all cases, although, as stated, many subjects are capable of remarkable adaption and may, within a fixed environment, lead a relatively normal existence.

Prognosis. Always very guarded to grave.

Treatment. There is no specific treatment in Great Britain, but hyperimmune serum may be used where available. Treatment is thus mainly supportive. Chloramphenicol has been claimed to be of value, but antibiotic therapy can only control secondary infection. Maintenance of body fluids by suitable infusions, usually glucose-saline subcutaneously, is essential. High potency vitamin preparations may be added. Good nursing is essential and should be undertaken by the owner to ensure maximum response by the patient. The cat should be kept at an even temperature in a well ventilated room. Vomitus should be cleaned from the mouth and face. Small quantities of fluid such as glucose water with or without a few drops of brandy, or egg white, glucose and brandy should be given at frequent intervals.

Prophylaxis. Modified live virus and inactivated virus vaccines are available. Both provoke good antibody response in fully susceptible subjects, the live virus after administration on a single occasion and the inactivated virus after two doses administered at 14 day intervals.Appreciable antibody levels may not be measurable until 7 days post vaccination, but an effective degree of protection is thought to exist within 3 days. Free living cats in endemic areas are likely to receive repeated exposure to virus and so to maintain high antibody titres, whereas isolated animals may require annual vaccinal boosting. Blanket recommendations for annual revaccination err on the side of safety since even dead viral vaccine is probably sufficiently antigenic to provoke life-long immunity [Povey (1973)]. Because passively acquired, maternally derived antibodies, transferred to kittens in colostrum, are likely to impair vaccinal response, a course of vaccination should not be completed before 12 weeks of age, by which time all kittens are thought to have lost the passive antibody. Since the degree and duration of protection conferred by the passive antibody is impossible to assess clinically, the requirements of a kitten in an endemic disease situation may best be served by repeated vaccination at intervals of 2 to 4 weeks from 8 weeks of age onward to 12 weeks.

Because of the known affinity of panleucopaenia virus for actively dividing cells, foetal tissues are particularly susceptible and the administration of live-virus vaccines during pregnancy is not considered advisable [Povey (1973)].

For convenient vaccination of groups of kittens placed in high risk situations, as at cat shelters, etc., the practicality of aerosol administration of vaccine has been demonstrated [Scott and Glauberg (1975)], although the technique is not in general use.

Note
During any acute local epidemic of feline enteritis it is wise to suspend all appointments for the castration and spaying of kittens. Even a brief sojourn in a waiting room or surgery into which infected patients are being brought may be sufficient to transmit infection to these kittens, which develop the disease in the post-operative period, often with a fatal outcome. Despite all explanations, this will be attributed by the owner to the neutering operation.

REFERENCES

Carpenter, J.L. (1971), *JAVMA,* **158, 857.**
Hammon, W.D., Enders, J.F., (1939), *J. exp. Med.,* **69,** 327.
Hindle, E. and Finlay, G.M. (1932), *J. comp. Path.* **45,** 11.
Johnson, R.H. (1966), *Res. Vet. Sci.,* 7, 112.
Johnson, R.H. (1969), *Vet. Rec.,* **84,** 19.
Kilham, L.; Margolis, G. Colby, E.D. (1971), *JAVMA,* **158,** 888.
O'Reilly, K.J. (1971), *JAVMA, * **158,** 862.
Povey, R.C. (1973), *JSAP,* **14,** 399.
Rohovsky, M.W. and Fowler, E.H. (1971), *JAVMA,* **158,** 872.
Scott, F.W. and Glauberg, A.F. (1975), *JAVMA,* **166,** 147.
Weipers, W.L. (1957), *Vet. Rec.,* **69,** 707.

SUGGESTED FURTHER READING

Feline Enteritis (Panleucopenia)
Sternfels, M. (1956) *Vet. Med.* **51,** 329. (Infectious enteritis and pneumonitis in cats.)

Newberne, J. W. *et al.* (1957) *South West. Vet.* **10**, 111. (Studies on clinical and histopathological aspects of feline panleucopenia (infectious enteritis).)

Noble, C. & Sim, M. (1958) *Vet. Rec.* **70**, 262. (A case of 'feline enteritis' treated with cortisone and ACTH.)

Christoph, H. J. & Vierneisel, H. (1961) *Kleintier-Praxis* **6**, 10. (Prognostic value of the white blood picture in feline enteritis.)

Vogel, A. (1961) *Kleintier-Praxis* **6**, 15. (The clinical picture of feline enteritis.)

Ulcerative Glossitis

This is a clearly recognised clinical entity, apparently infectious in nature, since a number of cases tend to be seen simultaneously in a district. It is usually regarded as of viral origin. Weipers (1957) postulates some relationship between ulcerative glossitis and feline enteritis since he has observed that cats recovered from the former disease appeared to be immune to the latter. It is certainly true that cases of both diseases do appear in a locality over a similar period of time. However it is probably wise to consider ulcerative glossitis as a separate entity.

Incidence. Variable. The disease usually occurs during young adult to early middle life, but is less common among kittens than feline enteritis. Cases occur sporadically or in minor local outbreaks, but the disease seldom attains true epidemic proportions. Special sources of infection have not been recognised. The morbidity rate is unknown. Mortality is very low.

Clinical Symptoms. Ulcerative glossitis is invariably a mild disease with a course of 5–9 days from the onset of symptoms.

Initially loss of appetite and slight depression are noticed. Within 12–36 hours a variable degree of salivation follows. Sometimes the lips are noted to be frothy, but copious salivation often results in strings of clear, watery slightly viscous secretion hanging from the mouth; pools may be formed where the cat has been sitting. The posture is usually a comfortable one with forelimbs flexed. Sneezing is slight, but spluttering attempts to rid the mouth of secretion are common. The nose and eyes are usually free of discharge. Washing and eating are in abeyance due to the soreness of the lesions on the tongue. Body weight and hydration are usually unaffected and though miserable, affected cats are not obviously ill.

Signs found on Examination. The temperature is slightly raised, usually to between 39·2° C. (102·5° F.) and 39·7° C. (103·5° F.). The appearance of the mouth is diagnostic. In the first 12–24 hours the whole buccal and glossal mucosa is congested; there is a tendency to frothiness rather than copious secretion at this stage. At 24–48 hours salivation increases and inflammatory changes are becoming localised to the tongue edges. From 48 hours onwards there is frank ulceration of the borders of the tongue with erosion extending from the edges over the dorsal surface. The ulcers are usually multiple and variable in size, and they may occasionally involve the hard and soft palates. Patients are frequently not presented until ulcers and salivation have developed, and it may be assumed that these are in the third or fourth day of illness. In most cases healing has commenced by the fifth day; ability to prehend food returns between the fifth and ninth days according to the severity of the ulceration. It is occasionally obvious that appetite has returned before painful symptoms have subsided.

Recovery is usually complete by the seventh to ninth day.

Diagnosis. Based on the clinical picture.

Differential diagnosis should exclude dental diseases which produce salivation (gingivitis, parodontal disease, foreign bodies) and the occasional case of ulceration of the hard palate unassociated with fever.

The characteristic distribution of ulcers differs from that of the randomly distributed ulcers of FCV infection and it is probable that a separate aetiological agent exists.

Prognosis. Good. Recovery within 10 days.

Treatment. There is no specific treatment. Antibacterial therapy is not usually indicated.

Advice on good nursing is valuable, including recommendations to keep the mouth free of discharges, the use of a simple mouthwash such as Compound Glycerin of Thymol, and maintenance of an even temperature. Forced feeding is rarely necessary and only advisable at the stage when appetite is clearly regained but lesions persist. The administration of fluids requiring any lapping movement on the part of the cat is not indicated: it is better to insert small pieces of soft solids, e.g. raw liver or meat, into the mouth between the pre-molar teeth. The cat will often chew them readily, as mastication is less painful than lapping. Since the cat is unable to wash itself, it will also be happier if its chin, neck and legs are kept dry. Vitamin therapy may be given when lesions commence to heal; a multi-vitamin preparation containing Vitamin C for parenteral use is preferable.

Prophylaxis. None available.

REFERENCES

Weipers, W. L. (1957) *Vet. Rec.* **69**, 707.

Feline Infectious Anemia.

This disease, sporadically reported in the United States and Great Britain, was initially described in S. Africa (Clark) in 1942. The causative blood parasite, variously designated Haemobartonella felis and Eperythrozoon felis, has been classified among the protozoa and the Rickettsia. Found in many animal species, these parasites are very host specific, are certainly transmitted by insect vectors and probably also by oral and transplacental infection. After a variable incubation period large numbers of organisms appear in blood as red cell parasites as a result of which haemolysis and anaemia occur. After subsidence of parasitaemia infection at low levels may persist, with occasional recrudescences. These parasites are sensitive to organic arsenicals and tetracyclines, but not to sulphonamides, penicillin or streptomycin.

Incidence. In spite of world wide distribution of the disease cases are rather infrequent since many infections are subclinical and unrecognized. In a review of 374 cases presenting routinely among, 43,514 feline cases in eleven American Veterinary School hospital clinics, the risk for males was seen to be some 2½ times that for females, with an age peak at from 4-6 years of age (Hayes and Priester (1973)). The condition is also often detected in cats presented for reasons other than anaemia, e.g. abscesses, suggesting that parasitism might predispose cats to such disease. Equally, severe and intractable infectious anaemia, positively diagnosed from blood smears, has been encountered in cats harbouring FeLV and it seems likely that the immunosuppressive effects of the viral disease may be responsible for the high incidence of anaemia as a major presenting symptom of FeLV infection, there may, inevitably, be problems of differential diagnosis in such cases.

Clinical Symptoms. As stated, some infections are inapparent, or symptoms are so mild as to attract no attention, but in others listlessness, anorexia, wasting and weakness may occur. Generally the disease runs a prolonged course of 2-3 weeks or more, but in some cases symptoms present precipitously and cats are presented in a collapsed or moribund condition.

Signs on Clinical Examination. Ectoparasitism may be evident. In some cases there may be mild pyrexia and in severe cases temperature may be subnormal, but in most cases it remains within normal limits. Conjunctival and buccal mucosae may be normal or pallid according to severity of anaemia and mild jaundice may occur. In some cases splenic enlargement is palpable.

Differentiation. Differentiating from the several other causes of anaemia in cats may be difficult especially in circumstances under which there may be suspicion of FeLV infection. If feline infectious anaemia is suspected a haematological examination must be made, but the parasites may be difficult to demonstrate with signs of haemolytic anaemia remaining the strongest suggestive evidence of infection.

Pathology. Blood may appear anaemic when withdrawn and haemoglobin level may be considerably reduced. Early smears may show leucocytosis, but anaemic changes usually occur after parasites have been demonstrable for some time and may include anisocytosis, polychromasia, normoblastosis and Howell-Jolly bodies. Parasites can be demonstrated in films prepared on clean slides and stained with Romanowsky or Giemsa stains. Care must be taken to avoid artefacts which may be mistaken for parasitic organisms. Most of the eperythrozoa occur on erythrocytes and are most easily seen on the tail (thin portion) of blood smears. The organisms are about 200 millimicrons in diameter, just visible with a light microscope, and may be seen singly or in small clusters on the surfaces of red cells. At the height of an infection 50 percent or more red cells may be infected, but in carrier states fewer than one red cell in a thousand may be involved. At autopsy the spleen may be enlarged and dark and lymph gland enlargement may also be presented. Paleness, wasting and jaundice of the carcass may also be evident, as may lesions of concurrent disease.

Prognosis. Depends on the state of the animal at the time of diagnosis and on the presence or absence of concurrent disease. In early subclinical or uncomplicated clinical cases prognosis is good, although total elimination of infection is difficult and recurrences may occur.

Treatment. With blood transfusion of citrated blood and supportive fluid therapy may be indicated in the severely ill patient. Organic arsenical drugs although effective against haemobartonella and eperythrozoa are more toxic than the tetracyclines which are therefore used in preference. Intermittent usage of arsenicals may be indicated in cases which have failed to respond to daily administration of tetracyclines, and chloramphenicol therapy may also be attempted.

Prophylaxis. Elimination of ectoparasites will help limit the spread from carriers and aseptic precautions should be observed for the same reason when injecting cats in colonies.

REFERENCES

Clark, R.J.S. (1942) *Afr. Vet. Med. Ass.* **13**, 15.
Hayes, H.M. and Priester, W.A. (1973) *JSAP,* **14**, 797

SUGGESTED FURTHER READING

Feline Infectious Anaemia
Flint, J. C. & McKelvie, D. H. (1956) *Proc. 92nd. Ann. Meet. Amer. Vet. Medical Association* 240. (Feline infectious anaemia—diagnosis and treatment.)
Splitter, E. J. *et al.* (1956) *Vet. Med.* **51**, 17. (Feline infectious anaemia.)
Schwartsman, R. N. & Besch, E. D. (1958) *Vet. Med.* **53**, 494. (Feline infectious anaemia.)
Flint, J. C. *et al.* (1958–59) *Amer. J. Vet. Res.* **19**, 164, **20**, 33. (Feline infectious anaemia. I. Clinical Aspects. II. Experimental cases.)
Inchii, S. *et al.* (1961) *Acta vet. jap.* **6**, 18. (In English.) (Experimental studies on feline infectious anaemia, haemobartonellosis.)

Feline Leukaemia Lymphosarcoma Complex

Feline Leukaemia Virus (Fe LV) Induced Disease.

The natural history of the feline leukaemia virus (Fe LV) has been thoroughly studied and reported in recent years [Cotter, Hardy & Essex (1975); Jarrett (1975); Mackey (1975)]. Debate on the zoonotic implications of feline viral infection and viral dissemination remains extant, though a balanced review by Hardy and his associates (1974) states them to be largely conjectural.

The results of virological surveys of domestic cats on both sides of the Atlantic (Cotter et. al. 1975. Jarrett 1975), have produced broadly complementary impressions of viral and disease distribution, although Cotter et. al., reporting surveys carried out in two distinctly different urban environments, emphasized that a preponderance of socially isolated subjects; e.g. single, flat-dwelling city cats, markedly reduces the incidence of Fe LV induced disease within that area.

Incidence. Subjects failing to develop effective resistance to Fe LV infection are liable, unless they become symptomless carriers, to succumb, after latency of sometimes several years duration, to disease of the lympho-reticular (reticulo-endothelial) system, which being a component of the connective tissues throughout all organ systems, results in a potentially widespread dissemination of disease symptoms. It was the prevalence within cat colonies of illnesses of this nature, either as true leukaemia or lymphosarcomatous tumour development, that initially led to an assumption of congenital transmission of the disease, with probable genetic implication. Observation of horizontal transmission; i.e. by contact, between unrelated colony members, however, led to a search for a transmissable agent as a result of which Fe LV was identified in tumour tissue and later isolated.

This oncorna virus has been grown in tissue culture of both human and feline origin, is known to multiply in a wide variety of tissues while causing damage only to cells of the lympho-reticular system, and to comprise at least three sub-groups not yet fully differentiated. Experimental investigation confirms the virus to be eliminated in saliva, respiratory mucous, urine and milk.

Reliable methods of detecting virus and antivirus antibodies in cats now exist and have faciliated epidemiological studies. Jarrett and co-workers presently prefer confirmation of virus infection to be by viral growth in tissue culture, but in the United States on-slide immuno fluorescent antibody tests, based on group specific internal virion antigens, are preferred. Confusion in the literature reporting serological surveys of the feline and human population appears to arise because neutralizing antibodies are produced to two other distinct antigens. One antibody produced specifically in response to the viral envelope antigen indicates the presence of Fe LV, the other produced in response to the antigen associated with new cell membranes manufactured to viral specification (known as feline oncorna virus cell membrane antigen or F.O.C.M.A.) but not themselves viral components, indicates that cell infection has occurred (Hardy 1974). Antibodies produced to F.O.C.M.A. enables cats to resist or reject virally induced tumours but to remain carriers of virus which is itself unaffected by the antibody.

The epidemiological studies reported suggest that beyond approximately five months of age, by which time the majority of free living and cattery cats will have been subjected to viral infection, the feline population is divisible into four groups. One group, containing neither virus nor antibody, represents all genetically resistant animals and a few fully susceptible animals which because of unnatural isolation have not met the virus. The major group, containing antibody but no virus, represents cats which are disease free, having met and rejected Fe LV. In both remaining groups, the cats harbour and excrete virus, in one group remaining disease free because of the presence of antibodies, but in the other having no antibody and eventually succumbing to symptoms of lympho-reticular disease.

In general, free living cats from single cat households are represented in the major group, having antibody but no virus. Conversely, multi-cat establishments, especially those imposing a restricted life style (i.e. catteries) yield a high proportion of viraemic cats, both symptomless and diseased, while the remainder of their inmates register high antibody titres. Present evidence suggests that prolonged exposure to virus may be necessary to establish infection in the face of the body's natural tendency to produce antibodies and reject the virus. For this reason, exposure at cat shows and during stud activities may be less hazardous than might at first be expected.

Clinical Symptoms. Inevitably variable since Fe LV infection results not only in disease of the tissues of the lympho-reticular system, but in a wider range of disease of the haematopoietic system, reproductive and renal systems and in illnesses induced by its immunosuppressive effects. Thus, an infected cattery may give rise to a large number of disease conditions before a typical leukaemia or lymphosarcoma occurs.

Frequently, the colony has a history of infertility and abortion among its females. Often foetuses palpable at four weeks are resorbed before the sixth week of pregnancy, sometimes with the accompaniment of a haemorrhagic vaginal discharge. Heavy losses of young stock, sometimes from relatively common and potentially minor infections, is attributable to an impaired ability to mount successful immune responses. Thus Fe LV infection may underlie apparently intractable septicaemuas, recurrent fevers, respiratory and enteric conditions which may sometimes mimic Panleucopaenia in severity.

Glomerulo nephritis has also been associated with Fe LV (Cotter et.

al. 1975), subjects presenting with persistent proteinurea, uraemia, hypoproteinaemia and oedema.

Isolation of Fe LV from a high proportion of cases of F.I.P. has led to diagnostic problems and confusion as to the true aetiology of F.I.P. (This is discussed more fully under the heading Feline Infectious Peritonitis).

Anaemia is a common presenting symptom of Fe LV infection, not necessarily associated with preceding leukaemic illness. Both haemolytic and aplastic anaemia may be attributable to Fe LV infection, the latter rapidly fatal and the former sometimes initially responsive to treatment. Excessively severe haemolytic anaemia attributable to Haemobartonella felis infection may also co-exist with Fe Lv infection. Lympho-reticular disease itself may present as 'true' leukaemia confined to the lymphoid cells of the bone marrow from which malignant cells seed out into circulation, or it may be multi-centric involving the reticulo-endothelial cells of many organ systems in the development of tumours. Distribution of tumours is variable and influences presentation of symptoms, but thymic masses causing respiratory distress and mesenteric or alimentary masses producing symptoms of alimentary disease are common. True multicentric lympho-sarcoma, presenting with enlargment of all peripheral lymph nodes also occurs but must be differentiated from the generalized lymphadenopathy relating to such infections as Toxoplasmosis.

In some cases presenting symptoms relate solely to the physical presence of an isolated tumour mass, as, for example, in the nasopharynx, in which cases symptoms are primarily those of nasal obstruction with occasional dysphagia.

Signs On Examination. Because of the complexity of this disease and the numerous organ systems occasionally involved, it is often impossible to achieve a diagnostic conclusion at first examination. Particular suspicion attaches to non-specific illnesses of young adult cats and especially to episodes of recurrent fever or lassitude and any sign of mucosal pallor. Unexpectedly severe illness of known aetiology must also be regarded with suspicion as must any record of unfertility.

Although Fe LV infection may most logically be suspected in subjects from multi-cat households, single households must not be overlooked, since many of these, especially pedigree varieties, may have emanated as kittens from an infected multi-cat situation.

Diagnosis. Changes in the haemogram are frequently inconclusive. Identification of the virus by the methods reported is necessary for positive diagnosis of any manifestation of the disease other than the classic multicentric lymphosarcoma in which case confirmatory biopsies may be obtained.

Treatment. Unsatisfactory and ill-advised. In some forms of the disease, as for example, early haemolytic anaemia, symptomatic treatment may affect transitory improvement. Temporary remission with some regression of tumour masses may be achieved by the use of cortio steroids and anti-tumour drugs like cyclophosphamide, but recorded results are discouraging (Henness & Crow 1977). At the present time there is no way to eliminate the virus from infected cats, and the majority of viraemic cats will eventually succumb to symptoms of disease.

At the present level of knowledge a viraemic cat remains under suspicion as a public health hazard (Hardy et. al. 1974), so that euthanasia is indicated even in the single cat household situation.

In a colony situation, viraemic animals constitute the reservoir for infection and euthanasia is essential since isolation of individuals is impossible. An erradication scheme with three-monthly retesting is recommended. In the case of particularly prized specimens a short period of isolation followed by a retest may be indicated on the basis that the animal may at initial test, have developed insufficient antibody to reject the virus. This is the most logically applied to the unexpected 'breakdown' case in a regularly tested colony in which case the duration of infection is known to be short.

A vaccine is in course of preparation, but is not yet clinically available.

Cotter S.M.; Hardy W.D.; Essex M. (1975) *J.A.V.M.A.* **166** 449.

Hardy W.D. (1974) *J.A.V.M.A.* **165** 316.

Hardy W.D.; McClelland A.J.; Hess P.W.: MacEwen E.G. (1974) *J.A.V.M.A.* **165** 1020

Henness A.M.; Crow S.E. (1977) *J.A.V.M.A.* **171** 263.

Jarrett O. (1975) *J.S.A.P.* **16** 409.

Mackey L.J. (1975) *Vet. Rec.* **96** 5.

Feline Infectious Peritonitis (F.I.P.)

Clearly recognizable as a clinical entity, this invariably fatal, chronic fibrinous peritonitis is apparently naturally infectious since simultaneous occurrences among members of the same household is frequently recorded. Experimental transmission by the injection of blood, urine, peritoneal fluid or tissue homogenates by several routes is recorded (Hardy & Hurvitz, *1971*), though occasionally with production of atypical disease symptoms (Ward, Gribble and Dungworth, *1974*), and particles of a filtrable virus-like agent have been indentified by electron microscopy in many induced and naturally occurring cases. This has recently been classified a Coronavirus (Horzinek M.C., Osterhaus A.D.M.E., Ellens D.J., *1977*).

Incidence. The disease occurs variably and morbidity is low. Felidae of all species and ages are susceptible, although the majority of recorded cases involve young domestic males of the "foreign" varieties. Though first described in domestics only as recently as 1963 (Holzworth) the disease has been known in the area of Davis, California since 1954 and New York City since 1956. It has since been sporadically reported outside the United States, although, on the basis of immunofluorescent assay techniques distribution of the virus is known to be widespread (Horzinek).

Clinical Symptoms. As originally described, symptoms are typified by persistent antibiotic resistant fever, often initially leading to suspicion of other diseases but subsequently associated with abdominal distension consequent upon copious peritoneal exudation. On the basis of experimental transmission studies an incubation of 2-14 days is postulated, but under field conditions, this may be as long as 4 months, because of the insidious nature of the disease, animals may initially be presented when exhibiting only symptoms of inappetance or lassitude prior to onset of more typical symptoms and the duration of identifiable illness may vary from one week to two months.

Signs Found on Examination. Early cases may be limited to lassitude, a variable pyrexia in the range 103°0-150°0°F (39°5-40°6°C) and in some cases slight abdominal tenderness with palpable enlargement of mesenteric lymph nodes. In more advanced cases, peritoneal effusion is the cardinal sign and may present as an initially pendulous abdomen or a tautly over-distended abdomen. Some subjects remain in this state for several weeks with development of a few additional symptoms, though terminal mucosal pallor and jaundice are common. Systolic murmurs may be associated with these terminal cardio-vascular symptoms (Robinson, Holzworth & Gilmore 1971) and symptoms of gastro-intestinal upset are also relatively common.

In less classic cases, symptoms of illness are associated with disease of other serosal surfaces, notably in chest and scrotum, Dyspnoea as a result of gross pleuritis with thoracic effusion may precede, follow or be concurrent with symptoms of abdominal distension and periorchitis and epididymitis may occur, though rarely with presentation of clinical symptoms. In a variant form (Slausson & Finn 1972, Legendre & Whitenack 1975) basic symptoms of anorexia, pyrexia, lassitude and deterioration with resistance to antibiotic therapy, are accompanied by symptoms arising from pyogranulomatous meningoencephalitis sometimes with panopthalmitis, rather than inflammation of serosal surfaces. Such animals present localized symptoms, including paresis, tremors and ocular lesions, sometimes with visible accumulation of purulent exudate in anterior eye chambers.

Diagnosis. Difficult because of the variety of presenting symptoms, although fever resistant to antibiotic therapy is a consistent feature.

In the more typically exudative cases, the nature of the exudate obtained by paracentesis is considered diagnostic, being an abundant bacteriologically sterile golden fluid of high specific gravity containing much protein and few cells, frequently flocculent in appearance and clotting on exposure to air. Thoracic and pericardial effusion, which may occur, present a similar appearance. Haemograms may reveal anaemia, neutrophilia and lymphopaenia.

Diagnostic Post-Mortem Features. Most consistently a focal or diffuse peritonitis with copious exudative fluid. In advanced cases, serosal surfaces have a greyish fibrinous texture, omentum may be thickened, opaque and patchily necrotic and there may be focal hepatic necrosis. Pleuritis is usually less severe, though there may be focal haemorhage, oedema and pneumonia in some cases. Orchitis and testicular enlargement may occur and granulomatous and suppurative meningitis may occur alone or in conjunction with other lesions.

Diagnostic Differentials. Include congestive cardiac failure, hepatic cirrhosis, chylothorax, pyothorax, aleukaemic lymphoma, tuberculosis, toxoplasmosis, feline infectious anaemia, pansteatitis and post-traumatic inflammatory changes.

Treatment. General supportive therapy using fluids, electrolytes, haematopoietics, steroids and antibiotics may prolong life for as long as the patient retains sufficient interest to feed, but relapse with dehydration and emaciation invariably leads to a fatal conclusion. A single case is reported to have responded to a regime of tylosin by mouth (50 mgm.t.i.d.) and intra peritoneally (200 mgm.) following paracentesis, together with prednisolone (Robinson et. al. 1971).

Prophylaxis. Preventative measures cannot be taken as long as the origin of infection and mode of natural transmission remain obscure. The aetiological agent is yet to be isolated, although viral particles have been described in experimental infection. The co-existence of FeLV infection in many subjects is considered to be more than coincidental (Hardy et. al. 1971), though precise aetiological significance is unclear.

REFERENCES

Hardy W.D.; Hurvitz A.I. (1971) *J.A.V.M.A.* **158**, 994.

Holzworth J. (1963) *Cornell Vet.* **53**, 157.

Horzinek. M.C., Osterhaus A.D. M.E., Ellens D.J. **1977** Zbl. *Vet. Med. B.* **24.**, p. 398-405).

Legendre A.M.; Whitenack D.L. (1975) *J.A.V.M.A.* **167**, 931

Robinson R.L.; Holzworth J.; Gilmore C.E. (1971) *J.A.V.M.A.* **158**, 981.

Slausson D.O.; Finn J.P. (1972) *J.A.V.M.A.* **160**, 729.

Ward, J.M.; Gribble D.H.; Dungworth D.L. (1974) *Am. J. Vet. Res.* **35**, 1271.

Additional reading: Wolfe, L.G.; Griesmer, R.A. (1971) *J.A.V.M.A.* **158**, 987. Feline Infectious Peritonitis: Review of Gross and Histopathologic lesions.

Tuberculosis

Infection with *Mycobacterium tuberculosis* was at one time a moderately common condition in the cat. The incidence was reported to vary between 2 and 13 per cent in autopsy cases (Francis). Cats are susceptible to the bovine strain but are comparatively resistant to the human. For this reason the incidence of tuberculosis in cats should be, and is, showing a marked decline following eradication of the disease from the national dairy herd. This contention is supported by figures for cats coming to autopsy at the Veterinary Hospital at Liverpool. In 1949 Jennings reported the unusually high incidence of 13 per cent, whereas for the seven year period 1957–63 only five cases (2 per cent) of tuberculosis were found in 235 cats at autopsy.

Although this trend is likely to continue it is still necessary for the veterinary surgeon to be aware of the possibility of tuberculosis as a disease in obscure syndromes in cats. Sporadic cases still arise in which it is impossible even to postulate a source of infection. The fact that some people believe the Siamese cat to be particularly liable to tuberculosis suggests the possibility of dormant infections in some communities such as breeding catteries.

It is not possible to describe any characteristic symptomatology. Symptoms are related to the organs infected and the usual conception of tuberculosis as being predominantly abdominal in the cat due to ingestion of infected animal products, milk or meat, is no longer true. In addition to infection of the abdominal lymph nodes (the ileo-colic node is commonly infected), infection of various other nodes has been found. This suggests that tuberculous lymphadenopathy is rather frequent in the cat. Less usual sites of infection are the thoracic organs and pleura, uterus and joints. In general it may be said that any disease in a cat which runs a sub-acute or chronic course (4 weeks to 4 months) and which is associated with wasting and a fluctuating or persistently elevated temperature should be critically reviewed with tuberculosis in mind. In addition any infected local lesion, especially if associated with a sinus, which shows no tendency to respond to routine treatment should be fully investigated bacteriologically. Sinuses of the neck region are traditionally suspect, and these too, should be carefully investigated for tuberculosis although most prove negative.

The undermentioned cases serve to emphasise the need for full investigation in animals with an unusual lesion and running an unusual course.

A $5\frac{3}{4}$ year castrated male cat showed lameness on the left forelimb which was localised to the carpus. Lameness persisted in variable degree for some months during which time pain could usually be elicited by flexion and extension of the carpus; the general health of the cat remained normal. Early in the fifth month a fluctuating swelling developed on the medial aspect of the carpus and temperature was raised to 39·4° C. (103° F.). There was no response to penicillin and the local lesion was opened and drained. Following surgery swelling spread from the lesion to involve the whole lower limb and foot; this was doughy and diffuse and suggested a cellulitis. Chlortetracyeline was prescribed; there was no response. The lesion showed no tendency to heal and radiography disclosed an arthritis; in view of the total absence of response to antibiotics a swab was taken for bacteriological examination. Tubercle bacilli were found and the cat was destroyed. At autopsy no other lesion was found in the body; the most likely explanation is that this infection was caused by a bite from another tuberculous cat. The organism was of the bovine type.

The second unusual case was a 9-months-old Siamese female presented with a vaginal discharge which had followed the first oestrus cycle. The owners refused advice to spay as they wished to breed from the cat. The cat was in moderate condition and temperature was slightly raised. There was no response to penicillin treatment. Discharge persisted and there was some loss of condition which caused the owners to agree to spaying. At operation the uterus was found to be markedly enlarged and thrown into curious spiral convolutions. The general condition of the cat improved considerably for some 2–3 weeks after operation but her condition then showed a general deterioration with recurrence of fever. In view of the failure of previous antibiotic therapy streptomycin was administered. There was a marked response, but an immediate relapse on withdrawal; this was regarded as highly suggestive of tuberculosis, and permission to destroy was eventually obtained. Postmortem examination confirmed the existence of advanced tuberculous peritonitis.

Diagnosis of tuberculosis presents much difficulty unless the organism can be demonstrated or isolated from suitable material such as pus or pleural and peritoneal effusions. The intradermal tuberculin test is not sufficiently evaluated in the cat and the subcutaneous test, unreliable at the best of times, is even less helpful in this species. The use of streptomycin (or other antitubercular drugs such as iso-nicotinic acid hydrazide) as a 'therapeutic-diagnostic' test is warranted and spectacular symptomatic response to specific therapy together with a suggestive clinical course may be taken as sufficient evidence to put a putative diagnosis strongly to owners.

Treatment is seldom justifiable in view of the risk of human infection, especially to children, and euthanasia is the usual course. In particular circumstances, and if strict isolation of the patient can be safely and effectively achieved, a line of treatment suggested and used by Smith (1964) in experimentally infected cats might be considered. An 8–12 week course of iso-nicotinic acid hydrazide punctuated by several 1-week courses of streptomycin is given, but Smith warns that one such treated cat yielded tubercle bacilli from a lymph node at autopsy, although apparently cured.

Although now rare, tuberculosis should be borne in mind by veterinary surgeons who have a serious public health responsibility in cases of this disease.

REFERENCES

Francis, J. (1958) *Tuberculosis in Animals and Man.* (Cassell).
Jennings, A. R. (1949) *Vet. Rec.* **61**, 380.
Smith, J. E. (1964) *J. Small An. Pract.* **5**, 517.

SUGGESTED FURTHER READING

Tuberculosis
Dobson, N. (1930) *J. Comp. Path.* **43**, 310.
Griffiths, A. S. (1926) *J. Comp. Path.* **39**, 71.
Innes, J. R. M. (1940) *Vet. J.* **96**, 96.
Lovell, R. (1930) *J. Comp. Path.* **43**, 205.
Lovell, R. & White, E. G. (1940) *Brit. J. Tuberc.* **34**, 117.
Lovell, R. & White, E. G. (1941) *Brit. J. Tuberc.* **35**, 28.
Goret, P. (1964) *Cah. Med. Vet.* **33**, 151. (In French).
Hawthorne, V. M. *et al.* (1957) *Brit. Med. J.* 675.

Hepatic-renal syndrome

This syndrome has been recognised regularly but not frequently in cats from 2½–7 years old, and is considered sufficiently characteristic to merit attention here in the hope that further investigation may be stimulated.

Symptomatically the disease has much in common with *Leptospira icterohaemorrhagica* infection in dogs but thorough investigation of a number of cases has eliminated leptospires as a possible cause. In this respect it should be noted that clinical disease due to leptospiral infection has not been reported in cats, although it appears likely that they could become infected with a wide variety of serotypes, especially those from small rodents. A serological investigation of about 100 cat sera demonstrated low titres of agglutinins to several leptospiral serotypes, but in no instance could clinical disease be correlated with these findings.

The hepatic-renal syndrome is characterised by a rather acute illness initially and owners seldom delay long before seeking advice. Symptoms include inappetence, dullness, vomiting and thirst. During the initial phase the temperature is always slightly raised to 39·2–40° C. (102·5–104° F.), and icterus is occasionally present from the outset.

On examination the raised temperature is noted and although there may have been no history of diarrhoea the faeces adhering to the thermometer are often changed, commonly being yellow-orange/red in colour and of semi-fluid consistency. The kidneys are painful on palpation and often noticeably enlarged; the liver is seldom enlarged. The urine is usually intensely coloured and appears concentrated (it is seldom possible at this stage to obtain a large sample); protein is often present and bile pigments are nearly always found in more than average concentration. If not icteric, the mucous membranes are normal. There may be slight dehydration.

Treatment. There is usually a definite response to penicillin, (600,000 units procaine penicillin intramuscularly once daily or 500,000 units crystalline penicillin subcutaneously initially in severe cases); temperature returns to normal, appetite is regained, kidney pain disappears and there is a general improvement in spirits. On the basis of this response, an infectious, probably bacterial aetiology is postulated.

Antibiotic treatment should be supported by the administration of glucose, adjustment of diet if necessary, and any other symptomatic therapy which may seem warranted, e.g. cholagogues.

Course. There is often apparent recovery within 1 week, including loss of icteric staining. In some cases, however, icterus persists despite the remission of symptoms; in one case symptomatic recovery occurred with return of appetite, fluid intake reduced to normal, cessation of vomiting and normal temperature but visible mucous membranes remained quite deep yellow. This state of affairs continued for several months before progressive weight loss commenced and destruction was eventually necessary.

In another case recovery from the original illness appeared to be complete, but over the next 2–3 years attacks of jaundice accompanied by some anorexia, occasional vomiting and dulness occurred at intervals of 3–4 months. In the interim the cat seemed normal. Increasing frequency of relapses and progressive loss of condition eventually led to euthanasia. As with other cases, post-mortem examination showed live cirrhosis: pancreatitis was also present.

Prognosis is thus reasonably good for the short-term but guarded to grave for long-term recovery. A small proportion of cases fail to recover from the initial illness.

SUGGESTED FURTHER READING

Fessler, J. H. and Morter, R. L. (1964) *Cornell Vet.* **54**, 115. (Experimental feline leptospirosis.)

Alston & Brown. *Leptospirosis in Man and Animals.* (E. & S. Livingstone.)

Van der Hoeden, J. (1958) *Adv. Vet. Sci.* **4**, 313. (Epizootiology of leptospirosis.)

Murphy, L. C. *et al.* (1958) *Cornell Vet.* **48**, 3. (The prevalence of leptospiral agglutinins in sera of the domestic cat.)

Vysotskii, B. V. *et al.* (1960) *Zh. Mikrobiol.* (Moscow) No. 2, 140. (Leptospirosis in cats.) Translation available.

Cryptococcosis

Although well recognised in some parts of the world cryptococcosis has not been widely considered in Great Britain as an important infection in cats. The recent description of two confirmed cases from widely separated geographical areas of this country suggests that more critical diagnostic methods applied to cases of chronic nasal discharge and/or the presence of granulomatous lesions associated with the nostrils and the area below the eyes might reveal a wider incidence of this infection than hitherto suspected.

The first reported case was that by Howell and Allan (1964), the salient features of which were snuffling of several weeks duration followed by ulceration of the nostril at the dorsal commissure; one week later an ulcer developed below the right eye and a mass of pale tissue protruded. *Cryptococcus neoformans* was cultured from biopsy material and the cat was destroyed.

The second case, reported by Fowler *et al.* (1965) had an ulcerating granulomatous lesion below the inner canthus of the right eye and a subcutaneous swelling adjacent to the right nostril. The causal organism was identified from post-mortem material.

The former authors emphasise the wisdom of eliminating cryptococcosis as a cause of chronic nasal discharge in cats before starting treatment in view of the grave nature of the disease in man.

Despite its rarity the public health duty of practising veterinary surgeons is such that this infection must be critically considered in the future as a possible zoonosis and all cases of granulomata, ulcerating lesions, and chronic nasal discharge in cats should be carefully investigated with this in mind.

REFERENCES

Howell, J. McC. & Allan, D. (1964) *J. Comp. Path.* **74**, 415.
Fowler, N. G. *et al* (1965) *Vet. Rec.* **77**, 292.

SUGGESTED FURTHER READING

Olander, H. J. *et al.* (1963) *J. Amer. Vet. Medical Association* **142**, 138, (Feline Cryptococcosis.)
Ainsworth, G. C. & Austwick, P. K. C. (1959) Review Series No. 6. Commonwealth Bureau of Animal Health; Weybridge. (Fungal diseases of Animals.)
Yamamoto, S. *et al.* (1957) *Jap. J. Vet. Sci.* **19**, 179. (Isolation of Cryptococcus neoformans from pulmonary granuloma of a cat and from pigeon droppings). In English.
Johnston, L. A. Y. & Lavers, D. W. (1963) *Aust. Vet. J.* **39**, 306. (Cryptococcal meningitis in a cat in North Queensland.)
Trautwein, G. & Nielsen, S. W. (1962) *J. Amer. Vet. Medical Association* **140**, 437. (Cryptococcosis in 2 cats, a dog and a mink.)

Holzworth, J. (1952) *Cornell Vet.* **42**, 12. (Cryptococcosis in a cat.)
Barron, C. N. (1955) *J. Amer. Vet. Medical Association* **127**, 125. (Cryptococcosis in Animals.)

Tetanus

This is an extremely rare condition in the cat due to the very considerable comparative resistance of the species to tetanus toxin. Were it not for this specific resistance the disease could be expected to be comparatively common consequent upon the accidental wounds so often sustained by cats. Records of tetanus in cats are few but these give such a clear picture of the condition that it is easy to compile a typical symptomatology.

Of the six case records studied four relate to the United Kingdom. In four cases (Fildes, Hare and Wright; Ludins; Kodituwakku and Wijewanta; Miller) a wound was present, in the other two tetanus followed within 2 weeks of castration. In two cases (Fildes *et al.* and Kodituwakku) *Clostridium tetani* was recovered, in the others the clinical picture was so classical that a firm diagnosis could be made. Two of these six cases recovered one in 17 days and the other in 25 days; the others died or were destroyed.

The symptoms comprised hyperaesthesia to sound and touch, tetanic spasms being easily provoked. The muscles of the limbs and trunk were stiff and even rigid, the membrana nictitans protruded, the tail was erect and in some cases there was opisthotonus. One interesting point is that in four cases trismus was absent only Hopson and Miller recording it as being present.

Treatment in the recovered cases differed owing to the drugs available at the particular time. Ludin's case in 1939 recovered when antitoxin alone was used, whereas in 1963 Miller successfully used penicillin, antitoxin and promazine. To judge from records in other species the ataractic drugs such as promazine and chlorpromazine are very valuable at least in relieving some of the distressing signs and it would thus seem that treatment should comprise penicillin, generous antitoxin and promazine or chlorpromazine repeated as required with parenteral administration of fluids in those patients in which trismus is present.

Whilst prognosis must always be very guarded it is clear that treatment is justifiable and should be attempted.

REFERENCES

Bateman, J. K. (1931) *Vet. Rec.* **43**, 805.
Fildes *et al.* (1931) *Vet. Rec.* **43**, 731.
Hopson, C. G. (1932) *Vet. Rec.* **44**, 302.
Kodituwakku, G. E. & Wijewanta, E. A. (1958) *Brit. Vet. J.* **114**, 48.
Ludins, G. H. (1939) *J. Amer. Vet. Medical Association* **231**.
Miller, E. R. (1963) *Vet. Rec.* **75**, 135.

SUGGESTED FURTHER READING

Mason, J. H. (1964) *J. S. Afr. Vet. Med. Ass.* **35**, 209. (Tetanus in the dog and cat; a review.)

Toxoplasmosis

Infection by the protozoan parasite Toxoplasma gondii is widespread in man and lower animals, though disease rarely occurs. Feline infection is of particular relevance since cats, though rarely exhibiting symptoms of illness, are established as definitive hosts of the parasite and as the only species to excrete potentially infective oocysts.

Though a wide range of disease symptoms have been associated with T. gondii infection, including hepatitis, myocarditis and pneumonia, the most important clinical entities are abortion in sheep, retino-choroiditis and encephalitis in man and, in the case of pre-natally acquired infection, vision impairment, encephalitis and mental retardation in man. Because of the risk of such congenital damage, the public health aspects of feline infection have excited considerable interest (Jones 1973).

Although it is likely that in many households both cat and man contract infection from the same source, usually undercooked sheep or pig meat, the possibility of transmission from cat to man cannot be overlooked. Pregnant women and neonates are most obviously at risk.

Fortunately, the majority of cats shed oocysts for relatively short periods of time following initial infection (Frenkel, Dubey & Miller 1970) though re-infection and further shedding by cats with toxoplasma antibody titres may sometimes occur. (Frenkel, Dubey 1972. Dubey 1976). The oocysts remain non-infective until sporulation occurs, which is usually within 1-5 days at room temperature (Dubey, Miller & Frenkel 1970). Effective control of spread from cat to man is therefore feasible as long as domestic hygiene is good and cat faeces are collected and removed before sporulation occurs. Practically, this entails daily attention to litter trays and a disinfection routine, during which the wearing of protective rubber gloves is a sensible additional precaution. Obviously, because of the particular hazard of pre-natal infection, pregnant women are advised to avoid participation in this routine. Additional sources of human infection are flowerbeds and sand pits contaminated by cats, so that the wearing of gardening gloves and the provision of sand pit lids is advisable.

Recommendation of such precautions assumes the inevitability of feline infection, a factor which can be reduced by the feeding of only well cooked foods and by the prevention of hunting; also all uncooked meat, whether for feline or human consumption, should be handled with hygienic precautions.

Serological testing of cats for toxoplasma antibodies is feasible some 8-10 days post infection (Krogstad, Juranek & Walls 1972) though cats develop lower titres and more slowly than other species.

Interpretation of test results is also somewhat speculative (Frenkel 1973) but positive diagnosis of active infection depends upon demonstration of rising antibody titres in samples collected at 14 day intervals.

Clinical Symptoms. Symptoms of illness very occasionally occur in cats. Commonest is a generalized lymphdenopathy easily mistaken for advanced multi-centric lymphosarcoma. Toxoplasma infections may also present symptoms confusingly similar to panleucopaenia and a progressive bronchopneumonia may also occur. Other symptoms may relate to cardiac, hepatic, renal or C.N.S. lesions.

Treatment. Available therapy is unreliable in its ability to prevent formation of oocysts (Dubey 1976). Pyrimethamine, though recommended, is reported toxic and unpalatable to cats in even small doses (Dubey). Best results are reported for sulphadiazine or triple sulphonamides administered in divided daily doses for up to 2 weeks. Research on the development of a vaccine is progressing.

REFERENCES

Dubey, J.P. (1976a) *Nature* **262**, *13*.

Dubey, J.P. (1976b) J.A.V.M.A. **169**, 1861.

Dubey, J.P.; Miller, N.L.; Frenkel, J.K. (1970) *J.A.V.M.A.* **157**, 1767.

Frenkel, J.K. (1973) in *"Opportunistic Pathogens"* Eds. Prier, J.E. & Friedman, H. University Park Press, Baltimore, Md.

Frenkel, J.K.; Dubey, J.P. (1972) J. *Infect. Dis.* **126**, 664.

Frenkel, J.K., Dubey, J.P.; Miller, N.L. (1970) *Science* **167**, 893.

Jones, S.R.(1973) *J.A.V.M.A.* **163**, 1038.

Krogstad, D.J.; Juranek, D.D.; Walls, K.W. (1972) *Ann. Int. Med.* **77**, 738.

Aujesky's Disease. (Pseudo-rabies) occasionally occurs in cats, and a case has recently been described in Britain in a cat on a pig farm where the disease had occurred (Dow & McFerran 1963). *Rabies* occurs in cats in countries in which the disease is endemic, but fortunately is no longer a problem in this country outside quarantine kennels and catteries. Although the virus does not apparently affect the cat which carries it, *Cat Scratch Fever*, as its name suggests, may occur in those scratched by cats.

REFERENCE

Dow, C. & McFerran, J. B. (1963) *Vet. Rec.* **75**, 1099.

SUGGESTED FURTHER READING

Toxoplasmosis

Petrak, M. & Carpenter, J. (1965) *J. Amer. Vet. Med. Ass.* **146**, 728. (Feline Toxoplasmosis.)

Cat scratch fever

Anonymous (1956) *Vet. Rec.* **68**, 186. (Cat scratch fever, a digest of some of the literature.)

Hinden, E. (1957) *Brit. Med. J.* **11**, 444. (Cat-scratch disease.)

For some infections not mentioned in the text

Robinson, E. M. (1963) *J. S. Afr. Vet. Med. Ass.* **34**, 45. (Biliary fever (metalliosis) in the cat.)

Burns, G. C. *et al.* (1959) *N. Z. Med. J.* **58**, 598. ('Cat bite' disease (Pasteurella septica infection).)

Buxton, A. (1955) *Proc. R. Soc. Med.* **48**, 636. (Salmonellosis, with mention of cats.)

Hemsley, L. A. (1956) *Vet. Rec.* **68**, 152. (Abortion in two cats, with the isolation of Salmonella cholerae-suis from one case.)

Habermann, R. T. & Williams, F. P. (1956) *J. Amer. Vet. Medical Association* **129**, 30. (Metastatic micrococci infection (botriomycosis) in a cat.)

Ainsworth, G. C. & Austwick, P. K. C. (1959) Commonwealth Animal Bureaux. (Fungal diseases of Animals.)

Langham, R. F. *et al.* (1959) *Mich. St. Univ. Vet.* **19**, 102 and 119. (Nocardiosis in the dog and cat.)

General

Newberne, J. W. *et al.* (1959) *Allied Vet.* **30**, 50. (Clinical differentiation of feline viral diseases.)

Bittle, J. L. *et al.* (1960) *Proc. Anim. Care Panel* **10**, 105. (Viral diseases of the laboratory cat.)

Kraft, H. (1961) *Tierarztl. Umsch.* **16**, 350. (Infectious diseases of cats—the clinical picture.)

Harding, S. K. *et al.* (1961) *Cornell Vet.* **51**, 535. (The transfer of antibodies from the mother cat to her newborn kittens.)

On general topics, e.g. laboratory techniques

Laboratory Aids to Clinical Diagnosis (British Veterinary Association.)

Manual of Veterinary Clinical Pathology. D. L. Coffin. (New York, Cornell University Press.)

Diagnostic Methods in Veterinary Medicine. G. F. Boddie. (Edinburgh, Oliver & Boyd.)

Pathology of the Dog and Cat. F. Bloom. (Illinois, American Veterinary Publications, Inc.)

The Urine of the Dog and Cat. F. Bloom. (New York, Gamma Publications, Inc.)

The Blood Chemistry of the Dog and Cat. F. Bloom. (New York, Gamma Publications, Inc.)

Chapter 20

SEPSIS

Septic Infections

The subject is of such tremendous clinical importance in everyday feline practice that it undoubtedly merits this separate section. In view of its ubiquity and frequency it is surprising that the subject has not received far more attention in small animal literature. Although the advent of antibacterial drugs, particularly the antibiotics, has literally revolutionised the treatment of cat sepsis it still remains a condition of importance and demands critical thought and careful attention if some of the more serious sequelae are to be avoided.

General Considerations

The vast majority of pyogenic infections in cats are the result of a bite from another cat. It is probably no exaggeration to say that this is true of 90 per cent of cases despite owner assertions that the cause has been rat, dog or other bites.

Bites are received during fighting or play; fighting may be to establish sexual superiority or in defence of territory. While entire male cats are most commonly involved, neuters of either sex may suffer attacks from entire males which mistakenly regard them as a threat in sexual persuits, or from entire males or neuters during protection of territory. The frequency with which entire males sustain cat bite wounds and their consequences is probably the strongest reason for advocating castration of tom kittens.

As has been noted elsewhere the feline skin is pretty tough and thus less easily torn than that of some other species consequently puncture wounds are extremely common. The normal flora of the cat mouth (dealt with below) is such that the puncture wound is virtually a subcutaneous or cutaneous inoculation with pyogenic bacteria and the nature of the lesion, i.e. no drainage, combines to make abscess formation and cellulitis very common sequels.

Bites may be received by aggressor or defender and it has been repeatedly noted that any one individual is likely always to sustain wounds in the same region of the body (e.g. always about the head and face, always base of tail, always limbs etc.) presumably due to that individual's method of fighting. Whilst this is not an invariable rule it is sufficiently common to warrant comment.

The frequency with which pyogenic infection complicates bites in cats makes prophylactic treatment with antibiotics a legitimate measure whenever it can be undertaken—this will be discussed in more detail below.

BACTERIOLOGY

It is essential for a proper evaluation of the subject that the bacteriology be considered and appreciated. For this reason the normal flora of the cats nose and throat is important since most sepsis lesions are due to endogenous infection. A survey by Smith (1964) shows that the commonest organisms isolated from nose and throat were *Pasteurella multocida* (found in 94 per cent of throats), alpha- and non-haemolytic *Streptococci* and *Escherichia coli*.

Pasteurellas are almost invariably present in septic lesions due to bites, often in association with beta-haemolytic *Streptococci* and anaerobic fusiform bacteria. The frequency with which Pasteurella occurs in the mouth and throat of cats makes cat bites in man always a potentially serious accident and it is essential that medical attention should be advised and sought as soon as possible after infliction if lymphangitis, lymphadenitis and abscess formation are to be avoided. The veterinarian has a clear public health duty to himself, his clients and his staff in this respect.

It is noteworthy that while Pasteurellas and Streptococci abound in the normal cat naso-pharynx Staphylococci are strikingly uncommon, Smith's survey showing one isolate of a haemolytic *Staphylococcus* (2 per cent) and seven non-haemolytic strains, all *Staph. albus*, i.e. 14 per cent. The relative rarity with which Staphylococci are associated with suppurating lesions may be the reason for the very good response of most cases to penicillin therapy.

SITES

Literally any part of the body surface can be the site of a cat bite but of the common ones some are listed below:

Head: Cheeks and temporal region.

Ears: Usually the lower part of the concha, the bite penetrating all tissues of the pinna. Also the base of the ear involving skin and entrance to auditory canal.

Forelimbs: Any part from scapula to pads; just below the elbow, forearm, carpus, metacarpus and feet are commoner.

Hindlimbs: Mainly from mid-thigh region downwards, especially around hock, metatarsals and feet.

Trunk: Any part, mainly dorsal aspects, base of tail area particularly common.

Tail: Usually near root.

It is often impossible to detect the original puncture and if the patient is not presented until a large abscess has developed the gravitation of fluid (pus) may change the apparent site of the lesion, e.g. a facial wound in the region of the cheek may gravitate and become inter-maxillary in position.

The Lesion

Always initially a puncture wound from a canine tooth. Frequently no second puncture is detectable although this would be expected. This primary lesion is often not detected but in cases presented early careful finger-tip palpation of the painful area may locate a minute speck of hardish material, dried blood or scab. It is obvious that numerous punctures do heal without any undue reaction but a very high proportion result in infection occurring, usually subcutaneously. The original puncture occasionally causes inflammation, pain and lameness or stiffness according to site but many are apparently quite painless until pyogenic infection is established.

To some extent subsequent developments depend on the site, related particularly to the amount and tension of subcutaneous tissues, e.g. bites around the forehead result in localised abscess formation but due to the lack of space under the skin the amount of pus accumulated before discharging is scanty while a puncture originally in the scapular area may give rise to a very large abscess gravitating to the axillary region which may contain upwards of 30 ml. pus.

Bites high in the forelimb often give rise to cellulitis rather than local abscess formation, the whole limb becoming grossly swollen.

In some cases the original puncture remains patent and the products of pyogenic infection are discharged through it from an early stage, i.e. a sinus is formed.

Abscesses

Abscess formation can arise at any site but will mainly occur where there is some loose connective tissue. The course is variable some cases being painful from the time the bite is sustained, some are only painful while pus is accumulating (usually 2–7 days after the injury) and others appear to be painless throughout and are presented for attention because a large swelling is present. Symptoms are also variable from quite marked malaise, inappetence and fever (T. 38·9–40·56° C. (102–104° F.)) to no signs at all other than an obvious lesion.

The pus is usually of a creamy consistence and varies in colour from creamy-white to sanguineous brown; the green pus associated with *Pseudomonas pyocyaneus* is rare as would be expected from the bacterial picture. Sometimes the pus is foul smelling, especially the reddish-brown type.

The natural course of the abscess varies with the site and relationship of the abscess cavity to the original puncture. If the cavity is above or level with the puncture discharge may occur through this at an early stage but will show no tendency to spontaneous resolution. If the cavity forms ventral to the puncture, drainage cannot occur unless natural pointing and bursting through the overlying tissues occurs; this in turn depends on the nature of the overlying skin, e.g. it is very difficult for an abscess to burst through the skin in the cheek region of an adult entire male cat due to the great thickness of the dermis in this region, which is a secondary sexual character. In some cases pointing and rupture takes place at a fairly high point in the lesion thus preventing adequate drainage unless a counter opening is provided.

It is unfortunate that owners are often lulled into a sense of false security and hence delay seeking attention because an abscess bursts and the lesion *apparently* resolves; this sequence of events may be repeated several times before professional advice is sought and a time lag of up to 12 weeks may have occurred since the original injury. In all delayed cases some thought should be given to complications which may have occurred, e.g. osteomyelitis, septic arthritis.

All the cardinal signs of abscess formation are not always present; swelling is usually detectable but pain is by no means invariable, heat is rarely very evident and reddening is not a characteristic of feline skin although gross discolouration of a purplish-red or even greenish-black nature may be found in necrotic skin about to slough.

Treatment. The bacteria associated with cat sepsis are, *in vivo*, sensitive to penicillin and the results of penicillin therapy instituted early and carried out vigorously are extremely good. Parenteral administration of antibiotics is preferable to ensure that the correct dose is actually received. Because of the good response to and comparative absence of toxicity of penicillin this, in the author's strong opinion, is the agent of choice. Streptomycin is best avoided on account of the cat idiosyncrasy to its toxic effects on the vestibular apparatus and resort to broad-spectrum antibiotics such as the tetracyclines and chloramphenicol is seldom necessary. Antibiotic therapy is advisable at any stage and considerably accelerates resolution even in ruptured lesions. The following approaches are suggested for some common types of lesion encountered:

1. Local pyogenic infection before frank pus formation has occurred. 600,000 units penicillin as procaine penicillin suspension, intramuscularly every 48 hours for 5–7 days; heat to be applied to the lesion. Frequently abscesses can be aborted in this way.

2. Small cavities draining through a small puncture. Parenteral penicillin as above, expression of contents of cavity and introduction of an intramammary preparation of penicillin, streptomycin or a combination of the two via the puncture. This procedure often obviates the need for lancing but the lesion *must* be carefully checked over a period of 6–10 days to be certain of complete resolution.

3. Larger cavities, no drainage. The lesion should be carefully examined to ascertain if there is any possibility of pointing and natural rupture at a place that will permit adequate drainage; if this seems likely pointing and rupture may be hastened by the application of local heat. Parenteral penicillin as before to limit bacterial multiplication. Such

cases must be re-inspected to ascertain (*a*) that bursting has occurred and (*b*) that drainage is adequate; if it is not, the opening must be enlarged as required.

If on examination natural rupture seems likely to be delayed or unlikely to occur due to thick overlying skin or if pointing is at a spot from which subsequent drainage is impossible then surgical incision is necessary without delay. This is preferably undertaken under general anaesthesia since in all the foregoing circumstances viable skin will be involved and pain inflicted during lancing; furthermore thorough cleaning of the cavity, exploration for foreign bodies and removal of the pyogenic membrane where indicated are greatly facilitated.

Lesions which are discharging through a superior opening will need a counter opening provided at a ventral spot suitable to permit adequate drainage. The old-fashioned trick of inserting a seton can still be very helpful in large lesions with widely separated openings and destruction of tissue can be minimised; a suitable length of bandage (1–2 inch width) previously sterilised and impregnated with an antibacterial dressing serves the purpose well.

In all cases simultaneous penicillin therapy is advisable over a period of 4–10 days.

It is often possible and certainly justifiable to adopt preventive measures. Owners of cats which have previously sustained septic lesions can often be persuaded to present such patients within 24 hours of knowing they have been involved in a fight. A single injection of 600,000 units procaine penicillin suspension prevents development of a septic focus. No evidence of the development of drug-resistance has been observed in the many cats subjected repeatedly to this routine.

It may be argued that these suggested lines of treatment are unnecessarily rigorous and prolonged but the greater is one's experience of cat sepsis lesions and possible sequelae the more is one convinced of the necessity for really thorough treatment in all, even the most trivial, cases.

Cellulitis

This diffuse inflammatory reaction of subcutaneous tissues arises most commonly in the forelimbs below the elbow. In these cases there is no localised pus formation although, of course, an area of cellulitis can arise adjacent to a septic focus in any locality.

The cat is usually severely lame and shows some general malaise including anorexia and disinclination to move. Temperature is frequently moderately raised, up to 39·7° C. (103·5° F.). The limb is diffusely swollen for the greater part or all of its length and the tissues have a doughy feel not unlike oedema. Pain on pressure is usually not severe.

Treatment should include penicillin to overcome bacterial activity together with application of heat to the limb. Corticosteroids may be incorporated from about the third day of antibiotic treatment and will hasten resolution.

276

The course is comparatively long, resolution occurring within 6–10 days. Prognosis is good. Rarely a small pus focus develops and discharges at a late stage in the course.

Local Infected Puncture

In some sites, especially the feet, small infected punctures occur without actual abscess formation or cellulitis. This is particularly liable to occur where tissue is dense, e.g. the pads, or where subcutaneous space is small such as below the carpus. These lesions are usually very painful on pressure and cause marked lameness. Signs are usually confined to the local lesion, fever and general malaise being uncommon.

Careful palpation of the affected limb, particularly the digits and pads, is essential. When located, a bead of pus may sometimes be expressed. Treatment is routine including soaking the affected foot in a suitable hot solution (e.g. strong solution of magnesium sulphate or sodium chloride) and needs to be continued until pain and lameness are abolished since these punctures may involve interphalangeal joints in some cases.

The following are some of the more serious effects of cat sepsis and occur sufficiently often to justify the vigorous treatment recommended above.

A. SEPTIC ARTHRITIS

This is particularly liable to occur where the puncture is adjacent to articulations which are virtually subcutaneous, i.e. carpus, tarsus and interphalangeal joints. In these circumstances although the initial lesion responds well to treatment lameness persists and pain can be elicited by pressure and/or movement of the associated joint; some swelling may persist especially around the carpus. Persistence of such signs beyond 7 days of the institution of ordinary treatment is an indication for more vigorous local therapy. Under general anaesthesia the area should be carefully explored for any suppurating focus and surgical drainage provided as necessary. In addition the local injection of suitable antibiotic and corticosteroid solution should be made around and, if possible, into the joint itself. Aqueous solutions of crystalline penicillin, procaine penicillin suspension, solutions of streptomycin, aqueous solutions of chloramphenicol succinate and suspensions of betamethasone are all suitable for use and should be used in high dosage, e.g. 500,000 units crystalline penicillin, 125 mg. chloramphenicol combined with moderate doses of corticosteroid, e.g. 0·25–0·5 ml. betamethasone suspension. Solutions of tetracyclines are unsuitable as they are painful.

A single treatment is often sufficient but if necessary may be repeated weekly until the joint returns to normal.

Similarly tendons may be involved in similar septic lesions and a tenosynovitis result. Augmentation of routine by the above local treatment is usually effective.

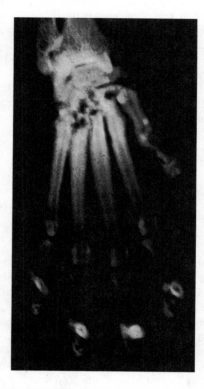

FIG. 34 Osteomyelitis of metacarpal bones several weeks after a cat bite injury. Cat lame

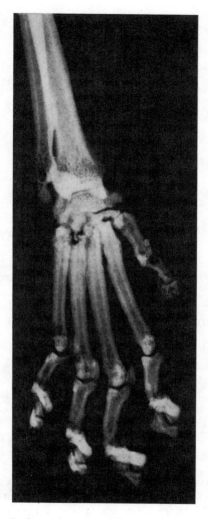

FIG. 35 Lesions of osteomyelitis greatly reduced following local infiltration with penicillin and betamethasome. Cat now sound

Should an infective arthritis persist abnormally, bacteriological investigation is desirable since, rarely, tuberculous arthritis may occur.

B. OSTEOMYELITIS AND OSTEITIS

These are not uncommon sequelae of infected or inadequately treated lesions of cat sepsis. The bones most commonly seen involved have been the ulna and metacarpals.

In any case in which persistent discharge of pus occurs in the forearm over any period of time—neglected cases may be presented after weeks or even months—the limb should be X-rayed to detect any bone involvement.

Extensive osteomyelitis and osteitis resulting in destruction of significant areas of bone have been seen, especially related to the ulna. The series of illustrations shows the progress of multiple lesions of osteomyelitis in the metacarpals of a cat which had a carpal infection of some duration.

In cases where a single sinus is associated with a bone and osteomyelitis is confirmed surgical intervention is required. The sinus should be explored and exposed; the bone should be exposed and examined and when possible, curetted and any cavity filled with a suitable antibacterial preparation.

C. SINUS FORMATION

This is very apt to occur when adequate drainage and/or vigorous antibiotic treatment have not been provided. It is most likely to arise in sites where muscle tissue is involved, e.g. the forearm or shoulder regions, or where drainage is difficult owing to the natural disposition of tissues, e.g. the ventral aspect of the neck.

Surgical treatment is necessary to explore and expose the sinus, to remove all diseased tissue and to provide adequate and continued drainage. When sinuses arise in the region of the neck consideration must be given to the possibility of a foreign body such as a needle being present and to tuberculous infections. The former is readily investigated by radiography, the latter is becoming less common, but bacteriological investigation is wise.

D. GENERALISED PYAEMIA

This can arise during the usual course of a case of cat sepsis but is more likely in neglected or inadequately treated cases. Multiple abscess formation occurs which may remain subcutaneous or involve internal organs.

In the former case cats are usually presented in poor condition, often off food and with a slightly raised temperature. A variable number of suppurating lesions is present and a very common site is the interdigital web and fossae. In many such cases the pus is of a rather thick consistense, yellow in colour and comparatively scanty in amount. Prognosis in most cases is grave. These patients are seldom fit for anaesthesia and surgery and in any event the multiplicity of lesions renders this impracticable.

When internal organs are involved there is quite serious illness the signs of which may be referable to the organs mainly involved, e.g. kidneys, liver.

In all pyaemic cases immediate resort to broad-spectrum antibiotics is advisable, e.g. chlortetracycline 100 mg. t.i.d. for 3 days reducing according to response. Supportive treatment by multi-vitamin therapy is required; the Vitamin B complex should in any case be provided when oral broad-spectrum antibiotics are in use.

Response is disappointing and even initial promise is usually followed by relapse.

On post-mortem examination pus foci may be found in a wide variety of sites.

E. PYOTHORAX

As previously described pyothorax seems to be a species tissue response with a number of possible aetiologies of which one is a previous septic focus anywhere on the body. The original lesion may have existed any time from 10 days to 6 weeks previously. Pyothorax has been dealt with in detail elsewhere but requires mention here as being one of the very serious sequelae of ordinary septic infections in cats.

F. PUS IN THE NEURAL CANAL

This extraordinary and disastrous sequel to cat sepsis has been seen on a number of occasions particularly in association with the common base of tail lesion.

The author has seen one case in a castrated male cat which sustained a bite near the base of the tail. Apparently adequate treatment with parenteral penicillin resulted in what appeared to be complete resolution. The cat remained to all intents and purposes normal until 24 hours before being presented with the history that it had then gone off food and a rapidly progressive paresis of hind limbs had occurred. When seen the cat was paralysed to the level of the mid-cervical region. It was destroyed. Post-mortem examination showed that the neural canal contained pus as far anteriorly as the cervical region; a small infected sinus was located which extended from the area of the original lesion to the spinal canal in the sacral region. Milnes records a similar case and also one in which pyogenic infection was more localised, a fat covered abscess occurring on the floor of the spinal canal over the body of the fourth lumbar vertebra—in this case the source of infection could not be traced.

Such instances, even if uncommon, emphasise the necessity for really adequate treatment of sepsis lesions, particularly those around the base of the tail.

Diagnosis in life is far from easy. A history of previous septic infection, absence of a history of accident and—as pointed out by Milnes—the presence of a femoral pulse differentiating from posterior aortic or iliac thrombosis.

At the risk of being accused of unnecessary exaggeration the importance of septic lesions in cats is once again emphasised. Any condition which occurs so commonly, indeed is an everyday occurrence in small animal practice, risks being dealt with and dismissed as boring routine and does not always receive the critical thought, thorough treatment and, when necessary, careful investigation which it demands. The younger clinician is often unaware of the impact of antibiotics on the problem of cat sepsis. In the pre-penicillin era veterinary surgeons' hospitals were full of cats with pyogenic lesions of one sort or another, often in a revolting state of non or slow healing; the local applications advocated were legion and only varying in their comparative ineffectiveness. Many cats died or were destroyed due to infections which today are dismissed with barely a second thought. Despite the penicillin revolution however, cat sepsis remains a problem demanding thoughtful therapy because of potentially serious sequelae in a proportion of cases.

REFERENCES

Milnes, D. M. (1959) *Vet. Rec.* **71**, 932.
Smith, J. E. (1964) *J. Small An. Pract.* **5**, 517.

Chapter 21

GERIATRIC CARE

The management of the aged cat comprises an important part of small animal veterinary practice. As already pointed out little is known of the average life span but it is perfectly clear that most cats may expect to enter a second decade and not a few complete it. In a table shown previously, twenty-six cats were 14 years of age or more. Recognising, then, that a pet cat may be a member of a household for 20-25 per cent of the natural life-span of man and hence become the object of very strong attachment by one or more members of a family the responsibility of the veterinary surgeon in providing attention needs no emphasis. This is particularly true of cats belonging to lonely persons who if themselves aged, may feel it unfair to take on a further pet when the present one dies.

Whilst many of the diseases occurring mainly in older age groups are not susceptible to cure it is often possible to adopt alleviative measures and to modify management, especially diet, in such a way that the progress of some diseases is retarded and that positive health is maintained at the highest possible level for the maximum time. Both dogs and cats adapt well to the limitations imposed by old age but whereas dogs become increasingly dependent, cats retain their inherent independence to the end which makes it impossible to protect them from hazards such as traffic. To compensate for this the special senses fail less readily than in the dog, senile defects of vision and hearing and locomotory handicaps such as osteo-arthritis being far less common.

Management of the ageing cat falls into two parts, owner responsibility and veterinary care but the veterinary surgeon has a duty in both respects since advice must be given to enable the owner to appreciate the part he has to play.

Owner Responsibility

(1) Diet.

A gradual return to the more frequent feeding methods used during kittenhood is often advisable. The number of meals should be increased to three or four daily giving appropriately reduced quantities at each feed. Food should be highly nutritious, digestible, as varied as possible and include a high proportion of fresh protein. Tinned foods should be decreased or even eliminated from the diet unless any of the special prescription formulae is advised. It is particularly important that food should be freshly prepared for each feed and temptingly presented. Whenever possible access to fresh greenstuff, especially grass, is desirable. Augmented vitamin intake, preferably by one of the balanced multi-vitamin preparations, is to be recommended. Any cat showing a tendency to any form of sluggish bowel action should receive a regular addition of a suitable bulk laxative or dietary additive (e.g. Vi-Siblin, Isogel, Bemax, All-Bran) preferably containing Vitamin B. It is essential that all foodstuffs and medicinal additions should be presented in a fully acceptable form. More harm than good can result from voluntary refusal of food by old animals and this applies even to prescription diets. It is no use treating a nephritic cat by insisting upon feeding only a prepared low protein diet and have an already ailing animal die of malnutrition rather than the disease from which it suffers!

(2) House Cleanliness

Although many old cats remain scrupulously clean to the end an early sign of senility in some is decreasing fastidiousness about both the place of excretion and its disposal. When an ageing cat starts to forget its house training it is not only useless, but wrong and even cruel, to punish it and worse still to keep it shut outside. When a cat is presented with the history that it is dirty in the house it must first be carefully investigated for disease which could result in increased urination (e.g. the polydipsia/polyuria of nephritis or diabetes) or defaecation (e.g. exogenous pancreatic deficiency, lymphosarcoma of intestine) and only after eliminating any such cause should the conclusion be drawn that it is due to senility. If the latter is the case it must be put clearly to the owner that not only is there no possibility of improvement but it is likely to get worse and the situation must be faced. If the owner cannot or will not tolerate the nuisance and unpleasantness involved then euthanasia should be firmly advised. If prepared to cope, an attempt should be made to persuade the cat to use a tray indoors, providing trays in several rooms. Some cats take to defaecating in a sink or wash-basin and it may be possible to leave one not used by the household accessible to the cat, e.g. leaving a cloak-room door open. This sort of situation may create friction in a family when one person who is extremely attached to a pet cat is prepared to put up with the unpleasantness when other members are not; this calls for a high degree of diplomacy by the attending veterinary surgeon who may at some point have to decide that consideration for human beings must transcend the wish to extend the life-span of a senile animal.

(3) Care of Coat

Another sign of age is decreased desire and sometimes decreased ability for self-grooming. At first the cat continues to wash itself but gradually confines this to easily accessible areas and subsequently licking becomes more feeble and useless. It is rarely that physical causes account for this but the mouth, tongue and pharynx should be examined for any visible lesion. It is then necessary for the owner to undertake regular grooming preferably using a metal comb. Obviously it is particularly necessary in long-haired cats but all types of coat require regular attention to remove dead coat and skin debris and to ensure that parasitic infestation does not occur. Regular careful inspection of the perinaeum is desirable (probably resented and resisted by the cat) particularly in hot weather to obviate the risk of blow-fly strike. Long-haired cats which are not regularly groomed may get large mats of dead coat which seem to accumulate in an incredibly short time; since general anaesthesia may be needed to deal with this, every effort should be made to avoid the eventuality as this is not a desirable exercise in the aged unless essential.

(4) Nails

Whether due to less exercising of nails by so-called 'sharpening' or to some atony of the retractor muscles of the claws it is often necessary to undertake regular nail clipping of old cats. The owner usually complains either that the cat is scratching legs and hands or furniture, or that it is continually getting a claw caught in the carpet or clothing. On extruding the nail it will be found that it is large and coarse with a long tapering point. The quick is easily seen but against this the nail has a marked tendency to split when cut. Strong scissors or nail clippers are equally suitable. If, as often happens, the nail splits the separated flakes should be removed. Periodicity varies with individuals, 3–6 months is an average interval.

(5) Decreased Body Heat

The hard winter of 1962–63 focused attention upon hypothermia as a cause of death in the elderly. All aged animals show some decrease in metabolic rate and this, coupled with diminution of activity and exercise, necessitates the provision of external warmth. Many old cats become very thin without there necessarily being systemic disease and this, too, necessitates provision of heat. Whenever possible boxes with a warm blanket or other bedding should be available in a sheltered place outside for any cat which spends much time out of doors. This is another reason why the shutting out of old cats cannot be condoned.

(6) Holidays

Care of the aged cat during its owner's absence from home is considerably more of a problem than for younger animals. Due to the need to ensure warmth and comfort the arrangement of having a neighbour put in food once daily becomes less satisfactory. Despite their independence old cats do tend to fret more when the owner is away and may refuse food in consequence. Temporary abstinence which may be of no consequence at all in a young animal can be serious in the old. For the same reason consignment to a boarding cattery may be unwise but if the animal has been used regularly to boarding then this is rarely a problem. Any change in routine involving a strange diet and lack of freedom may have an adverse effect and can even cause serious disorientation.

These, then, are some of the points the veterinary surgeon may have to discuss with owners in deciding upon the future of an aged cat. What is obvious to the trained mind is often not plain to even an intelligent owner hence the need for full advice from the small animal practitioner.

Veterinary Care

Comparatively few of the diseases of age are completely curable but many can be alleviated and expectation of life considerably increased by regular veterinary attention. It is in the old animal that regular health checks are of value and when possible 3 monthly clinical examination preferably augmented by 6 (or at most 12) monthly urine analyses should be instituted. This routine is by no means pandering to the client nor can it be criticised as having a mercenary implication; it is a means by which certain diseases, e.g. diabetes mellitus, may be recognised at an early stage when treatment is most likely to be beneficial.

Diseases likely to be encountered in the old cat have been fully dealt with in preceding chapters but for convenience of reference they are again systematically grouped and outlined here.

Alimentary System

1. TEETH

Dental calculus, parodontal disease and alveolitis occur increasingly in the older age groups. Regular dental checks are most helpful and occasional dental attention under anaesthesia can be undertaken at appropriate intervals. In any cat in which soft calculus is deposited rapidly, and especially if associated with halitosis, urine analysis is essential to assess pancreatic and kidney function. Tooth scaling and extractions are often needed; multiple extractions may be undertaken fearlessly in cats which are otherwise in good health. Naturally anaesthesia is an increasing hazard with advancing age but the careful use of intravenous thiopentone sodium at double the usual dilution is usually satisfactory.

2. THE TONGUE

The ventro-lateral aspects of the frenum lingui and root of the tongue should be inspected regularly to detect inflammatory or neoplastic lesions at an early stage. Biopsy is a valuable diagnostic aid subject to the reservations expressed earlier regarding the difficulty of differentiation. Antibiotic and subsequently antibiotic/steroid therapy should be commenced before any histological report is received. If carcinoma is confirmed euthanasia must be recommended as soon as clinical signs are evident.

3. PHARYNX

This should be inspected carefully and if clinical signs exist indicating some lesion in the area it may need to be carried out under general anaesthesia. The presence of an enlarged mandibular or retropharyngeal lymph node is also an indication for such examination. It is often wise to obtain permission to destroy while under anaesthesia should any incurable lesion be found. Lesions which may be detected are tonsil carcinoma and neoplasms (lymphosarcoma or carcinoma) involving root of tongue, tonsillar area and retropharyngeal tissues.

4. OESOPHAGUS

Carcinoma is the commonest abnormality in old cats. The characteristic symptomatology of increasingly frequent regurgitation after solid food, and later progressive emaciation, usually cause the owner to seek advice. Should the lesion be proliferative and sited anterior to the first pair of ribs it may be palpable but in the more usual intrathoracic site between, or just posterior to, the first ribs then investigation under general anaesthesia is necessary. The lesion may be proliferative or erosive in type and is often annular in distribution causing progressively severe stenosis of the lumen of the oesophagus; these can usually be recognised by endoscopy. Advanced lesions are often demonstrable by radiography using a contrast medium which may indicate the narrowed lumen of the gullet or outline the irregular tissue of the tumour. If these examinations are negative the possibility of a space-filling lesion pressing on the oesophagus must be considered, e.g. lymphosarcoma of mediastinal lymph nodes. In all such conditions euthanasia is required.

5. STOMACH

This organ is not particularly subject to senile lesions although it may be the site of lymphosarcomatosis. Neither Cotchin nor Head list gastric carcinoma in their series.

6. SMALL INTESTINE

Rather similar to the stomach but lymphosarcoma involving small intestine is quite common. Mucoid adenocarcinomata have also been reported; the associated syndrome is of a progressively obstructive nature. Chronic diarrhoeas are fairly common in aged cats but, with the exception of diffuse lymphosarcomatosis, are more usually due to disease in other organs, e.g. pancreas, liver, heart. In older cats having persistently changed faeces examination should include trypsin estimations and evaluation of liver and cardiac function. Even the empirical use of pancreatin and bile salts is likely to prove more useful than loading with antibiotics.

The atonic colon often arises in middle life but is likely to worsen with age. Bulk laxatives, high residue food and augmented Vitamin B intake will keep episodes of impaction to the minimum; if severe, impaction may demand manual relief under anaesthesia.

Incarceration of a knob of hard faecal material between external and internal anal sphincters is not uncommon and can be relieved digitally as though emptying anal sacs.

Associated Digestive Organs

Pancreas

Exogenous and endogenous deficiencies occur and the associated syndromes are important in geriatric practice as both respond to replacement therapy.

Exogenous deficiency is characterised by increased appetite (anorexia may occur in the late stages), loss of weight and faeces of a persistently fluid or semi-fluid consistence. Although occasionally the classically described bulky, pale, greasy and foetid stools are seen the change is more often to a stool of creamy consistence and varying shades of brown in colour. Trypsin estimations should be repeated as wide normal variations occur. The typical signs plus a regularly low titre or absence of trypsin warrants a firm diagnosis. Treatment is by replacement, and hence life-long, using keratin coated tablets or granules of pancreatin, preferably with bile salts. Satisfactory treatment can only be maintained in cats which can be regularly and easily dosed if tablets are used; granules may be taken mixed with food if the patient is not too fastidious a feeder.

Diabetes mellitus is associated with an increased water intake but, depending on the individual cat's habits, this may not always be observed, hence the value of regular routine urine analysis. Other signs include an early increase and later decrease in appetite, loss of weight, diminution of energy and, uncommonly, lens opacities. Glycosuria regularly found on re-check of carefully collected specimens warrants diagnosis. Insulin therapy may prolong life for a number of years. The dose usually lies between 5 and 11 units daily of Protamine Zinc Insulin or Insulin Zinc Suspension. The maintenance of 'clinical balance' as estimated by body weight and water intake is more important than a regularly negative urine. Diabetes is commoner than usually believed in older cats, thus any patient with any increase in water intake should be fully investigated with this in mind.

The Liver

Both degenerative conditions such as cirrhosis or fatty infiltration and neoplasia may occur. The differentiation of liver changes is not easy and laboratory techniques are not yet fully evaluated for this species. Clinical signs of liver disease other than palpable enlargement are indefinite and seldom even remotely diagnostic. Anorexia and weight loss predominate in the cat although vomiting and depression are also often seen. Depression is perhaps less profound than in similar conditions in the dog. Nausea may often be deduced by an apparent eagerness for food which rapidly becomes rejection and distaste when eating is attempted. Ascites may be present in advanced liver disease. Treatment of most senile liver conditions is unrewarding. The use of cholagogues and a diet augmented by readily available carbohydrate such as glucose may afford temporary symptomatic improvement.

Spleen

A condition of splenomegaly due to massive mast cell infiltration occurs as referred to elsewhere and has been seen in cats of 7–15 years. The syndrome is mildly obstructive in nature with weight loss and anaemia in some cases. The organ is easily palpated and splenectomy is very well tolerated and results excellent.

The spleen is also often a site of lymphosarcoma deposits, it has been noted as involved in a case of lymphatic leukosis also as the primary site of reticular cell sarcoma and carcinoma metastases. In all cases of enlarged spleen every endeavour should be made to decide if this is the primary lesion since decision as to treatment will rest on this.

Respiratory System

Whilst it may reasonably be assumed that the old cat has a pretty solid acquired immunity to panleukopenia this is not necessarily true of the respiratory viruses due both to the multiplicity of strains and the transience of immunity, therefore any aged cat exposed to infection, especially a severe challenge such as an epidemic in boarding kennels, may well become infected. Infections of normally low pathenogenicity may be far more serious in age due to less reserve to combat debility and a general lack of physical and mental resistance to the unpleasant symptoms, hence elderly patients may succumb quite unexpectedly to an infection normally regarded as not serious. Correspondingly greater nursing effort is required and a good nutritional state must be maintained from an early stage; forced feeding may be indicated far sooner than in young vigorous animals. Considerable time and patience is needed to keep such cats comfortable and free from discharges and to maintain morale.

Chronic nasal catarrh and even sinusitis may supervene in any cat but is more likely in the elderly. In such cases the history of a previous illness and the bilateral nature of the nasal discharge serve to differentiate it from the far more disastrous carcinoma of the nasal cavity which is not a rare lesion in these age groups. Diagnosis of the latter condition is not easy, since radiological changes are not invariable but the persistence of unilateral nasal discharge, often blood-tinged, in a progressively wasting old cat is characteristic and warrants a recommendation of euthanasia.

Bronchi and Lungs

Bronchitis and pneumonia are not particularly geriatric problems, nor is pyothorax which may arise in any age group.

Pulmonary congestion and pleural effusion are seen in association with left side heart defects but clinical signs are often not observed until the cat is in failure when response to therapy is extremely poor and is rendered very difficult owing to the feline intolerance of digitalis glycosides.

Chronic cough and the typical double expiratory effort of pulmonary emphysema have not been noted.

Cardiovascular System

Arterial thrombosis is not essentially a problem of age but recovered cats may be left with defects due to infarction which may be of clinical significance in later life; examples include renal insufficiency due to infarcts and myonecrosis followed by fibrosis in muscles deprived of a blood supply.

Heart disease is not uncommon but, as previously noted, may not be detected until the cat is in failure since the owner seldom sees any signs demanding veterinary attention. Murmurs are occasionally detected during routine clinical examinations but often no overt clinical signs attributable to cardiac incompetence are found. Tachycardia is likewise a common clinical finding but again no significant correlation has been recognised.

Most cases of heart disease seen in practice are old cats with a history extending over only a few days, as seen by the owner. Onset is apparently acute with rapidly decreased exercise tolerance, maintenance of sternal recumbency with elbows abducted for long periods of time and the development of dyspnoea and cyanosis on minimal exertion. A fluid line can often be easily detected following the rapid accumulation of transudate in the pleural cavities. Prognosis is grave.

Routine examination of the old cat should include a superficial assessment of blood quality as anaemia is not uncommon. Tongue colour is often a better guide than the normally rather pallid gums and conjunctivae. Haematological examination should be undertaken if any doubt exists. Unfortunately the anaemia may be non-specific and secondary to disease elsewhere, especially kidneys and liver. Some aged cats with no obvious primary disease elsewhere respond well to a regular (2–4 weekly) injection of liver extract or cyanocobalamin.

Locomotor System

Locomotor ataxias are quite common in aged cats and in most cases aetiology is unknown. Steps should be taken to exclude conditions such

290

as otitis media (vestibular signs are not usually prominent) or space occupying lesions in brain or cord, the latter are, as previously noted, conspicuously rare as clinical entities. Intervertebral disc protrusions may be demonstrated but evidence of clinical correlation is lacking.

The signs are usually confined to the hind limbs and posterior lumbar region and comprise a swaying gait and increasing weakness occasionally with knuckling of toes. There is often a marked lack of muscle tone and volume. In a few cases there is response to vitamin therapy, especially high potency B complex, which may be associated with a mild thiamine deficiency. In some patients spontaneous remissions occur after periods of quite severe inco-ordination and paresis usually followed by relapse after variable intervals of up to one year; in this sense—and it is not suggested that the conditions are analogous—there is some resemblance to multiple sclerosis in man.

Arthritis is not common but does occur. Osteo-arthritis may be associated with obesity and hence is usually seen in neuters. The vertebral column is often involved in osteo-arthritic changes and any old cat showing skeletal pain and disinclination to move which is not clearly attributable to a local lesion should be subjected to radiographic examination.

'Rheumatoid arthritis' has been seen mainly in patients over 8 years. Criteria include polyarthritis, joint pain, swelling and tenderness especially of the smaller articulations, e.g. phalanges, carpus, tarsus, and often associated malaise. Radiography shows changes to be peri-articular. This is not a disease which should be lightly diagnosed and a very critical assessment is necessary before applying this label. In milder cases cats may be maintained symptom free for several years on low dosage of corticosteroids; withdrawal results in return of symptoms.

Malignant bone tumours are lesions of the older cat as a rule, all age groups 6 years+, but may arise also in younger animals. Any old cat showing lameness which cannot be easily ascribed or a firm swelling associated with bone in any area should be investigated radiographically.

Central Nervous System

Epileptiform convulsions have been seen in cats in middle or old age. Every care should be taken to differentiate so-called fits from any form of circulatory failure, not an easy matter since the veterinary surgeon rarely sees an episode and has to rely on owner description; hospitalization for observation may entail a stay of several weeks which is not always feasible or desirable. Treatment with primidone or potassium bromide often gives good results but needs to be maintained over long periods of time. Adequate Vitamin B intake should be ensured.

Sudden hemiplegic episodes are a regular occurrence in aged cats; they are analogous to 'stroke' in man and many milder cases recover spontaneously.

Skin

Most of the common skin diseases are not associated with age but as mentioned earlier in this chapter problems of grooming do arise and blow-fly strike is more likely in aged cats which do not keep themselves clean and which sleep heavily thus allowing egg-laying by the fly to proceed undisturbed.

Tumours of skin tend to arise in age groups 7 years+ and have a widely varied pathology.

Surgical excision is usually required; histo-pathological examinations are highly desirable and are helpful to prognosis.

Reproductive System

Female: Pyometra is essentially a disease of the older barren cat and is usually acute in onset demanding prompt surgical intervention. Ovaro-hysterectomy is so well tolerated in this species that attempted operation is warranted at almost any age if the physical condition is otherwise reasonable.

Endometritis may arise in non-breeding or breeding females. It is less acute than pyometra and not associated with marked uterine distension. In breeding queens it is the later stage of the syndrome comprising reduced litter size → still births → abortions → endometritis. Again operation in even aged subjects is to be advocated.

Mammary neoplasia is less common than in bitches and another contrast is that it is commoner in regular breeders. Tumours are often malignant and metastasis has often occurred by the time advice is sought hence careful examination of drainage lymph nodes and lungs is essential prior to a decision regarding surgery. Prognosis is always guarded. Vaginal tumours in entire females have also been recorded. Male: Often absent! Neoplasia of testes is extremely rare as is prostatic disease; both have been seen.

Urinary System

Kidneys: Chronic interstitial nephritis is quite common with the typical syndrome of polydipsia/polyuria, anorexia, dulness and weight loss. Vomiting occurs but is not invariable. Ulceration of mucosa of mouth and pharynx occurs in advanced cases but is often not visible on examination of the conscious cat since the lesions are usually pharyngeal rather than buccal in situation. Any old cat presented with a history of dysphagia, salivation and foul breath odour should have renal function carefully assessed particularly if any form of dental treatment under anaesthesia is envisaged. Reliance should not be placed upon chemically impregnated paper strips for detection of proteinuria in this species in which they are very unreliable. Abdominal palpation of kidneys is usually easy in the cat and a small, indurated kidney with an irregular surface can often be recognised.

Diet often has to be adjusted to reduce protein intake and this presents considerable problems in an aged cat in poor health. It is difficult and may be impossible to persuade such a patient to accept a changed diet especially when the constituents are not those normally preferred. Rather than risk increasing a state of lowered nutrition and possibly dehydration it is better to permit some food which is acceptable even if theoretically contra-indicated. If forced feeding becomes necessary hydrolysed protein is valuable; it is occasionally voluntarily taken alone or mixed with milk or water.

The kidneys are often the site of neoplasia, especially the lymphosarcoma complex, and routine examination of old cats should include abdominal palpation with special reference to kidney size. Lymphosarcoma often causes gross enlargement of one or both kidneys and occasionally irregularities of contour can be felt. In this connection it is important to remember that the kidneys of the entire male cat are normally far larger than those of females or neuters and that in middle-aged or old cats, especially in summer at the end of the breeding season, these organs can not only be very easily felt but even seen as a high lateral swelling at and behind the last rib; a hasty diagnosis of neoplasia is thus not wise in tom cats unless there is clear-cut clinical correlation.

The kidneys are also occasionally the site of metastatic deposits from another primary site.

The bladder and urethra do not pose special geriatric problems.

Lymph Nodes

Lymphoid tissue is involved in a wide variety of diseases but the most significant in the older cat are lymphosarcoma and lymphatic leukosis, the latter relatively uncommon.

The clinical signs will depend to some extent on mechanical interference with other organs by pressure (e.g. mediastinal and bronchial nodes on oesophagus) as well as the symptoms related to the primary neoplastic process.

Euthanasia is almost always necessary.

The Eye

This is not a frequent site of senile changes, cataract being comparatively uncommon and causing little interference with vision. Senile corneal dystrophy is remarkably uncommon. Lens luxation is occasionally seen but not specifically in the aged animal. Lymphosarcoma deposits have been seen in the iris.

General

Many old cats show a progressive tissue wasting not referable to any specific organic disease. They eat well and are reasonably active; careful observation suggests that they still enjoy life. 'Neighbour euthanasia' is the worst problem in such cases, well-meaning friends(?) delighting in painting lurid pictures of wasting disease and suffering to the owner who may, as a result, request euthanasia before this is remotely necessary.

In such cases the veterinary surgeon's duty lies in firstly satisfying himself that no organ failure or neoplastic disease is present and then affording the owner moral support in rebutting uninformed advice. Should progressive fatal disease or irreversible organ failure be confirmed the advice to destroy must be firmly and fearlessly given.

Euthanasia

Humane destruction of the aged and feeble cat can present some difficulty. The restraint essential to precise venepuncture in this species is often resisted violently and the vein itself is often small and atonic. If intravenous injection of pentobarbitone is selected the use of syringe and needle in perfect condition is vital.

Intrathoracic and intraperitoneal injection of triple strength solution 200 mg. per ml. (3 gr. per cc.) pentobarbitone is usually easily administered, only slightly resented and usually quickly effective. The occasional stormy induction with inco-ordination, narcotic excitement and even crying out remains a hazard and can cause much distress to the owner. Sometimes a violent spasm of coughing is provoked when anaesthetic solution enters a bronchiole or bronchus. These routes will fail in subjects with pleural or peritoneal effusions and are thus quite useless. Cats in circulatory failure may have a greatly prolonged induction time due to slow absorption. In such circumstances intracardiac administration should be attempted and if this fails the use of a gaseous agent by face mask (e.g. halothane) or in a lethal cabinet (e.g. coal-gas or chloroform) may be the only reasonable solution.

Induction by open mask with halothane may well prove the solution to many difficulties although even this may be resented. The expense involved in using such a drug is not significant; few owners quibble at the fee for the most satisfactory method of providing this last veterinary service to an aged pet.

SUGGESTED FURTHER READING

Joshua, J. O. (1964) *J. Small An. Pract.* **5**, 525. (Feline Geriatrics.)
Whitehead, J. E. (1963) *J. Amer. Vet. Medical Association* **142**, 144. (Feline Geriatrics.)

Chapter 22

SOME COMMON ACCIDENTS AND INJURIES

The extreme agility of cats and the traditional 'nine lives' tend to foster a general opinion that they seldom become involved in accidents and that if they do, they usually escape injury. Both these premises are untrue. Not only are they frequently involved in accidents but some of the lesions sustained are decidedly bizarre. Cats fall off roofs and through greenhouses or cold-frames, or else they end up in a heap of quicklime or a pool of paint or turpentine, they manage to get hit by air-gun pellets and caught in wire snares and they often dash out of garden hedges and collide with the hub-cap of a passing car. They ingest toxic dressings by constant licking, they turn on gas taps in play and gas themselves; there is no limit to the variety of accidents which befall felines and small animal practitioners cease to be surprised at anything.

Most of the skeletal injuries have been dealt with fully in their respective sections but a reiteration of some of the more frequent may be helpful.

Fractures of the hard palate and jaws are common. The nasal bones are often damaged in addition with variable haemorrhage and severe dyspnoea. Most such cases are susceptible to treatment.

Skull fractures are uncommon but a curious fracture has been seen due to penetration of the roof of the cranium (and the cerebral hemisphere) by a sharp foreign body; how such an injury could be sustained other than maliciously is a mystery.

Fracture of the cervical spine may result from a cat colliding head-on with something such as the hub-cap of a passing car; fractures of the thoracic and lumbar spine are more usually due to crushing, e.g. a car wheel passing over the trunk. Sacrococcygeal injuries result from blows from behind or a fall on the base of the spine.

Limb fractures occur in all types of accident; epiphyseal separations (e.g. of top of tuber calcis or lower end femur or tibia) often result when the kitten has been suspended in some way—this may happen when descending from a tree or shrub. Radial paralysis can arise from similar causes.

Pelvic fractures are common sequelae of street accidents; they heal extremely well but some deformity is usually left which is important in entire females.

Soft tissue injuries are legion and diverse. The feline skin is tough and not easily torn other than when pierced by a sharp object such as glass or a protruding nail. Muscle contusions and tears are common, the latter particularly so in the abdominal wall giving rise to ventral herniae. Tendons are usually damaged during attack by another animal, often a dog; the gastrocnemius tendon is the most usual site of such a lesion. The cruciate ligaments of the stifle very occasionally rupture due to external violence or a hanging accident.

The diaphragm may be ruptured in crushing street accidents resulting in herniation of abdominal organs into the chest.

Haemorrhage into pleural or peritoneal cavities results from ruptured viscera, abdominal organs being most common. The somewhat elastic rib-cage seems to protect the lungs but the pliable and soft abdominal wall offers little resistance and serious damage to liver and kidneys is not unusual.

Less usual causes of damage include:

(a) Air-gun pellets

Rather surprisingly cats often sustain air-gun shot wounds usually due to thoughtless 'pot-shots' from children but occasionally from adults exasperated either by the prolonged caterwaulings of courtship or repeated damage to cherished gardens. Unless obvious lesions arise, such as in the eye, it may be difficult to determine the type of accident and that a foreign body has penetrated somewhere. Radiography may well be required. When the eye is penetrated a rapidly developing pan-ophthalmitis is usual necessitating early enucleation; the pellet is usually found in the posterior chamber.

Freak (personal communication) records a case in which the air-gun pellet punctured the abdominal wall, traversed liver and duodenum, travelled along the edge of the pancreas and came to rest in the omentum; the duodenal puncture allowed escape of ascarids into the peritoneal cavity. The track taken by the pellet was clearly demarcated by embedded fur. Routine surgical repair was successful.

(b) Other penetrating foreign bodies

Thorns occasionally enter the eye embedding themselves in the cornea. Provided the posterior chamber is not entered tissue reaction may be remarkably slight. In one case a thorn $\frac{1}{2}$ inch long penetrated the cornea, crossed the anterior chamber and its tip entered the crystalline lens. Reaction was minimal; after removal a small opaque spot persisted for several months in the lens but eventually resolved completely.

Pieces of glass, sometimes of considerable size, may be found in incised dissecting wounds especially of axillary and groin regions. The lesion may appear superficially small and insignificant but if there is any evidence that it is of a dissecting nature careful exploration is advisable.

(c) Wire Snares

Even in this enlightened day and age wire snares are still occasionally laid and cats are trapped. Usually the cat is presented after an absence from home of variable duration often with the wire loop still *in situ* or with the characteristic lesions if it has escaped from the snare or been released. The forelimbs below the carpus are the more usual sites. There is always interference with circulation and according to the duration of the injury, oedema, necrosis and/or gangrene may be present in the limb distal to the snare. Despite the apparent extent of tissue damage, which will always involve skin and subcutaneous tissue and often extend to tendons and even bone, resolution often takes place to a remarkable degree and most cases merit attempted treatment; this is on routine lines and includes removal of the wire if still present, careful cleansing and débridement of damaged tissues (preferably all under general anaesthesia if the condition of the cat permits) and followed by penicillin and subsequently combined penicillin/corticosteroid therapy. Surgical repair of individual tissues such as severed tendons is seldom called for, the end result of natural repair aided by antibacterial drugs being usually surprisingly good.

POISONING, INCLUDING TOXICITY FROM DRUGS

The average household pet cat is usually a well fed and fastidious feeder hence the direct ingestion of poisoned bait put down for rodents is not a common happening but there are various indirect ways in which toxic matter may be taken. These include drugs used therapeutically whether due to idiosyncracy, e.g. streptomycin and antihistamines, or to ingestion of substances applied topically or their absorption through the skin. Falling into materials such as paint or turpentine with subsequent ingestion due to attempted self-cleaning by licking is another source. Cats rarely eat rodents already dead but may well catch rats or mice which have taken poisoned bait and are in the early stages of poisoning and thus easy prey, e.g. warfarin and zinc phosphide, and thus ingest poison themselves. The ingestion of birds which have themselves fed on seed or vegetation dressed with toxic compounds such as the chlorinated hydrocarbons is so indirect that it is unlikely that toxic quantities will be absorbed.

1. Toxic Signs from Systemic Administration of Some Common Drugs Used Therapeutically

A. Antibiotics

Penicillin. This is not only a very effective but also a very safe antibiotic. A very small number of cases has been seen in which a violent dermatitis has followed injections of penicillin. In one case the allergic response followed a second course of penicillin, the first having been given some weeks previously. The signs are those of intense pruritus, erythema and heat of large areas of skin and rapid hair loss. The pruritus may be intense enough to cause some general malaise. Response to therapy is extremely slow.

Streptomycin, (including dihydrostreptomycin)

Nausea, vomiting and ataxia are not uncommon following within 1–2 hours of administration of streptomycin in normal therapeutic doses. Usually no more than an attack of vomiting occurs which ceases spontaneously within a few hours. Whenever possible streptomycin treatment should be instituted gradually using initially a low average dose and increasing to full therapeutic levels if no adverse signs are recorded. It is appreciated that this is contrary to the principle of using high initial dosage to avoid development of drug resistance but the toxic effects can be sufficiently serious to merit this unorthodox approach. In overdosage the above signs are followed by collapse and loss of consciousness and death can ensue on rare occasions. Warmth and anti-histamine drugs are the only possible lines of treatment.

Chronic toxicity also occurs and high dosage should not be maintained for more than 3–4 days. Streptomycin, to which cats are the most sensitive of all animals (Garner), mainly attacks the cochlear division of the eighth cranial nerve causing vestibular signs with loss of balance which in some cases is irreversible. Dihydrostreptomycin mainly attacks the auditory division of the eighth cranial nerve and permanent deafness may result without other evidence of toxicity (Daykin). Since subjective signs are not available in animals this is a very real danger in cats in which species deafness cannot always be appreciated early. The use of a combination of streptomycin and dihydrostreptomycin minimises the risk from either.

B. Antihistaminics

Mepyramine maleate. Grossly abnormal response to therapeutic doses has been seen. Signs are of loss of balance and general disorientation. Affected cats not only become ataxic but are restless and often cry repeatedly in a distressing manner; varied abnormal movements and postures are common including attempts to climb non-existent objects, creeping into corners of furniture and somersaulting when trying to jump or move. In severe cases signs may persist 36–48 hours after withdrawal of the drug but spontaneous recovery is usual. Whenever possible the cat should be removed to a hospital cage where it will not only be less likely to damage itself but unnecessary anxiety for the owner can be avoided as these side-effects are very distressing to watch.

C. Ataractics, Narcotics, Sedatives, Anaesthetics

Chlorpromazine, promazine and trimeprazine are fairly widely used in cats, the two former as part of pre-anaesthetic medication or to facilitate handling and restraint; the latter mainly for its antipruritic action.

Chlorpromazine is hepato-toxic in man and may cause blood

298

dyscrasias but it is seldom used over long periods in cats so these effects are of little practical significance. Immediate side effects are occasionally seen due either to idiosyncracy or an insufficiently accurately assessed dose; they comprise ataxia, loss of balance and mental disorientation. Untoward signs usually pass off in a few hours; if serious distress is caused a *small* dose of pentobarbitone sodium may be given intravenously.

Promazine appears to be less liable to cause similar side-effects. One case has been seen of restlessness, disorientation, distressed crying and attempts to climb walls in a cat on thrice daily dosage (10 mg.) of trimeprazine for a skin condition. Spontaneous recovery occurred in 36–48 hours following withdrawal.

As a group narcotics are singularly useless in the cat. With the exception of pethidine, morphine and its related substances (including substitutes such as thiambutene) cannot be used in the cat as they all cause hyperaesthesia which can become maniacal or even convulsive.

Pethidine is well tolerated but overdosage causes hyperaesthesia and convulsions; in one cat given the usual 10 mg./kg. (5 mg./lb.) by the intramuscular rather than subcutaneous route these symptoms were caused—they were easily controlled by intravenous pentobarbitone under which surgery was performed and recovery was normal.

Of the commonly used sedatives chlorbutol is the one most likely to cause trouble as the cat is highly susceptible to its toxic effects—it is best avoided.

Acetylsalicylic acid. (Aspirin)

Many generations of veterinary surgeons have used aspirin as an analgesic or mild sedative agent in the cat especially for short periods and, to judge by the paucity of reports of toxicity, without untoward effects. Although the irritant effect of acetylsalicylic acid on the gastric mucosa is well recognised the comparative infrequency of vomiting following its therapeutic use in the cat has appeared to indicate that this species is not unduly sensitive to this action. The report of Larsen (1963) provides a rude and probably salutary shock.

In an experimental study using twelve cats three groups were studied: four controls, four on low dosage, i.e. 120 mg. (2 gr.) daily as a single dose for 35 days and four high dose, i.e. 300 mg. (5 gr.) daily until death (an average of 12 days). Summarised the results showed that clinical signs of toxicity—which in some cases appeared after only one or two doses —included depression, anorexia, vomiting, weight loss and death in the higher dose group. Gastric lesions, toxic hepatitis and suppression of erythropoiesis in bone marrow occurred in several cats. The low dose induced toxic hepatitis in two of the four low dose group.

In view of these findings and despite the apparent rarity of adverse effects from normal clinical use it is clear that the greatest caution must be used in the exhibition of aspirin in cats. In the light of this published evidence a veterinary surgeon might be held culpable if serious side-effects arose in patients if no warning or guarding statement had been given to the owner.

Barbiturates

Apart from respiratory or cardiac failure during anaesthesia by volatile agents the barbiturates are most likely to cause concern due to idiosyncracy, overdosage or—very commonly—the unwise use of augmenting doses. The last is most likely to arise when anaesthesia is induced with thiopentone or pentobarbitone for investigation, e.g. radiography, and is followed within a few hours by the re-induction or deepening to surgical anaesthesia for operation. Prolonged recovery, hypothermia and respiratory depression are all likely. Some cases have been seen in such circumstances when recovery to normality has taken 4–6 days and has necessitated the repeated use of bemegride and subcutaneous infusions of glucose saline to achieve it. The practice of re-inducing or deepening barbiturate anaesthesia in cats without allowing an interval of complete normality is to be deprecated.

Bemegride sodium is to be preferred in the treatment of delayed recovery from barbiturate anaesthesia although repeated doses are necessary since the duration of action is only about 30 minutes. Picrotoxin has been known to cause a prolonged convulsive state and even death from exhaustion in this species.

Toxicity from topically applied therapeutic drugs

Toxicity may arise from ingestion due to licking of dressed areas or by absorption through the skin. Most such incidents are likely to arise during treatment for skin disease, particularly parasitic infestation.

Derris is usually a very safe ectoparasiticide for cats and even kittens provided normal discretion is observed and it is used as a dry dusting powder. One case has been seen in which profound depression verging on coma followed the use of derris in water suspension as for the dog. Recovery was spontaneous.

Benzyl benzoate is usually said to be totally contra-indicated in the cat and it should certainly never be dispensed for application by owners. Its occasional use by the veterinary surgeon as a dressing for otacariasis has, in the author's hands, always been safe.

Gamma benzene hexachloride (Gammexane) is very safe as a dry dusting powder properly used and has proved safe when applied repeatedly (weekly) as 0·05 per cent washes (half the concentration used for dogs) in the treatment of miliary exzema.

Toxic signs are similar to dicophane.

Whenever anti-parasitic or other agents are used for the treatment of skin disease in cats it is the veterinary surgeon's duty to ensure that the owner understands how to use it. Advice should always be given to remove any excess of powder (whether applied dry or in suspension) from the surface of the coat by lightly dusting down, rubbing with a towel or brushing lightly after treatment; this will minimize risks from ingestion.

Bromocyclen (Alugan—Hoechst) a powerful insecticidal coat dressing is available in aerosol spray for use in cats and kittens although its use as a bathing agent is contra-indicated. Ingestion of toxic quantities results in symptoms of vomiting and diarrhoea and finally convulsions and coma. Atropine may be antidotal.

Dichlorvos (Nuvantop—Ciba-Geigy) is similarly available as aerosol coat dressing for use in all except very young kittens. This is a cholinesterase inhibitor and symptoms of toxic overdosage (listed below) may be treated with atropine to counteract muscarinic effects of acetyl choline.

Methyl violet as a 1 per cent solution is occasionally used in the treatment of labial ulcers. One case has been seen in which too generous application of the dressing and consequent licking resulted in a serious and intractable chemical pharyngitis.

Toxicity from Orally Administered Insecticides and Vermifuges

Systemic insecticides **Ronnel** (Ectoral C-Vet) and **Cythioate** (Cyflee-Cyanamid) and vermifuge **dichlorvos** (Task—T.V.L.) as cholinesterase inhibitors are toxic in overdosage. Symptoms including salivation, vomiting, diarrhoea, abdominal pain, midriasis, excess lacrimation, loss of sphincter control, shallow respiration, cyanosis, bradycardia, muscle twitching, opisthotonus and convulsions may be treated with repeated injection of atropine, preferably intravenously, together with supportive nursing including saline purgation when possible.

Accidentally Acquired Systemic Poisons

The average household cat is unlikely to have ready access to, or to ingest, many toxic substances and the decreasing use of the more distasteful methods of pest control, e.g. by strychnine, many now prohibited by law, makes this increasingly improbable.

The most likely source of such poison is rats or mice dying of warfarin poisoning when they are slow and thus easily caught. However, in most cases repeated small doses are necessary to produce poisoning although the resistance of cats to single doses is extremely variable. According to Garner toxicity in cats and dogs may arise from the ingestion of rats dead from warfarin poisoning if the diet consists of practically nothing else for 4–10 days. Warfarin is an anticoagulant hence signs of toxicity are those of internal haemorrhage; evidence of subcutaneous haemorrhage is not necessarily seen. The author has seen one case of an old cat which died after an undiagnosed illness comprising weakness and lethargy lasting a few days; post-mortem examination showed extensive haemorrhages suggestive of warfarin poisoning but the source of this could not be ascertained.

The work of Clark and Halliwell (1963) on the treatment of warfarin poisoning in the dog is a valuable indication of what may be equally effective in the cat. They found that the water soluble analogues were of little or no value and that preparations of Vitamin K_1 were necessary and proved a valuable antidotal treatment. Of the preparations they used some caused severe transient side-effects necessitating the previous administration of a suitable antihistaminic; whether similar reactions might occur in the cat is problematical, however, it would probably be wise to select the preparation they found free from such effects, viz. Mephyton up to a dose rate of 5 mg./kg. (2 mg. per lb.).

The authors recommend a dose for the dog of 1–2 mg./kg. (0·5–1 mg. per lb.) by intramuscular, or in very acute cases intravenous, injection at 24-hour intervals for a minimum of 4 days. Based on these findings suggested treatment for an average cat would be 5–7 mg. Vitamin K_1 intramuscularly every day for 4 days at least.

Although the cat is a fastidious and discriminating feeder, random cases of poisoning with a wide range of toxic agents have been recorded, including even maliciously administered barbiturates and accidentally ingested corrosive disinfectants.

The increasing agricultural use of highly concentrated insecticides and weedkillers has resulted in cases of poisoning due to skin absorption of cholinesterase inhibitors and due to accidental ingestion of the dipyridilium compound paraquat. Symptoms of presumed paraquat poisoning include vomiting, anorexia, lethargy and bradycardia with subsequent dyspnoea, tachycardia, cyanosis and death. There is no treatment.

Fluoroacetamide is no longer available for use as an insecticide, but poisoning may still associate with its use as a potent rodenticide. Little is known of the mode of action of this drug which is a CNS and cardiovascular stimulant. Symptoms of poisoning include hyperexcitability and convulsions prior to death due to respiratory and cardiac failure.

Food Preservatives

Benzoic acid, a commonly used meat preservative has been demonstrated experimentally in cats (Bedford and Clarke 1972) to induce symptoms of hyperaesthesia with aggression, convulsions, buceal ulceration and centrilobular hepatic necrosis. The cumulative effects of this drug at lower dose level are considered responsible for a clinical syndrome characterised by aggression and hyperaesthesia, although its precise mode of action is unknown.

Local toxic substances accidentally acquired

Cats may fall into or be forced to walk through a wide variety of materials which can cause local or general signs. The tendency for cats to clean themselves vigorously by licking, no matter how noxious the substance, predisposes them to absorption.

Phenol. It is probably proper to include under this heading the improper use of dressings or washes containing phenol or cresols applied by laymen, obviously without professional guidance. Such substances should never be used on cats, which are highly susceptible to their toxic actions but owners will occasionally, in a panic, bath a cat found to have ectoparasites using a phenol or cresol preparation.

Symptoms of acute poisoning arise due both to ingestion from licking and absorption through the intact skin; they comprise convulsions and coma with death from respiratory paralysis.

Antidotal measures are symptomatic by demulcents; lavage may be attempted; further absorption is prevented by washing the cat in warm soapy water. The usual anti-shock measures are necessary.

Paint, tar, paraffin, turpentine etc.

Cats not infrequently become widely contaminated by any of the above substances from falling or jumping into builder's yards etc. Although in most cases the irritant nature of the contaminant will prevent or at least limit attempted self-cleaning by licking, some cats will persist despite the unpleasantness and may thus ingest significant amounts.

Ingestion of lead paint could presumably cause lead poisoning but no such case has come to the author's notice.

Ingestion of tar, paraffin, turpentine, etc., will cause chemical stomatitis, pharyngitis, oesophagitis and gastritis. Symptomatic treatment with demulcents is required.

More commonly, however, the veterinary surgeon is required to give advice regarding the safe removal of contaminants and may be called upon to treat local lesions such as pedal dermatitis due to the chemical.

Care must be exercised in the choice of solvents for paint and tar. Probably the safest procedure is to use lavish applications of butter or margarine to the affected area of coat massaging well in to dissolve the paint which is then removed by repeated washing in copious soapy water or detergent solutions. Soapy water and detergents may be used directly for removal of paraffin and turpentine. The propensity for some detergents to cause contact dermatitis must be remembered.

Treatment for shock may be necessary; shock may be provoked as much by the procedure necessary to remove the contaminant as from the incident itself!

Unwillingness to walk or a tentative, gingerly gait ('cat on hot bricks') is an indication for careful examination of the feet when a dermatitis of the interdigital web and even erosion of the keratin covering of the pads may be found. Causes include paraffin, turpentine and quick lime. Treatment is symptomatic and may include corticosteroids to reduce inflammation if all precautions regarding bacterial infection are observed. Healing is satisfactory but slow.

Carbon monoxide poisoning

Accidental poisoning from gas or boiler fumes is by no means uncommon. Apart from accidental escapes of gas, cats shut in kitchens or sculleries for the night may turn on gas taps themselves by jumping on the cooker (if the taps are not of the safety type) and inadequate ventilation when a solid fuel boiler is in use is also a cause of accidental gassing. Usually the cat is found semiconscious or unconscious first thing in the morning. On receipt of such a call immediate advice to put the animal outside in the open air should be given no matter how inclement the weather.

Early symptoms include vertigo and muscular weakness but most animals are already comatose when found. Diagnosis is usually self-evident.

Administration of oxygen is helpful and respiratory stimulants such as nikethamide and leptazol may be used. Cylinders of oxygen can usually be obtained from local chemists and administration in emergency can be simply by connecting the cylinder to an enamel, glass or plastic funnel by rubber tubing.

Recovery takes place within a few hours. Comben (1949) records temporary deafness following recovery in two cats; hearing returned within 21 days. The same author also gives an indirect report of a cat being both blind and deaf after coal gas poisoning, again spontaneous recovery occurred within 10 days.

REFERENCES

Bedford, P.G., Clarke, E.G. (1972) *Vet. Rec.* **90**, 53.
Clark, W. T. & Halliwell, R. E. W. (1963) *Vet. Rec.* **75**, 1210.
Comben, N. (1949) *Vet. Rec.* **61**, 128.
Daykin, P. W. (1960) *Veterinary Applied Pharmacology and Therapeutics* (Bailliere, Tindall and Cox.)
Freak, M. J. (1962) Personal communication.
Garner, R. J. (1963) *Veterinary Toxicology* (Bailliere, Tindall and Cox.)
Larson, E. J. (1963) *J. Amer. Vet. Medical Association* **143**, 837.

SUGGESTED FURTHER READING

Easton, K. L. (1961) *Canad. Vet. J.* **2**, 310. (Chlordane poisoning in a cat.)
Ernst, M. R. *et al.* (1961) *J. Amer. Vet. Medical Association* **138**, 197. (Susceptibility of cats to phenol.)
Tapernoux, A. *et al.* (1964) *Rev. Méd. Vét.* **115**, 114. (Frequency of metaldehyde poisoning in dogs and cats.) (In French.)
Sturtevant, F. M. & Drill, V. A. (1957) *Nature, Lond.* **179**, 1253. (Tranquilising drugs and morphine-mania in cats.)
Bell, R. R. *et al.* (1955) *J. Amer. Vet. Medical Association* **126**, 302. (Toxicity of malathion and chlorthion to dogs and cats.)
Pile, C. H. (1956) *Aust. Vet. J.* **32**, 18. (Thallium poisoning in domestic felines.)
Tessang, A. A. *et al.* (1958) *Commun. Vet. Bogor.* **2**, 71. (Aldrin, dieldrin and endrin intoxication in cats.)
Hadlow, W. J. (1957) *J. Amer. Vet. Medical Association* **130**, 296. (Acute ethylene glycol poisoning in a cat.)
Cross, R. F. & Folger, G. C. (1956) *J. Amer. Vet. Medical Association* **129**, 65. (The use of malathion on cats and birds.)

Weights and Measures—Dose Equivalents

The following tables are intended solely for converting doses in the Imperial system into equivalent doses in the metric system, or vice versa. The equivalence is approximate only, and the values are not accurate enough for formulating, analytical and similar purposes.

POUNDS AND OUNCES			PINTS AND FLUID OUNCES		
Pounds	Ounces	Grammes	Pints	Fluid Ounces	Litres
$1\frac{1}{2}$	24	700	2	40	1·2
1	16	500	$1\frac{3}{4}$	35	1
$\frac{3}{4}$	12	350	1	20	0·6
$\frac{1}{2}$	8	250	$\frac{3}{4}$	15	0·4
$\frac{1}{4}$	4	125	—	6	0·175
—	$3\frac{1}{2}$	100	—	4	0·12
—	2	60	—	2	0·06

MINIMS OR GRAINS					
Minims or Grains	Millilitres or Grammes	Minims or Grains	Millilitres or Grammes	Minims or Grains	Millilitres or Grammes
480 (1 fl. oz.) ⎱	30	90	6	8	0·5
450 (1 fl. oz.) ⎰		75	5	$7\frac{1}{2}$	0·45
		60	4	6	0·4
375	25	45	3	5	0·3
300	20	40	2·4	4	0·25
		30	2	3	0·2
240 ($\frac{1}{2}$ fl. oz.) ⎱	15	25	1·6	$2\frac{1}{2}$	0·15
225 ⎰		20	1·2	2	0·12
150	10	15	1	$1\frac{1}{2}$	0·1
120	⎰ 8 ⎱ 7·5	12	0·8	1	0·06
		10	0·6		

FRACTIONS OF A GRAIN					
Grains	Milligrams	Grains	Milligrams	Grains	Milligrams
1	60	$\frac{1}{8}$	⎰ 8 ⎱ 7·5	$\frac{1}{100}$	0·6
$\frac{3}{4}$	50	$\frac{1}{10}$	6	$\frac{1}{120}$	0·5
$\frac{3}{5}$	40	$\frac{1}{12}$	5	$\frac{1}{130}$ ⎱	
$\frac{1}{2}$	30	$\frac{1}{15}$	4	$\frac{1}{150}$ ⎰	0·4
$\frac{2}{5}$	25	$\frac{1}{20}$	3	$\frac{1}{160}$	
$\frac{1}{3}$	20	$\frac{1}{24}$ ⎱ $\frac{1}{25}$ ⎰	2·5	$\frac{1}{200}$	0·3
$\frac{1}{4}$	15	$\frac{1}{30}$	2	$\frac{1}{240}$	0·25
$\frac{1}{5}$	12·5	$\frac{1}{40}$	1·5	$\frac{1}{300}$ ⎱ $\frac{1}{320}$ ⎰	0·2
$\frac{1}{6}$	10	$\frac{1}{50}$	1·25	$\frac{1}{400}$	0·15
$\frac{3}{20}$	9	$\frac{1}{60}$	1	$\frac{1}{480}$ ⎱ $\frac{1}{500}$ ⎰	0·125
		$\frac{1}{75}$	0·8	$\frac{1}{600}$	0·1
		$\frac{1}{80}$	0·75		

The following table gives the approximate equivalents per pound body-weight of doses per kilogram body-weight.

Milligrams per kilogram body-weight	Milligrams per pound body-weight	Grains per pound body-weight	Milligrams per kilogram body-weight	Milligrams per pound body-weight	Grains per pound body-weight
0·1	0·05	$\frac{1}{1400}$	50	23	$\frac{3}{8}$
0·25	0·1	$\frac{1}{600}$	60	27	$\frac{2}{5}$
1·0	0·45	$\frac{1}{140}$	70	32	$\frac{1}{2}$
1·5	0·7	$\frac{1}{100}$	75	34	$\frac{1}{2}$
2·0	0·9	$\frac{1}{72}$	80	36	$\frac{1}{2}$
2·5	1·0	$\frac{1}{60}$	90	41	$\frac{2}{3}$
3	1·4	$\frac{1}{50}$	100	45	$\frac{3}{4}$
4	1·8	$\frac{1}{36}$	120	54	$\frac{4}{5}$
5	2·3	$\frac{1}{28}$	150	68	1
6	2·7	$\frac{1}{24}$	200	91	1$\frac{2}{5}$
7	3·2	$\frac{1}{20}$	220	100	1$\frac{1}{2}$
8	3·6	$\frac{1}{18}$	250	110	1$\frac{3}{4}$
9	4·0	$\frac{1}{16}$	300	135	2
10	4·5	$\frac{1}{14}$	400	180	3
15	7	$\frac{1}{10}$	500	225	3$\frac{1}{2}$
20	9	$\frac{1}{7}$	600	270	4
25	11	$\frac{1}{6}$	700	320	5
30	14	$\frac{1}{5}$	800	360	5$\frac{1}{2}$
40	18	$\frac{1}{4}$	900	410	6
45	20	$\frac{1}{3}$	1 gramme	450	7

CONVERSION FACTORS*

To convert:
  milligrams per kilogram to milligrams per pound, multiply by 0·45
  milligrams per kilogram to grains per pound, multiply by 0·007
  milligrams per pound to grains per pound, multiply by 0·015
  grains per pound to milligrams per pound, multiply by 65
  grains per pound to milligrams per kilogram, multiply by 143

* The factors are approximate, but sufficiently accurate for dosage purposes.

Tables taken from British Veterinary Codex 1965.
Reproduced by courtesy of the Pharmaceutical Society of Great Britain.

INDEX

Streptococcus, 12
  in septic infections, 273
Streptomycin, side effects, 299
Stroke, 239
Sutures, 21

T

Tachycardia, 166
Taenia taeniaformis infestation,
  133, 134
Tail, fractures, 222
Talus, 27
Tar, removal from body, 303
Tarsus, 27
  dislocation, 223
  fracture, 220
Tartar deposits, 100, 102
Teeth, carious, 101
  carnassial, 39
  disorders, 98
  in old age, 286
  extraction, 102
  root extraction with abscess
    or sinus, 103
  tartar deposits, 100, 102
Temper in cats, 12
Temperament, 73
Temperature taking, 63, 74
Temporo-mandibular joint,
  luxation, 80
Testes, 47
  disorders, 195
Tetanus, 268
Tetany, lactation, 183
Thiamine deficiency, fits due
  to, 238
Thiopentone sodium, 68
Thrombosis, arterial, 157
Thymus, 36
Thyroid tumours, 122
Tibia, 26
  fractures, 220

separation of lower epiphysis,
  220
Ticks, infestation with, 201
Tongue, 39
  disorders in old age, 286
  examination, 75
  ulceration, 106
Tonsils, 36
  examination, 75
  neoplasia, 118
Tonsillitis, 118
Toxacara cati infestation, 133,
  134
Toxacaris leonina infestation,
  133, 134
Toxoplasmosis, 269
Trachea, 38
Transportation of cats, 13, 14
Travelling, 13, 14
  sedation for, 15
Trichlorethylene, 69
Trichophyton infection, 207
Trombicula autumnalis infestation, 202
Tuberculosis sinus of neck, 121
Tumours of bone, 225
  of central nervous system, 241
  of colon, 132
  of cranium, 83
  of ear, 110
  of eye, 96
  of kidney, 165
  of liver, 141
  of lung, 154
  of mammary gland, 195
  of nasal cavity, 82
  of oesophagus, 122
  of pancreas, 141
  of skin, 214
  of small intestine, 129
  of stomach, 124
  of tonsils, 120

of uterus and vagina, 195
ventro-lateral to frenum
linguae, 106
Turpentine, removal from skin,
303
Tympanic bullae, 21

U
Ulcer, labial, 83
Ulna, 23
fractures, 221
Umbilical hernia, 198
Ureters, 46
Urethra, 46
obstruction, 168
Urethrostomy, ante-pubic, 173
Urinary bladder, 46
Urinary calculi, 173
system, diseases, 163-175
in old age, 292
Urine, collection for examina-
tion, 63
Urolithiasis, feline, 168-175
Uterine inertia, 181
Uterus, neoplasma, 195

V
Vagina, neoplasia, 195
Vein, hepatic portal, 44
Vertebrae, cervical, 21
lumbar, 23
sacral, 23
thoracic, 23
Vertebral column, 21
Vestibule, 47
Villi, 44
Viruses, respiratory, 243
vaccination against, 16
Visceral pleura, 38
Vulva, 47

W
Warfarin poisoning, 301
Washing and ill health, 72
Weights and measures, conver-
sion tables, 305
Wire snares, injuries due to,
296

X
Xylazine, 66

Z
Zimmer finger splint, 217